PROSTATE BIOPSY

CURRENT CLINICAL UROLOGY™

Eric A. Klein, SERIES EDITOR

PROSTATE BIOPSY

INDICATIONS, TECHNIQUES, and COMPLICATIONS

Edited by

J. STEPHEN JONES, MD

Chairman, Department of Regional Urology
Cleveland Clinic Glickman Urological
*   and Kidney Institute*
Associate Professor of Surgery (Urology)
Cleveland Clinic Lerner College of Medicine
*   at CWRU*
Cleveland, OH

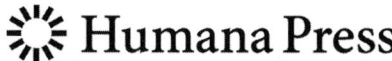 Humana Press

Editor
J. Stephen Jones, MD
Chairman, Department of Regional Urology
Cleveland Clinic Glickman Urological and Kidney Institute
Associate Professor of Surgery (Urology)
Cleveland Clinic Lerner College of Medicine at CWRU
Cleveland, OH, USA

Series Editor
Eric A. Klein, MD
Section of Urologic Oncology
Glickman Urological Institute
Cleveland Clinic Foundation
Cleveland, OH, USA

ISBN: 978-1-58829-790-7   e-ISBN: 978-1-60327-078-6
DOI: 10.1007/978-1-60327-078-6

Library of Congress Control Number: 2007931649

Cover illustration: Figure 3, Chapter 17, "Pathologic Implications of Prostate Biopsy," by Ming
Zhou and Cristina Magi-Galluzzi.

Printed on acid-free paper

9 8 7 6 5 4 3 2 1

springer.com

For my mother, whose wisdom and integrity inspired me to a wonderful life.

—J. Stephen Jones

Preface

Prostate biopsy has progressed over the past century from an era of significant morbidity to the point where it can be performed in an office setting with low morbidity. The original description was an open perineal prostate biopsy performed as the first stage of a perineal prostatectomy. In contrast, major complications are now uncommon and prostate biopsy is one of the most common procedures performed by urologists.

Interest in the topic has increased dramatically in recent years as evidenced by the number of publications in the peer-reviewed literature by year of publication shown in Figure 1. This indicates that the topic will continue to grow as prostate cancer becomes more prevalent in an aging population.

Much of this recent interest relates to efforts to increase cancer detection, but there is increasing emphasis on improved instrumentation and technology. In addition, biopsy is now utilized to enhance evaluation of cancer quality relating to active surveillance for patients foregoing treatment because of the morbidity of prostate cancer treatments. However, the most significant increase in interest has been in the area of management of pain issues as evidenced by the number of peer-reviewed publications, which has exploded since the year 2000 (Figure 2).

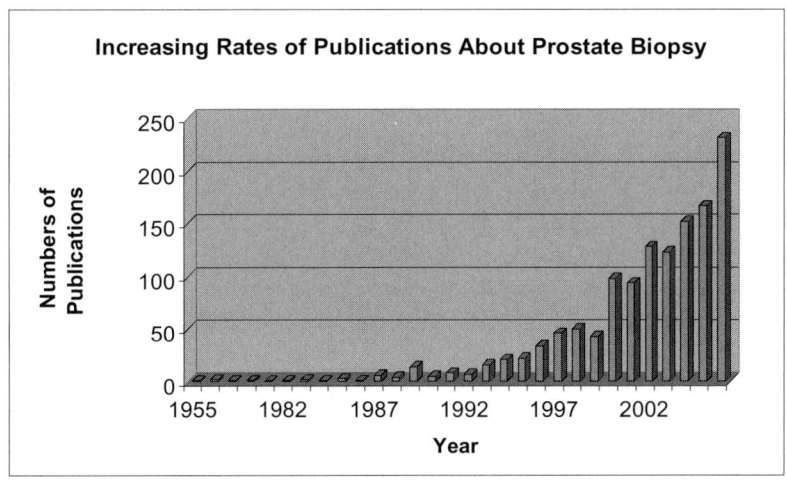

FIGURE 1.

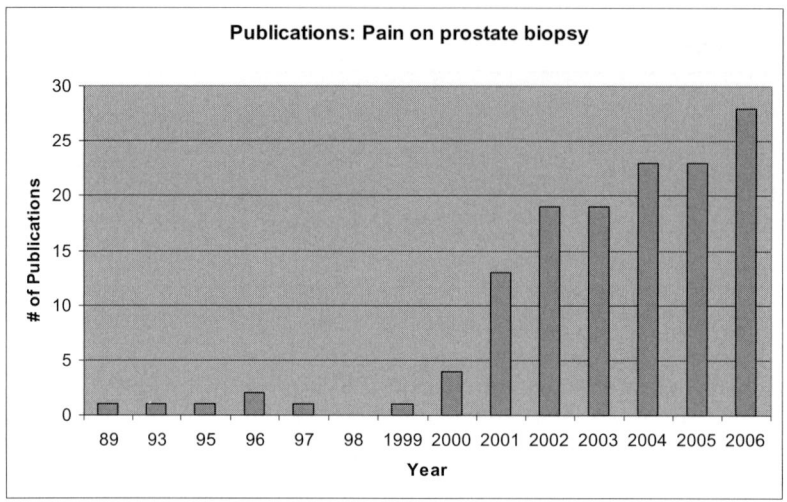

F<small>IGURE</small> 2.

The authors in this book have been carefully chosen as they represent the highest levels of expertise in this field. Browsing the list of authors involves recognition of those who have defined the science of prostate cancer diagnosis and those who continue to improve it. Taken together, their work shapes the state of the art in prostate biopsy and all topics related to prostate cancer diagnosis. The book includes intentional overlap of several chapters to acknowledge the existence and controversial nature of differing viewpoints by authorities considered the masters of their fields. Upon completion of this text, the reader will possess the most current understanding of this field.

J. Stephen Jones, M<small>D</small>

Contents

Contributors

LIONEL L. BAÑEZ, MD • *Center for Prostate Disease Research, Uniformed Services University of the Health Sciences, Rockville, MD*

TIMOTHY C. BRAND, MD • *Department of Urology, University of Texas Health Science Center, San Antonio, TX*

EDUARDO I. CANTO, MD • *Antilles Research Institute, San Juan, PR, and Baylor Prostate Center, Scott Department of Urology, Baylor College of Medicine, Houston, TX*

H. BALLENTINE CARTER, MD • *James Buchanan Brady Urological Institute, John Hopkins School of Medicine, Baltimore, MD*

WILLIAM J. CATALONA, MD • *Department of Urology, Feinberg School of Medicine, Northwestern University, Chicago, IL*

SAM S. CHANG, MD • *Department of Urologic Surgery, Vanderbilt University Medical Center, Nashville, TN*

MICHAEL S. COOKSON, MD • *Department of Urologic Surgery, Vanderbilt University Medical Center, Nashville, TN*

BOB DJAVAN, MD, PhD • *Department of Urology, University of Vienna, Vienna, Austria*

PAOLO EMILIOZZI, MD • *San Giovanni Hospital and Vincenzo Pansadoro Foundation, Rome, Italy*

NICHOLAS J. FITZSIMONS, MD • *Division of Urologic Surgery and Duke Prostate Center, Duke University Medical Center, Durham, NC*

SCOTT M. GILBERT, MD • *Department of Urology, University of Michigan, Ann Arbor, MI*

MISOP HAN, MD • *Department of Urology, Feinberg School of Medicine, Northwestern University, Chicago, IL*

J. STEPHEN JONES, MD • *Department of Regional Urology, Cleveland Clinic Glickman Urological and Kidney Institute, and Cleveland Clinic Lerner College of Medicine at CWRU. Cleveland, OH*

PIERRE I. KARAKIEWICZ, MD • *Cancer Prognostics and Health Outcomes Unit, University of Montreal Health Center, Montreal, Quebec, Canada*

MICHAEL W. KATTAN, PhD • *Department of Quantitative Health Sciences, Cleveland Clinic, Cleveland, OH*

STACY LOEB, MD • *Department of Urology, Georgetown University, Washington, DC*

CRISTINA MAGI-GALLUZZI, MD, PhD • *Departments of Anatomic Pathology, Urology, and Cancer Biology, Cleveland Clinic, Cleveland, OH*

SIBYLLE MARIHART, MD • *Department of Urology, University of Vienna, Vienna, Austria*

JUDD W. MOUL, MD • *Division of Urologic Surgery and Duke Prostate Center, Duke University Medical Center, Durham, NC*

ALAN M. NIEDER, MD • *Department of Urology, University of Miami Miller School of Medicine, Miami, FL*

MATTHEW E. NIELSEN, MD • *Brady Urological Institute, Johns Hopkins University School of Medicine, Baltimore, MD*

ROSALIE NOLLEY, MD • *Department of Urology, Stanford University Medical Center, Stanford, CA*

VITO PANSADORO, MD • *San Giovanni Hospital and Vincenzo Pansadoro Foundation, Rome, Italy*

ALAN W. PARTIN, MD, PhD • *Brady Urological Institute, Johns Hopkins University School of Medicine, Baltimore, MD*

JOSEPH C. PRESTI, JR., MD • *Stanford University School of Medicine, Stanford Cancer Center, Stanford, CA*

WAEL SAKR, MD • *Wayne State University School of Medicine, Detroit, MI*

RAJAL B. SHAH, MD • *Department of Urology and Pathology, University of Michigan, Ann Arbor, MI*

KATSUTO SHINOHARA, MD • *Department of Urology and Mt. Zion/ Comprehensive Cancer Center, University of California, San Francisco, San Francisco, CA*

KEVIN M. SLAWIN, MD • *Antilles Research Institute, San Juan, PR, and Baylor Prostate Center, Scott Department of Urology, Baylor College of Medicine, Houston, TX*

MARK S. SOLOWAY, MD • *Department of Urology, University of Miami Miller School of Medicine, Miami, FL*

THOMAS A. STAMEY, MD • *Department of Urology, Stanford University Medical Center, Stanford, CA*

LEON L. SUN, MD • *Division of Urologic Surgery and Duke Prostate Center, Duke University Medical Center, Durham, NC*

MARTHA K. TERRIS, MD • *Medical College of Georgia, Augusta, GA*

IAN M. THOMPSON, MD • *Department of Urology, University of Texas Health Science Center, San Antonio, TX*

DOROTHEA TORTI, MD • *Department of Urology, Stanford University Medical Center, Stanford, CA*

ALON Z. WEIZER, MD • *Department of Urology, University of Michigan, Ann Arbor, MI*

DAVID P. WOOD, JR., MD • *Department of Urology, University of Michigan, Ann Arbor, MI*

MING ZHOU, MD, PhD • *Departments of Anatomic Pathology, Urology, and Cancer Biology, Cleveland Clinic, Cleveland, OH*

1
Defining the Problem: From Subclinical Disease to Clinically Insignificant Prostate Cancer

Wael Sakr

Abstract

The widespread use of prostate-specific antigen testing and the increasing rate of prostate needle biopsies with recent refinement of sampling approaches have led to a dramatic increase in the diagnoses of small-volume, early-stage prostate cancer and premalignant lesions (prostatic intraepithelial neoplasia). The Wayne State autopsy study has shown the prevalence of subclinical prostate cancer and prostatic intraepithelial neoplasia to be much higher than previously reported, with a steady increase with advancing age. The findings of this and other studies raise challenges regarding the potential relationship of subclinical cancer to minute cancer foci detected in biopsies. The clinical management of patients diagnosed with such cancers is becoming more controversial because the progression potential of clinically detected small cancer foci is difficult to predict.

Keywords: "subclinical prostate cancer," autopsy, prevalence, screening

Compared with other solid tumors, prostate cancer is rather unique in its epidemiologic characteristics and the marked variations in the progression potential for patients clinically diagnosed with the disease.[1-4] Over the last decade, the debate regarding this cancer focused mainly on aspects of screening/early detection approaches in terms of defining serum prostate-specific antigen (PSA) values that are "abnormal" to trigger a biopsy, and more recently, on the number and location(s) of needle biopsies deemed adequate to establish a pathologic diagnosis of cancer. An equally important issue in this debate is the controversy regarding the "clinical significance" of at least a proportion of the cancers discovered through

From: *Current Clinical Urology: Prostate Biopsy: Indications, Techniques, and Complications*
Edited by J.S. Jones © Humana Press, Totowa, NJ

screening/early detection efforts and, finally, the impact of these efforts on disease-specific mortality.

This introductory chapter offers an overview of the epidemiology/prevalence of early neoplastic transformation of prostatic epithelium resulting in carcinoma and/or prostatic intraepithelial neoplasia (PIN). It also attempts to relate the concept of "latent/subclinical disease" to that of clinically diagnosed cancer by focusing on questions such as the following:

Is subclinical disease the precursor for what is to become clinically evident cancer? If so, why does the latter show more than 30-fold differences in incidence among different geographic populations and ethnicities whereas the prevalence of the undetected disease is reported to be remarkably less variable?

What about the potential precursor role for recently defined epithelial alterations such as PIN?

How long is the "latency" period, and what determines the progression subsets of subclinical tumors to manifest clinically?

From a practical standpoint, does the growing category of men who have small-volume, often low-grade cancers in radical prostatectomy specimens suggest that our detection methods have started to tap into the huge pool of prostate cancer historically kept "undisturbed"?

The preference to use the term "subclinical" cancer (rather than latent, incidental, or histologic) to characterize prostate cancer discovered in postmortem settings, reflects a conceptual approach to a "biologic continuum" of what is largely a slow progressing disease that encompasses a relatively small subset with a more aggressive course. These views offered are influenced by the trends in prostate cancer demographics during the last two decades and by observations gathered from a rather unique autopsy study the author has been involved with. The intent is to try to reconcile observations from these two phases of the disease to better understand the natural history of prostate cancer and hopefully to offer insight into reasonable management approaches.

How Prevalent Is "Subclinical" Prostate Cancer?

Although the incidence of clinically diagnosed prostate cancer has increased markedly since the introduction of PSA testing and, subsequently, the evolving biopsy approaches, the prevalence of the subclinical form of the disease discovered in prostates of autopsied men remains by far remarkably higher. The microscopic changes required to fulfill the criteria needed to characterize a prostatic epithelial lesion as carcinoma are exceedingly prevalent. Historically, this form of prostate cancer, often referred to as "latent" cancer, has been reported to be present in approximately 30% of men older than 50 years of age upon postmortem examination.[5,6] More recently, however, data from Sakr et al.[7] have indicated that histologically evident malignant transformation starts as early as the third decade of life and that 25%–30% of men younger than 50 years of age harbor foci of prostate cancer in their glands.

The high prevalence of preclinical cancer is reported to be universal with relatively mild geographic and ethnic variability. Whereas the prevalence is reported to be highest in the Western hemisphere, autopsy data derived from different geographic regions indicate a limited two- to threefold variation worldwide. There is the potential to underestimate variations in subclinical disease because these are related to the age range and ethnicity of the cohort studied and very importantly to the thoroughness of tissue sampling, and to an extent, the diagnostic criteria.

In a comparative study of the frequency and characteristics of "latent" carcinoma of the prostate involving populations from seven geographic areas (total of 1327 men from two Chinese populations, Sweden, Germany, Jamaica, Israel, and Uganda), Breslow et al.[8] reported 350 (12%) postmortem cancers overall with a prevalence that showed no association with age or ethnicity, although the authors reported that the rates of larger latent tumors increased with age. They also noted that the small cancers were almost exclusively situated in the outer half of the prostate.

In 1980, Guileyardo et al.[9] reported the results of a study of prostate glands from 500 autopsied African American and Caucasian men from New Orleans in which the authors found similar prevalence of latent cancers between the two racial groups with a higher prevalence of what they termed "latent infiltrative" tumors in African American men. Those tumors were also larger compared with the "latent noninfiltrative" category.

There are several limitations when one evaluates published studies addressing the prevalence of subclinical prostate cancer. These stem from the notions that:

- The majority of these data are extracted from relatively older, pre-PSA-era reports. There are scarce data based on contemporary international prostate cancer autopsy studies with inclusions of different geographic regions and ethnic populations. The latter is particularly true for groups in which the incidence and mortality rates of clinically detected prostate cancer are sharply discrepant.
- The sampling methods used in some of the frequently cited reports were partial examination and, in some cases, very limited representation of the glandular tissue subjected to microscopic evaluation.
- The microscopic criteria used for diagnosis and grading were variable and the currently adopted Gleason system was not used to grade these tumors. Precursor lesions were not documented in the majority of these reports.
- Most autopsy studies evaluated prostate glands from older men who died in hospital settings and often had comorbidities of chronic diseases.

In attempt to address some of these concerns, Wayne State University and the Medical Examiner's Office of Wayne County, both located in Detroit, Michigan, collaborated to form a contemporary autopsy study, the results of which were last updated in a 2005 report. The most recent set comprises 1027 prostate glands obtained from consecutively autopsied African American and Caucasian men from 20 to 80 years of age through the Medical Examiner's Office between the years 1992–2001. The glands were step-sectioned perpendicular to the posterior rectal surface at intervals of 2.5 mm and the resulting tissue slices were embedded as whole-mount paraffin blocks from which 5-micron hematoxylin and eosin–stained sections were obtained.

Microscopic evaluation entailed a thorough analysis of the entire gland for the presence of adenocarcinoma. The foci of carcinoma were mapped on individual specimen diagrams with the Gleason score of each focus (including the primary and secondary patterns if applicable), recorded, and the microscopic dimension of the focus was documented using a micrometer. The total cancer volume in glands harboring adenocarcinoma was then calculated by adding the volume of the individual foci. A collective final Gleason score was also documented for such specimens.

In addition, areas of high-grade PIN (HGPIN) were identified and mapped on the diagram. The degree of involvement by HGPIN was classified (graded) as focal, multifocal, or extensive, based on whether the lesion was present in 1–2 foci, 3–5 foci, or more than 5 foci, respectively. The focus of HGPIN was determined to be spatially associated with carcinoma if the two were present within one 10× microscopic field from each other.

The anatomic "zonal" distribution of the foci of cancer and HGPIN and their distance from the prostatic capsule and prostatic urethra were also documented in a large subset of the study cohort. Results of these studies were reported in a series of publications focusing on different aspects of the analysis.[7,10–13]

The major findings of the Wayne State autopsy study were:

- The prevalence of subclinical prostate cancer was much higher than previously reported with an overall rate of 34% including a large proportion of male cohorts in their 20s and 30s, an age group accounting for more than 40% of the entire study sample.
- The age was the most predictive factor for increasing prevalence as subclinical prostate cancer increased steadily from 7% to 23%, 39%, 44%, 65%, and 72% of men in their third, fourth, fifth, sixth, seventh, and eighth decades, respectively.
- Whereas the collective mean tumor volume was exceedingly small for the entire cohort (median 0.047 cc, mean 0.13 cc), the volume of subclinical prostate cancer increased significantly across the age brackets of the study, achieving a mean of 0.51 cc in men in their 70s.

- Tumor multifocalty (defined as a prostate gland harboring three or more anatomically separate tumor foci) also increased with age. There was a statistically significant difference in the number of tumor foci between men younger and older than 50 years of age.
- Gleason score was also a parameter that showed significant increase with advancing age with only a rare encounter (1.6%) of tumors harboring any pattern 4 component in men younger than 50 years of age compared with 10%, 14%, and 21% in men in their 50s, 60s, and 70s, respectively.
- There were no significant differences in these parameters between the Caucasian and the African American cohorts of the study, although within the older age groups in which the sample size became smaller (in a medical examiner–based study), the tumors found in the glands of African American men in their 50s and especially in their 60s and 70s, tended to be more multifocal, larger, with a higher proportion of foci harboring a Gleason pattern 4 component.
- With respect to HGPIN, the lesion also started to appear at a surprisingly young age with a prevalence that increased steadily as men became older. HGPIN was identified in 7%, 26%, 46%, 72%, 75%, and 91% of African Americans between the third and eighth decades compared with 8%, 23%, 29%, 49%, 53%, and 67% for Caucasian men.
- The overall prevalence of HGPIN was generally higher in the glands of African Americans compared with Caucasians but the statistically significant difference was established when the lesion was semiquantitated using a scale based on the extensiveness of its distribution in the gland. African Americans, particularly younger than age 60, had a higher proportion of extensive glandular involvement compared with their Caucasian counterparts.
- The topographic distribution of the microscopic foci of carcinoma and those of HGPIN was interesting: Close to 90% of these foci were identified in the outer peripheral zone, within 5 mm from the capsular surface/ anatomic boundaries of the gland. This phenomenon was true for both racial groups and within the spectrum of age brackets included in the study. The distribution was also evident regardless of the size "volume" of the prostate. Whereas the latter also increased consistently with older age reflecting primarily expansion of the transition zone by benign prostatic hyperplasia, the location of the small neoplastic foci remained overwhelmingly peripheral. This observation is of importance because it relates to the improved yield of the "extended" biopsy approach based on targeting of the outer lateral gland and on obtaining more biopsy cores.
- The relationship between foci of carcinoma and HGPIN was complex and variable. This encompasses the presence of one lesion or two lesions in the same gland, whether the "extensiveness" of HGPIN relates to the

likelihood of the gland harboring carcinoma, and the spatial association between the two lesions, i.e., presence within the same microscopic vicinity defined in this study as being within one 10× microscopic field. The presence of carcinoma or HGPIN in isolation of each other, meaning glands harboring one of the two lesions only, was more evident in the younger age group of the study in both races with 17% of microscopic cancers identified in men younger than 50 years of age occurring in glands with no evidence of HGPIN. This phenomenon practically disappeared in older men in whom nearly all glands with cancer were found to harbor HGPIN in a close or distant anatomic site. Identifying HGPIN in isolation of cancer, however, was more common and less confounded by age with an overall 29% of HGPIN lesions present in glands in which carcinoma was not identified. The extent of HGPIN within the prostate correlated significantly with the likelihood of the gland harboring carcinoma: Prostates with focal, multifocal, and extensive HGPIN were found to contain carcinoma in 26%, 49%, and 74% of the cases, respectively.

Although the study has the advantage of accounting for detailed documentation of the earliest neoplastic transformation of prostatic epithelium in a large, racially mixed cohort of a wide age spectrum, it has the limitations of not having access to information on risk factors, personal or family history, or PSA levels.

Another recent report from the University of Iowa focused mainly on the changing prevalence of latent (subclinical) prostate cancer found at autopsy before and after the wide utilization of PSA. Konety et al.[14] reviewed institutional autopsy records from two periods: 1955–1960 (pre-PSA, total 3307 men) and 1991–2001 (after the introduction of PSA, total 2938 men). Each cohort had an adequate number of men at risk for prostate cancer, defined as being older than 40 years.

The authors calculated the age-based incidence of subclinical cancer in an at-risk population of men (older than 40 years) and compared Gleason grade distribution and the proportion of locally advanced stage (cT3 or greater) between the two periods of the study. They reported a prevalence of subclinical prostate cancer of 4.8% for the 1955–1960 period compared with 1.2% prevalence for 1991–2001. The proportion of autopsy-detected cancers in relation to all prostate cancers reported to the author's institutional tumor registry between 1955 and 1960 was 76 of 1195 (6.3%) compared with 6 of 2187 (0.73%) between 1991 and 2001. The proportion of subclinical cancers detected at autopsy and reported to the statewide registry was 0.4% (96 of 25,238) between 1991 and 2001.

Seventeen of 76 (22%) of the cancers detected between 1955 and 1960 were classified as stage cT3 whereas none of the cancers detected at autopsy in the 1991–2001 period were found to extend grossly beyond the prostate. The proportion of lower-grade tumors (Gleason ≤6) was reported to be significantly higher during the more recent period of the study.

The study conclusions suggest that the more widespread use of PSA for screening contributed to a threefold decrease in the prevalence of latent prostate cancer with the effect most pronounced in men older than 70 years and that both the stage and the grade of tumors discovered during the PSA era were lower compared with those detected before PSA use.

Other recent reports suggested similar effect of decreasing subclinical and incidental cancer rates during the last 15 years as a direct link to PSA screening. In a similar study, Zigeuner et al.[15] evaluated the impact of PSA testing on the rate of incidental prostate cancer in patients undergoing surgery for obstructive symptoms caused by presumed benign prostatic enlargement. Whereas incidental cancer was found in 13% of the 2422 patients, only 6.4% of patients had both negative age-specific PSA levels and negative digital rectal examination findings. The authors concluded that in the PSA era, the rate of incidental prostate cancer decreased by more than 50%. The findings based on the Utah Cancer Registry reported by Merrill et al. also suggest that age-specific transurethral resection of the prostate–detected cancer rates were flat between 1980 and 1990, decreased through 1994, and then leveled off. The authors also attributed the decrease to PSA screening.

Despite the significant limitations related mainly to the incompleteness of tissue sampling for pathologic examination, most evident in the study by Konety et al., the report of the Iowa group raises the possibility that a significant proportion of tumors that would have been detected historically in a postmortem setting only are being diagnosed during the lifetime of men subjected to PSA screening.

Whereas a study by Yatani et al.[16] indicated a decrease in the volume of subclinical cancer in Japan when the two periods of 1965–1979 and 1982–1986 were compared, Konety et al. conversely reported an increase in the prevalence of subclinical cancer in Japan between the two periods of their study. The variables in this study, however, are difficult to compare with those of the study by the Iowa group in terms of ethnicity, single versus multiinstitutional cohorts, and also regarding the pathologic terminology used.

Winkler et al.[17] designed a study to investigate the relationship between PSA level and tumor volume for incidental prostate cancer found in cystoprostatectomy specimens and to identify the prevalence of clinically significant cancers in such specimens. Microscopic evaluation was performed entirely on submitted prostates removed during cystoprostatectomy for urothelial carcinoma. The authors found incidental prostate cancer in 58 of 97 (60%) specimens with 31 (53%) defined as significant (>0.5 cc and/or with a component of Gleason pattern 4). The correlation between tumor volume and PSA level was weak with median PSA level for patients with and without cancer being 3.1 and 1.1 ng/mL, respectively (p = 0.06). The authors defined more than half of the cancers discovered as clinically significant, and concluded that PSA in asymptomatic healthy men is largely produced by benign prostatic hyperplasia and is therefore a poor screening tool in such men.

If PSA screening is indeed decreasing the pool of what traditionally was considered subclinical prostate cancer, does that mean that PSA testing is more likely to detect tumors with low progression potential and that some of those may not need to be discovered or treated? More specifically, has PSA screening begun to detect a growing subset of clinically insignificant cancers?

In a recent report, Graif et al.[18] attempted to quantify the rates of over- and underdiagnosed prostate cancer in a cohort of 2126 men with clinical stage T1c cancer treated with radical prostatectomy and divided into three subsets based on treatment periods (1989–1995, 1995–2001, and 2001–2005). The authors defined "overdiagnosed" cancers as pathologically organ confined, Gleason score ≤6, volume of ≤0.5 cc, and negative surgical margins. Underdiagnosed tumors were characterized as nonorgan confined, pathologic stage T3 or greater, or with positive surgical margins. Based on these definitions, the authors found 1.3%–7.1% of the cancers to be overdiagnosed compared with an underdiagnosed rate of 25%–30%.

Younger men (≤55 years) were significantly more likely to meet the authors' criteria for overdiagnosed cancer. Their results also indicate that lowering PSA threshold for biopsy from 4.0 to 2.5 ng/mL reduced the rate of underdiagnosed tumors from 30% to 26% whereas it increased the proportion of tumors characterized as being overdiagnosed from 1.3% to 7.1%. Changing the PSA threshold for biopsy also increased the 5-year progression-free survival rate from 85% to 92%.

Using similar criteria to define over- and underdiagnosed cancer, Pelzer et al.[19] investigated this concern in two cohorts with two PSA ranges of 2.0–3.9 (lower range) and 4.0–10.0 ng/mL (higher range) of an asymptomatic screening population. The authors found 19.7% and 16.5% overdiagnosis rates in the lower and upper PSA ranges, respectively, whereas the corresponding figures for the underdiagnosed tumors were 18.9% and 36.7%, respectively.

The findings of a similar cohort reported by Makarov et al.[20] indicated more favorable pathologic features for patients biopsied and diagnosed based on a lower PSA threshold. Of the 2896 men with clinical stage T1c disease treated with radical prostatectomy between 1985 and 2004, two subsets with prebiopsy PSA of 2.6–4.0 (784) and 4.1–6.00 (2112) ng/mL were identified. Using a lower PSA threshold for biopsy resulted in significantly decreased odds of Gleason score 7 or greater, positive surgical margins, and extraprostatic extension in the radical prostatectomy specimen. Only a trend for decreased risk for biochemical progression was associated with using lower versus higher PSA for biopsy (relative risk 1.48, 95% confidence interval 0.69–3.19, $p = 0.31$, statistically insignificant). A study by Krumholtz et al.[21] also found that the use of a 2.6 ng/mL PSA threshold for screening resulted in more frequent detection of small, organ-confined tumors without overdetecting possibly clinically insignificant ones.

Even if PSA is "neutralized" as a factor in determining the need for biopsy, the likelihood of discovering clinically unsuspected prostate cancer remains alarmingly significant. The concern is further compounded by the notion that a subset of the cancers discovered in the absence of "abnormal" PSA values, including men with levels of PSA less than 2.00 and even 1.00 ng/mL were potentially progressive cancers with a proportion containing a Gleason grade 4 component.[22–25]

However, the sextant needle biopsy technique, which has dominated the earlier phase of the PSA era as the primary sampling approach for prostate cancer detection, has been largely abandoned. It became increasingly evident over the last decade that sextant biopsies are associated with a "false-negative" rate reported to range from 20% to 73%. This concern is supported by studies using data based on findings of repeat biopsies, computer simulation, and correlation with tumor presence/distribution in radical prostatectomy specimens. The "underdetection" of the sextant likely reflects the limitation of the sampling method and the notion that a significant proportion of the larger tumors have been discovered during a decade of testing, making it more difficult to detect smaller cancers using the same numbers of biopsies/sampling approaches.[26–30] Furthermore, investigators have shown that the sextant protocol tends to undersample certain areas of the prostate such as the anterior "horns" and the most lateral "outer" aspects of the peripheral zone.

The combination of increased number of core biopsies obtained routinely (replacing the six-core sextant approach by an average of 8–14 cores) with targeting the most outer peripheral zone compartment including the "apical/anterior horn of the prostate," has increased the efficiency of detecting smaller tumors at the offset and improved the ability to confirm cancer diagnosis in patients who had repeat biopsies for a variety of reasons. It can be argued that the refinement of the biopsy approach has the benefits of increasing detection particularly as specific recommendations are considered for patients with larger glands and those who require more than one biopsy set, including the smaller proportion of patients subjected to saturation biopsies.[31]

Summary

There is some validity, however, to the notion that our "perfection" of cancer detection by identifying the patients at higher risk for prostate cancer based on ethnicity, age, and family history, lowering PSA threshold for biopsy, and increasing and better targeting of sampling has resulted in an increasing proportion of patients who have potentially "clinically insignificant" tumors. Are we contributing to an expanded area of overlap between the subclinical and the clinically evident phases of the disease?

From a pathologist's perspective, this new phase of the disease introduces certain diagnostic challenges as the determination is based on increasingly smaller cancers, often limited to a few malignant acini that are present in only one of the multiple cores obtained. In a proportion of these early cases, definitive diagnosis cannot be established on the original hematoxylin and eosin slides requiring further efforts of leveling, immunoperoxidase staining, and expert opinion. The proportion of cases showing earlier and preinvasive neoplastic changes also increases.

Perhaps the more important challenge is that posed to the newly diagnosed patient and his managing clinician(s): What is the management of a less than 1-mm Gleason score 6 carcinoma identified in one of 10 cores in a patient with a biopsy PSA of 2.4 ng/mL? It is difficult to answer this question with any absolute certainty despite the knowledge we managed to expand regarding the ubiquitously prevalent subclinical disease, the striking stage shift in the clinically diagnosed/treated disease, and the diminishing risk of both progression (biochemical recurrence) and decreasing disease-specific mortality. The "statistical" knowledge that the greatest majority of prostate cancers are slow-growing nonthreatening cancers does not preclude the "individual" reality of our limited ability to predict the biologic course of a particular small, low-grade cancer discovered in increasingly younger, healthier patients with longer life expectancy.

References

1. Boyle P, Severi G, Giles GG. The epidemiology of prostate cancer. Urol Clin North Am 2003;30(2):209–17.
2. Delongchamps NB, Singh A, Haas GP. The role of prevalence in the diagnosis of prostate cancer. Cancer Control 2006;13(3):158–68.
3. Quinn M, Babb P. Patterns and trends in prostate cancer incidence, survival, prevalence and mortality. Part I: international comparisons. BJU Int 2002;90(2):162–73.
4. Nelen V. Epidemiology of prostate cancer. Recent Results Cancer Res 2007; 175:1–8.
5. Franks LM. Latent carcinoma of the prostate. J Pathol Bacteriol 1954;68(2): 603–16.
6. Holund B. Latent prostatic cancer in a consecutive autopsy series. Scand J Urol Nephrol 1980;14(1):29–35.
7. Sakr WA, et al. The frequency of carcinoma and intraepithelial neoplasia of the prostate in young male patients. J Urol 1993;150(2 Pt 1):379–85.
8. Breslow N, et al. Latent carcinoma of prostate at autopsy in seven areas. The International Agency for Research on Cancer, Lyons, France. Int J Cancer 1977;20(5):680–8.
9. Guileyardo JM, et al. Prevalence of latent prostate carcinoma in two U.S. populations. J Natl Cancer Inst 1980;65(2):311–6.
10. Sakr WA, Grignon DJ, Haas GP. Pathology of premalignant lesions and carcinoma of the prostate in African-American men. Semin Urol Oncol 1998; 16(4):214–20.
11. Sakr WA, et al. Age and racial distribution of prostatic intraepithelial neoplasia. Eur Urol 1996;30(2):138–44.

12. Sakr WA, et al. Epidemiology of high grade prostatic intraepithelial neoplasia. Pathol Res Pract 1995;191(9):838–41.
13. Sakr WA, et al. Epidemiology and molecular biology of early prostatic neoplasia. Mol Urol 2000;4(3):109–13; discussion 115.
14. Konety BR, et al. Comparison of the incidence of latent prostate cancer detected at autopsy before and after the prostate specific antigen era. J Urol 2005;174(5):1785–8; discussion 1788.
15. Zigeuner RE, et al. Did the rate of incidental prostate cancer change in the era of PSA testing? A retrospective study of 1127 patients. Urology 2003;62(3): 451–5.
16. Yatani R, et al. Trends in frequency of latent prostate carcinoma in Japan from 1965–1979 to 1982–1986. J Natl Cancer Inst 1988;80(9):683–7.
17. Winkler MH, et al. Characteristics of incidental prostatic adenocarcinoma in contemporary radical cystoprostatectomy specimens. BJU Int 2007;99(3):554–8.
18. Graif T, et al. Under diagnosis and over diagnosis of prostate cancer. J Urol 2007;178(1):88–92.
19. Pelzer AE, et al. Under diagnosis and over diagnosis of prostate cancer in a screening population with serum PSA 2 to 10 ng/ml. J Urol 2007;178(1):93–97.
20. Makarov DV, et al. Pathological outcomes and biochemical progression in men with T1c prostate cancer undergoing radical prostatectomy with prostate specific antigen 2.6 to 4.0 vs 4.1 to 6.0 ng/ml. J Urol 2006;176(2):554–8.
21. Krumholtz JS, et al. Prostate-specific antigen cutoff of 2.6 ng/mL for prostate cancer screening is associated with favorable pathologic tumor features. Urology 2002;60(3):469–73; discussion 473–4.
22. Thompson IM, et al. Screening for prostate cancer: opportunities and challenges. Surg Oncol Clin North Am 2005;14(4):747–60.
23. Bozeman CB, et al. Prostate cancer in patients with an abnormal digital rectal examination and serum prostate-specific antigen less than 4.0 ng/mL. Urology 2005;66(4):803–7.
24. Gosselaar C, et al. Screening for prostate cancer at low PSA range: the impact of digital rectal examination on tumor incidence and tumor characteristics. Prostate 2007;67(2):154–61.
25. Thiesler T, et al. Patients with low prostate-specific antigen levels (≤4 ng/ml) would benefit from a twelve-core biopsy protocol for prostate cancer detection. Urol Int 2007;78(4):318–22.
26. Becopoulos T. Clinically significant and nonsignificant prostate cancer: an ongoing question. Acta Chir Iugosl 2005;52(4):27–9.
27. Djavan B, Margreiter M. Biopsy standards for detection of prostate cancer. World J Urol 2007;25(1):11–7.
28. Miyake H, et al. Increased detection of clinically significant prostate cancer by additional sampling from the anterior lateral horns of the peripheral zone in combination with the standard sextant biopsy. Int J Urol 2004;11(6):402–6.
29. Presti JC Jr. Prostate biopsy: how many cores are enough? Urol Oncol 2003;21(2):135–40.
30. Stamatiou K, et al. Impact of additional sampling in the TRUS-guided biopsy for the diagnosis of prostate cancer. Urol Int 2007;78(4):313–7.
31. Stewart CS, et al. Prostate cancer diagnosis using a saturation needle biopsy technique after previous negative sextant biopsies. J Urol 2001;166(1):86–91; discussion 91–2.

2
What Every Patient Should Know about Prostate Cancer Before He Submits to Biopsy of His Prostate

Thomas A. Stamey, Rosalie Nolley, and Dorothea Torti

Abstract

Prostate cancer increases with each decade of life. Eight percent of men have invasive prostate cancer in their 20s; 80% of men have invasive prostate cancer in their 70s. Prostate cancer is easily cured and the actual death rate is very low. The common development of prostate cancer with aging and low death rate should be explained to every patient before he undergoes biopsy.

Keywords: screening, clinically insignificant, prostate biopsy

Every man should recognize two facts before he submits to biopsy of his prostate. First, almost all men develop prostate cancer, albeit age dependent. Beginning in 8% of men in their 20s, prostate cancer increases with each decade of life until 80% of men (both black and white) in their 70s have an invasive prostate cancer.[1] Second, despite this astonishing ubiquity of prostate cancer, the death rate is extraordinarily small at 226 per 100,000 men 65 years and older, which is about 0.002%.[2] This small risk of dying from prostate cancer should be explained and emphasized to every man *before* he undergoes biopsy of his prostate. Because essentially all men develop prostate cancer as they age, this very small risk (0.002%) of dying from prostate cancer is obviously important. It is irrelevant—although often pointed out—that prostate cancer is the second most common cause of cancer death in men (lung cancer from cigarette smoking is the most common). The irrelevance derives from the facts that very few men are cured of lung cancer whereas most men are easily cured of prostate cancer or live to die of some other, more serious disease.

From: *Current Clinical Urology: Prostate Biopsy: Indications, Techniques, and Complications*
Edited by J.S. Jones © Humana Press, Totowa, NJ

Positive biopsy rates for prostate cancer are largely determined by the patient's age at the time of biopsy, how many biopsies are taken by the urologist (an average of 23 biopsies are taken at one famous institution), and whether the cancer was palpable on digital rectal examination of the prostate, i.e., felt like one of the knuckles of your clenched fist. If the cancer is large enough to be felt by the finger on examination of the prostate, it is usually large enough to warrant treatment, i.e., surgery, radioactive I^{125} seed implantation, or external beam radiation therapy. When performed by experienced clinicians, the cancer cure rates are reasonably similar for all three of these major modalities of treatment.

We believe that every man should recognize two biologic facts *before* submitting to biopsy of his prostate. First, prostate cancer is unique among all human cancers in that almost all men develop it with increasing age. Sakr's autopsies performed on 525 black men and white men accidentally killed on the streets of Detroit (314 black men and 211 white men) show that an invasive prostate cancer is present in 8% of both black and white men in their 20s but increases with each passing decade until 80% of both races have prostate cancer in their 70s.[1] In addition to the ubiquity of prostate cancer (all men get it if they live long enough), it is very important to recognize that the death rate from prostate cancer as determined by the National Cancer Institute is astonishingly small: about 0.002%.[2] Thus, even though most men will develop prostate cancer with aging, fortunately, the actual death rate from prostate cancer is very, very small. It is true that prostate cancer is the second largest cause of cancer death in the United States, with lung cancer from smoking cigarettes being the number one cause; the tragedy of this comparison is that lung cancer is almost exclusively caused by smoking cigarettes and therefore is essentially preventable. This information, in our opinion, should be carefully and fully explained to every man before he submits to a biopsy of his prostate. It is most important to understand that the death rate from prostate cancer is very small, i.e., only 226 per 100,000 men over 65 years old.

References

1. Sakr WA, Grignon DJ, Haas GP, Heilbrun LK, Pontes JE, Crissman JD. Age and racial distribution of prostatic intraepithelial neoplasia. Eur Urol 1996;30:138–144.
2. Ries LAG, Eisner MP, Kosary CL, et al. SEER Cancer Statistics Review, 1975–2000, National Cancer Institute. Bethesda, MD. Available at: http://seer.cancer.gov./csr/1975_2000. 2003.

3
Prostate-Specific Antigen and Prostate Cancer Screening

Stacy Loeb, Misop Han, and William J. Catalona

Abstract

Although the Food and Drug Administration recommends a prostate-specific antigen (PSA) threshold of 4 ng/dL as abnormal, investigations into the use of lower thresholds have shown substantial positive predictive value. The authors recommend that screening for prostate cancer begin at age 40 years. Initial PSA value should be assessed in respect to the median PSA level for the patient's age group. If findings on digital rectal examination are suspicious for prostate cancer or the total PSA is greater than 2.5 ng/dL, a 12-core transrectal ultrasonography–guided biopsy should be strongly considered. Both patient and physician should maintain a PSA flow chart that records all PSA values, the date of measurement, and the PSA assay used. Patients with persistent elevated PSA levels may benefit from further evaluation using other PSA parameters to improve prostate cancer detection and assessment of aggressiveness before biopsy. Parameters described in this chapter include percent free PSA, age-specific PSA levels, complexed PSA levels, PSA density, PSA transition zone density, PSA velocity, PSA doubling time, pro-PSA, and human glandular kallikrein.

Keywords: PSA, percent free PSA, PSA density, PSA velocity, screening

Prostate-specific antigen (PSA) was initially described in forensic medicine as a marker for human semen and, thus, initially was called gamma-seminoprotein.[1] It was later recognized as a marker for prostate diseases. Wang et al.[2] purified PSA in 1979 and developed PSA-specific antisera for

From: *Current Clinical Urology: Prostate Biopsy: Indications, Techniques, and Complications*
Edited by J.S. Jones © Humana Press, Totowa, NJ

use in subsequent studies. They found immunoreactive PSA in all samples of normal prostate, benign prostatic hyperplasia (BPH), and prostate cancer; whereas, the PSA antisera had no reactivity with extracts from other, nonprostatic tissues. Additional studies by these authors suggested the presence of PSA in higher concentrations in the serum of prostate cancer patients but not in those of healthy controls, leading them to suggest that "this prostate antigen, although a eutopic component of the prostate, may play a role in the detection of prostate cancer."[2] However, because of the substantial overlap between serum PSA levels of patients with BPH or prostatitis and those with prostate cancer, it was initially believed that PSA could not be used as a screening test for prostate cancer.

Over the next two decades, considerable research was undertaken to further elucidate the properties of PSA. PSA is a member of the human kallikrein family of proteins.[3,4] It is a serine protease produced by the prostatic acinar and ductal epithelium. Some PSA is also demonstrable immunohistologically in the periurethral glands. The biologic function of PSA is believed to be to liquefy the seminal coagulum.[5] Under normal physiologic conditions, PSA is secreted in a polar manner away from the basement membrane of the prostatic acini almost entirely into the prostatic acinar lumen and ducts in concentrations of up to 1,000,000 ng/mL or more, with minimal diffusion into the systemic circulation (approximately 1 ng/mL). However, the serum level of PSA may be increased in clinical diseases and with manipulation of the prostate gland, including prostate cancer, BPH, prostatitis, after ejaculation, and clinical manipulation or instrumentation of the prostate gland, such as urethral catheterization, cystoscopy, transrectal ultrasonography (TRUS), and digital rectal examination (DRE).

It has been reported that prostate cancer tissue releases approximately 10-fold more PSA into the serum than does benign prostate tissue.[6] Although PSA exists in several different forms in the circulation, the majority is "complexed" to its natural substrates, such as α-1-antichymotrypsin.[7,8] Commercial immunoassays for total PSA detect both this complexed form and the unbound ("free") isoforms of PSA.

Stenman et al.[7] and Lilja et al.[8] reported that the relative proportion of free PSA was lower in association with prostate cancer than with BPH. This observation led to the paradigm that the percentage of free PSA could be used as a serum marker to help discriminate between prostate cancer and BPH.[9]

Subsequently, Mikolajczyk et al.[10] identified three isoforms of free PSA. Two of these, called "B" (BPH)-PSA and "i" (inactive) PSA seem to be increased with BPH; whereas, several different proenzyme "pro"-PSA isoforms are present in increased concentrations with prostate cancer (see Figure 3.1). These recently discovered PSA isoforms also might prove useful in the detection of prostate cancer and in the assessment of its potential aggressiveness.

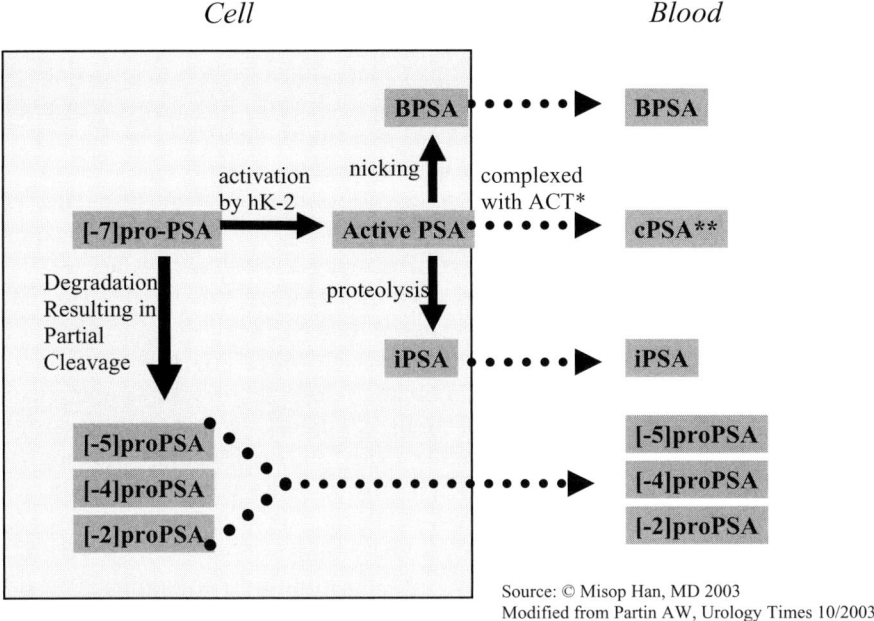

FIGURE 3.1. Prostate-specific antigen (PSA) isoforms in cells and blood. *ACT = a1-antichymotrypsin. **PSA-ACT is immunoreactive, but not PSA-a2-macroglobulin. hK-2 = human glandular kallikrein, BPSA = benign prostate-specific antigen, iPSA = initial prostate-specific antigen, cPSA = complexed prostate-specific antigen. (Adapted from Partin AW, Gretzer MB. Molecular forms of PSA: what does the future hold? Urology Times 10/2003.)

Uses of Total Prostate-Specific Antigen

PSA was first approved as a serum tumor marker by the United States Food and Drug Administration (FDA) in 1986, for monitoring patients with documented prostate cancer. However, the 1980s also marked the beginning of considerable research into the possible role of PSA in prostate cancer screening and detection. In 1990, Cooner et al.[11] reported on studies from their private practice in which PSA levels were recorded in men who were evaluated for prostate cancer and biopsied exclusively for abnormalities on DRE or suspicious findings on TRUS. These studies revealed a strong association of PSA levels with the finding of prostate cancer on biopsy.

Catalona et al.[12] initiated a longitudinal community-based prostate cancer screening study that ultimately enrolled more than 36,000 men and lasted for 12 years. They reported that PSA could be used as a first-line screening test for prostate cancer and that, in this regard, PSA was more accurate than DRE for detecting prostate cancer. These screening studies also demonstrated that PSA-based screening nearly doubled the detection rate of organ-confined prostate cancer, leading to the cancer detection in an earlier, more curable stage.[13,14] Based on a national, multiinstitutional study in 1994, the FDA approved PSA as an aid to the early prostate cancer detection, using a threshold of 4.0 ng/mL for recommending biopsy.[15]

Since that time, however, there has been investigation into the use of lower PSA thresholds for biopsy or, alternatively, for the use of a sliding scale approach including PSA information for assessing prostate cancer risk.[16] A substantial proportion of prostate cancers can be detected by biopsy in men with PSA levels less than 4 ng/mL. In a population of men with benign findings on DRE, Krumholtz et al.[17] found a positive predictive value of 26% in the PSA ranges between 2.6 and 4.0 ng/mL, as compared with 31% for PSA levels greater than 4.0 ng/mL. Subsequently, using regression analysis to correct for verification bias, Punglia et al.[18] estimated that many prostate cancers are missed if only patients with a PSA >4 ng/mL undergo prostate biopsy. In the Prostate Cancer Prevention Trial, men in the placebo group who had a benign DRE and a PSA level <4.0 ng/mL during the 7-year study period were invited to undergo an empiric end-of-study biopsy. In this group of patients, as the PSA level ranged from <0.5 to 4 ng/mL, the cancer detection rate steadily increased from 6.6% to 26.9%.[19] Yet, even at these relatively low PSA levels, the prostate cancer detection rate is directly correlated with the serum PSA level across all clinically relevant PSA levels. Nevertheless, a potential problem with lowering the PSA threshold below 4 ng/mL is that it would lead to an immediate increase in the number of prostate biopsies recommended.[20] However, longitudinal screening studies have shown that approximately 50% of men with PSA levels >2.5 ng/mL have their PSA levels increase above 4 ng/mL within 5 years and thus would be advised to have prostate biopsy at a later time anyway.[21] For these men, lowering the threshold merely moves the biopsy forward in time.

Not only is PSA used to detect the current presence of prostate cancer, but it has also been shown to predict future prostate cancer risk.[22] Gann et al.[23] reported that men with a higher baseline PSA level are significantly more likely to be diagnosed with prostate cancer many years after the initial PSA measurement, findings which were based on men in the Physician's Health Study with at least 10 years of follow-up after an initial PSA measurement but who were not part of a formal screening protocol. For example, compared with men with a baseline PSA level <1 ng/mL, single baseline PSA measurements of 1.01–1.5, 1.51–2.0, 2.01–3.0, 3.01–4.0, 4.01–10.0, and >10 ng/mL were associated with 2.2-, 3.4-, 5.5-, 8.6-, 22.2-, and 145.3-fold increased relative risk of prostate cancer detection in the next decade. Similarly, Whittemore et al.[22] reported that PSA levels measured in sera of men in their 30s were significantly associated with the risk of being diagnosed with prostate cancer many years later. For example, men in their 30s

with PSA levels >0.55 ng/mL had a 5.7-fold increased risk of being diagnosed with prostate cancer as compared with comparably aged patients
whose levels were <0.24 ng/mL.

Variations on Prostate-Specific Antigen to Improve the Accuracy of Prostate-Specific Antigen Testing

To minimize confounding of PSA-based prostate cancer screening by
benign conditions and to avoid some unnecessary biopsies in men with
intermediate total PSA levels, other PSA-based parameters have been
proposed to improve the specificity of PSA for prostate cancer detection
and assessment of aggressiveness.

Percent Free Prostate-Specific Antigen

The percentage of free PSA in serum is increased in men with BPH,
because the transition zone of the prostate, where BPH predominantly
occurs, contains increased levels of free PSA isoforms, that diffuse into the
circulation. In contrast, the percentage of free PSA generally is lower in
men with prostate cancer. Catalona et al.,[9] in a multiinstitutional study,
demonstrated that measurements of the percentage of free PSA could help
discriminate between cancer and benign prostatic disease in men whose
PSA ranges between 4 and 10 ng/mL. In this study, the risk for finding
cancer on biopsy was 8% in men with >25% free PSA as compared with
56% in those with <10% free PSA. Based on these studies, in 1994 the FDA
approved the free PSA test as an aid to early prostate cancer detection.
The percent free PSA also is helpful in determining the need for performing
a repeat prostate biopsy in patients whose initial biopsies are negative for
cancer.[24]

Age-Specific Prostate-Specific Antigen Reference Ranges

Age-specific PSA cutoffs for recommending biopsy have been proposed as
a means to increase the specificity of PSA in older men and to increase the
sensitivity of PSA testing in younger men. For example, Oesterling et al.[25]
proposed a cutoff of 2.5 ng/mL for men aged 40–49, 3.5 ng/mL for men aged
50–59, 4.5 ng/mL for men aged 60–69, and 6.5 ng/mL for men aged 70–79.
Morgan et al.[26] also factored in race, and proposed threshold values of
2.0 ng/mL for black men aged 40–49, 4.0 ng/mL for black men aged 50–59,
4.5 ng/mL for black men aged 60–69, and 5.5 ng/mL for black men aged
70–79. Although these reference ranges would substantially decrease the
overall number of negative biopsies, they would miss or delay the detection
of prostate cancer in older men.

Recent studies have shown that age-specific cutoffs based on the median PSA value for the age group in men without clinical evidence of prostate cancer also are strongly associated with the risk for prostate cancer. For example, among a large population of screened community men, the median PSA was 0.7 ng/mL for men in their 40s, 0.9 ng/mL for men in their 50s, and 1.5 ng/mL for men aged 60 and older.[27] Men whose PSA levels are above the median for their age group are at increased risk for subsequently being diagnosed with prostate cancer and for having aggressive prostate cancer. Overall, these data highlight that any man with a PSA level higher than 2.5 ng/mL, or with a PSA level above the age-specific median, is at high risk of prostate cancer.

Complexed Prostate-Specific Antigen

Some authors have proposed the use of assays measuring complexed PSA (cPSA) in screening for prostate cancer. There are limited clinical studies assessing risk for prostate cancer based solely on the serum concentration of cPSA. Brawer and his collaborators reported that, in a heterogeneous multiinstitutional patient cohort, cPSA had a greater specificity for prostate cancer than either total PSA or the percentage of free PSA (areas under receiver operating curves = 0.772, 0.688, and 0.689, respectively).[28] Studies of other patient populations generally have not confirmed this observation. Because the total PSA equals the sum of free PSA and cPSA, no one measurement should provide more predictive information than the other two. From a practical standpoint, the main information yielded from the cPSA measurement is that the total PSA concentration is equal, slightly higher, or substantially higher. cPSA testing has not received widespread use in clinical practice.

Prostate-Specific Antigen Density

PSA density is calculated by dividing the serum PSA level by the estimated volume of the prostate gland. Veneziano et al.[29] first reported a mean PSA/ volume index of 1.73 in men diagnosed with prostate cancer, 0.107 in men with prostatitis, and 0.0946 in patients with BPH. Benson et al.[30] reported that the PSA density (using the radical prostatectomy specimen weight) in 41 men with prostate cancer (0.581) was higher than in 20 comparison patients with BPH (0.044, using prostate volume measurements from magnetic resonance imaging).

One limitation of PSA density is the requirement for TRUS measurements to estimate prostate volume. To evaluate the accuracy of the prostate volume estimation, Terris and Stamey[31] compared 15 different mathematical formulas. They concluded that the elliptical formula was most accurate in men with a prostate gland weighing less than 80 grams, whereas the spherical formula performed better in larger glands. Our research group reported a correlation coefficient of 0.65 between TRUS volume estimations and the weight of the surgical specimen.[32] In addition to its suboptimal accuracy, the routine use of TRUS for the sole purpose of estimating prostate volume adds cost and patient discomfort to the screening process. Nevertheless, when TRUS measurements are available, PSA density is useful for discriminating between cancer and benign disease as the cause of an elevated PSA and for assessing the potential aggressiveness of the cancer, as PSA density correlates with prostate cancer volume.

Prostate-Specific Antigen Transition Zone Density

PSA transition zone density, or PSAD-TZ, is a variation of PSA density calculated by dividing the serum PSA by the volume of the transition zone estimated by TRUS. Similar to the total prostate volume, the volume of the transition zone is estimated using the prolate ellipsoid formula. Zlotta et al.[33] reported an average PSAD-TZ of 1.03 ng/mL/cc in men with prostate cancer, as compared with 0.21 ng/mL/cc in men with biopsies negative for prostate cancer. Unfortunately, as with PSAD, the calculation of PSAD-TZ requires both the use of TRUS and the ability to accurately estimate the volume of the transition zone (not always clearly demarcated on TRUS in all prostate glands).

Prostate-Specific Antigen Velocity and Prostate-Specific Antigen Doubling Time

PSA velocity (PSAV) is the term used to describe the rate of change of PSA over time. Carter et al.[34] first demonstrated in a small, nonscreened population that the PSAV was significantly greater in men with prostate cancer (0.75 ng/mL/year) than in controls. Smith and Catalona[35] subsequently examined the role of PSAV in prostate cancer detection in a large community-based screening population. Prostate cancer was detected in 47% of men with a PSAV greater than 0.75 ng/mL/year, compared with 11% of participants with a lower PSAV.

PSA measurements in individual patients have a considerable short-term physiologic variability, as well as additional variability attributable to benign conditions that can confound the accurate calculation of PSAV and variability attributable to differences in assay standardization and differential measurement of PSA isoforms by antibodies used in commercial assays. Roehrborn et al.[36] reported on 291 men who underwent repeat PSA measurements less than 90 days apart. In 30% of these men, the PSA values differed by greater than 1 ng/mL, which in some cases may have altered the recommendation for biopsy based on which value was used. Thus, for

PSAV to be meaningful, there must be a sufficient time interval between the component PSA measurements. In patients who have fluctuating PSA levels with "peaks" and "valleys" in plots of their PSA over time, plots of the "valleys" may be more meaningful in assessing the general PSAV trend. PSA kinetics measurements also can be confounded by high-grade prostate cancers that do not produce much PSA.

Although men who develop prostate cancer may have a greater PSAV many years before prostate cancer diagnosis,[37] the PSAV during the year before diagnosis has been reported to have a significant prognostic value for treatment outcome. For example, D'Amico et al.[38] examined the PSAV in the year before diagnosis in 1095 men who underwent radical prostatectomy for clinically localized prostate cancer. A PSAV greater than 2 ng/mL/year was significantly associated with lymph node metastases, advanced pathologic stage, high-grade disease, biochemical progression, cancer-specific mortality (nearly 10-fold higher), and overall mortality after radical prostatectomy. In a later study, D'Amico et al.[39] evaluated the association between pretreatment PSAV and outcome in 358 men undergoing external beam radiation therapy for prostate cancer. A PSAV greater than 2 ng/mL/year was similarly associated with a significantly greater risk of progression, cancer-specific mortality, and overall mortality after radiotherapy.

PSAV is significantly associated with the total PSA level. Men with higher total PSA levels are significantly more likely to have a high PSAV. Furthermore, the higher the total PSA level, the greater the proportion of patients who have a life-threatening PSAV >2 ng/mL/year.

PSA doubling time (PSADT) is another measurement of PSA kinetics that has been used to assess the risk for prostate cancer and the prognosis for recurrent disease. PSADT is the time it takes for the PSA concentration to increase twofold. Because cancer grows by one cell giving rise to two, the PSADT is a function of the logarithm to the base 2. Another way to express the PSADT is the reciprocal of the PSAV weighted by the total PSA level ($PSADT = 1/PSAV \times PSA$). For instance, a tumor that would increase the serum PSA concentration by 1 ng/mL per year would have a PSADT of 1 year if the man's baseline PSA was 1 ng/mL per year. However, the PSADT of the same tumor in a man with a baseline PSA of 4 would be 4 years, because it would take 4 years for the serum PSA to increase to 8 ng/mL/year. PSADT is therefore more highly dependent on the baseline PSA value than PSAV. Thus, to compare the aggressiveness of different tumors with PSA kinetics, PSAV may be more useful in the pretreatment setting involving patients with different baseline PSA levels; whereas, PSADT (using posttreatment PSA measurements) might be more useful in comparing the aggressiveness of recurrent tumors among men who all start out with a very low baseline PSA after radical prostatectomy or radiotherapy. In patients with the same baseline PSA levels, PSAV and PSADT provide the same predictive information.

Pro–Prostate-Specific Antigen

As discussed earlier, the proportion of total PSA that circulates in the "free" form has been used in prostate cancer screening and detection. Similarly, the proportion of free PSA that is in the "pro" isoforms (the pro-PSA to free PSA ratio) may be useful to distinguish men with prostate cancer from those with benign disease, and to distinguish those men with more aggressive disease.[40,41] Mikolajczyk et al.[10] reported that pro-PSA comprised a median of 33% of free PSA in men with prostate cancer, as compared with 25% in men without cancer. Moreover, in a separate study involving 1091 serum samples, pro-PSA detected nearly all extracapsular and high-grade tumors, suggesting that it may have selectivity for more advanced or aggressive prostate cancer.[40] Further clinical studies are necessary to evaluate pro-PSA as a possible prostate cancer biomarker.

Human Glandular Kallikrein

Human glandular kallikrein (hK2) is another member of the human tissue kallikrein family to which PSA belongs. Finlay et al.[42] demonstrated that the levels of hK2 are elevated in the serum of men with prostate cancer. The relationship between levels of hK2 and free PSA has also been examined as a tool for prostate cancer screening.[43,44] Kwiatkowski et al.[3] reported that the ratio of hK2 to free PSA was more specific than the free to total PSA ratio in a small cohort of men.

One practical limitation of using hK2 as a clinical serum marker is that the levels in serum are far lower than PSA.[4] For example, Kwiatkowski et al.[3] reported that the serum levels of hK2 were approximately 2% of the total PSA concentration.

The Results of Prostate-Specific Antigen Screening

Epidemiologic studies have used the trends in prostate cancer mortality over several decades to assess whether PSA-based screening decreases prostate cancer-specific mortality rates. According to the United States Surveillance, Epidemiology and End Results (SEER) program, the proportion of newly diagnosed prostate cancers that are metastatic at presentation have decreased by 75% in the PSA era (since 1992). The overall 5-year relative survival rate for prostate cancer (compared with men without prostate cancer) improved from 75% between 1983 and 1985, to 99% between 1995 and 2000, representing the greatest improvement for any tumor.[45] Accompanying this, there has been approximately a 4% annual reduction in the prostate cancer mortality rate, amounting to a total 25% reduction in the prostate cancer mortality rate between 1995 and 2002, which is continuing to the time of this writing. Prostate cancer has now gone from being the second-leading cause of cancer deaths in men to the third-leading cause—after colorectal and lung cancer. Additional epidemiologic evidence was reported in Tyrol, Austria, where PSA screening was offered free of charge to all men aged 45–75 years beginning in 1993.[46] Bartsch et al.[46] reported that the prostate cancer mortality rate was 55% lower in Tyrol than in the remainder of Austria, where screening was not as widely utilized at that time.

There are currently two ongoing large, randomized trials of PSA screening. The European Randomized Study of Screening for Prostate Cancer (ERSPC) is currently being conducted in eight European countries, with the goal of enrolling 180,000 men. In the United States, the National Cancer Institute initiated the Prostate, Lung, Colorectal, Ovarian Cancer Screening Trial (PLCO). From 1992 to 2001, 155,000 men and women with no history of prostate, lung, colorectal, or ovarian cancer were recruited. Participants were randomized either to the control arm (involving routine healthcare by their primary doctor) or the screening arm (where they received annual screening at 1 of 10 screening centers nationwide). Men randomized to the screening arm received a PSA and DRE at study entry, followed by annual PSA measurements for 5 additional years, and annual DRE for 3 years. However, no recommendations for performing a prostate biopsy were given to the research participants. The results of these trials will be available in the next several years, and will provide additional insight on the effect of population PSA screening on prostate cancer–specific mortality.

Recommendations for Prostate-Specific Antigen–Based Prostate Cancer Screening

The senior author (W.J.C.) recommends that screening for prostate cancer begin at age 40 with a serum total PSA determination and a DRE. The initial PSA value should provide an important risk assessment. If the PSA is higher than the median for the age group (0.7 ng/mL), the patient is at increased risk for having prostate cancer or for developing it in the future. If the findings on DRE are suspicious for prostate cancer (induration or irregularity) or if the total PSA is >2.5 ng/mL/year, a 12-core TRUS-guided biopsy of the prostate should be strongly considered. However, sudden elevations in PSA may represent prostatitis and can be further assessed through repeat measurements after an empiric course of antibiotics. If the PSA levels remain elevated, further evaluation with other PSA parameters (such as the percent free PSA and PSA density) may be useful. Particularly if the percentage of free PSA is low (~10%) or the PSA density is high (>0.10 ng/mL/cc), biopsy should be considered.

Both the patient and the physician should maintain a PSA flow chart that records all PSA values, the date of measurement, and the PSA assay used.

If the patient is younger than 60 years of age or has a total PSA <4 ng/mL, but it is increasing at >0.3–0.5 ng/mL/year, biopsy should also be considered. If the total PSA is >4 ng/mL/year and a prior prostate biopsy was negative for cancer, a PSAV cutoff of 0.75 ng/mL/year is a more appropriate cutoff for recommending a repeat biopsy. In the preoperative setting, PSAV may be more meaningful than PSADT, because it is less influenced by the baseline PSA level.

References

1. Hara M, et al. [Immunoelectrophoretic studies of the protein components in human seminal plasma (especially its specific component). (Forensic immunological study of body fluids and secretions. VI)]. Nippon Hoigaku Zasshi 1969;23(2):117–22.
2. Wang MC, et al. Purification of a human prostate specific antigen. Invest Urol 1979;17(2):159–63.
3. Kwiatkowski MK, et al. In prostatism patients the ratio of human glandular kallikrein to free PSA improves the discrimination between prostate cancer and benign hyperplasia within the diagnostic "gray zone" of total PSA 4 to 10 ng/mL. Urology 1998;52(3):360–5.
4. Black MH, et al. Development of an ultrasensitive immunoassay for human glandular kallikrein with no cross-reactivity from prostate-specific antigen. Clin Chem 1999;45(6 Pt 1):790–9.
5. Lilja H. A kallikrein-like serine protease in prostatic fluid cleaves the predominant seminal vesicle protein. J Clin Invest 1985;76(5):1899–903.
6. Stamey TA, et al. Prostate-specific antigen as a serum marker for adenocarcinoma of the prostate. N Engl J Med 1987;317(15):909–16.
7. Stenman UH, et al. A complex between prostate-specific antigen and alpha 1-antichymotrypsin is the major form of prostate-specific antigen in serum of patients with prostatic cancer: assay of the complex improves clinical sensitivity for cancer. Cancer Res 1991;51(1):222–6.
8. Lilja H, et al. Prostate-specific antigen in serum occurs predominantly in complex with alpha 1-antichymotrypsin. Clin Chem 1991;37(9):1618–25.
9. Catalona WJ, et al. Use of the percentage of free prostate-specific antigen to enhance differentiation of prostate cancer from benign prostatic disease: a prospective multicenter clinical trial. JAMA 1998;279(19):1542–7.
10. Mikolajczyk SD, et al. Proenzyme forms of prostate-specific antigen in serum improve the detection of prostate cancer. Clin Chem 2004;50(6):1017–25.
11. Cooner WH, et al. Prostate cancer detection in a clinical urological practice by ultrasonography, digital rectal examination and prostate specific antigen. J Urol 1990;143(6):1146–52; discussion 1152–4.
12. Catalona WJ, et al. Measurement of prostate-specific antigen in serum as a screening test for prostate cancer. N Engl J Med 1991;324(17):1156–61.
13. Catalona WJ, et al. Detection of organ-confined prostate cancer is increased through prostate-specific antigen-based screening. JAMA 1993;270(8):948–54.
14. Smith DS, Catalona WJ. The nature of prostate cancer detected through prostate specific antigen based screening. J Urol 1994;152(5 Pt 2):1732–6.

15. Catalona WJ, et al. Comparison of digital rectal examination and serum prostate specific antigen in the early detection of prostate cancer: results of a multicenter clinical trial of 6,630 men. J Urol 1994;151(5):1283–90.
16. Lujan M, et al. Prostate cancer detection is also relevant in low prostate specific antigen ranges. Eur Urol 2004;45(2):155–9.
17. Krumholtz JS, et al. Prostate-specific antigen cutoff of 2.6 ng/mL for prostate cancer screening is associated with favorable pathologic tumor features. Urology 2002;60(3):469–73; discussion 473–4.
18. Punglia RS, et al. Effect of verification bias on screening for prostate cancer by measurement of prostate-specific antigen. N Engl J Med 2003;349(4):335–42.
19. Thompson IM, et al. Prevalence of prostate cancer among men with a prostate-specific antigen level ≤4.0 ng per milliliter. N Engl J Med 2004;350(22): 2239–46.
20. Welch HG, Schwartz LM, Woloshin S. Prostate-specific antigen levels in the United States: implications of various definitions for abnormal. J Natl Cancer Inst 2005;97(15):1132–7.
21. Smith DS, Catalona WJ, Herschman JD. Longitudinal screening for prostate cancer with prostate-specific antigen. JAMA 1996;276(16):1309–15.
22. Whittemore AS, et al. Prostate specific antigen levels in young adulthood predict prostate cancer risk: results from a cohort of Black and White Americans. J Urol 2005;174(3):872–6; discussion 876.
23. Gann PH, Hennekens CH, Stampfer MJ. A prospective evaluation of plasma prostate-specific antigen for detection of prostatic cancer. JAMA 1995;273(4): 289–94.
24. Djavan B, et al. Optimal predictors of prostate cancer on repeat prostate biopsy: a prospective study of 1,051 men. J Urol 2000;163(4):1144–8; discussion 1148–9.
25. Oesterling JE, et al. Serum prostate-specific antigen in a community-based population of healthy men. Establishment of age-specific reference ranges. JAMA 1993;270(7):860–4.
26. Morgan TO, et al. Age-specific reference ranges for prostate-specific antigen in black men. N Engl J Med 1996;335(5):304–10.
27. Loeb S, et al. Baseline prostate-specific antigen compared with median prostate-specific antigen for age group as predictor of prostate cancer risk in men younger than 60 years old. Urology 2006;67(2):316–20.
28. Brawer MK, et al. Complexed prostate specific antigen provides significant enhancement of specificity compared with total prostate specific antigen for detecting prostate cancer. J Urol 2000;163(5):1476–80.
29. Veneziano S, et al. Correlation between prostate-specific antigen and prostate volume, evaluated by transrectal ultrasonography: usefulness in diagnosis of prostate cancer. Eur Urol 1990;18(2):112–6.
30. Benson MC, et al. Prostate specific antigen density: a means of distinguishing benign prostatic hypertrophy and prostate cancer. J Urol 1992;147(3 Pt 2):815–16.
31. Terris MK, Stamey TA. Determination of prostate volume by transrectal ultrasound. J Urol 1991;145(5):984–7.
32. Loeb S, et al. Accuracy of prostate weight estimation by digital rectal examination versus transrectal ultrasonography. J Urol 2005;173(1):63–5.

33. Zlotta AR, et al. Prostate specific antigen density of the transition zone: a new effective parameter for prostate cancer prediction. J Urol 1997;157(4): 1315–21.
34. Carter HB, et al. Longitudinal evaluation of prostate-specific antigen levels in men with and without prostate disease. JAMA 1992;267(16):2215–20.
35. Smith DS, Catalona WJ. Rate of change in serum prostate specific antigen levels as a method for prostate cancer detection. J Urol 1994;152(4):1163–7.
36. Roehrborn CG, Pickens GJ, Carmody T 3rd. Variability of repeated serum prostate-specific antigen (PSA) measurements within less than 90 days in a well-defined patient population. Urology 1996;47(1):59–66.
37. Carter HB, Ferrucci L, Metter EJ. PSA velocity and risk of prostate cancer death in the Baltimore Longitudinal Study of Aging. J Urol 2005;173(Suppl 4):257, abstract 951.
38. D'Amico AV, et al. Preoperative PSA velocity and the risk of death from prostate cancer after radical prostatectomy. N Engl J Med 2004;351(2): 125–35.
39. D'Amico AV, et al. Pretreatment PSA velocity and risk of death from prostate cancer following external beam radiation therapy. JAMA 2005;294(4):440–7.
40. Catalona WJ, et al. Serum pro-prostate specific antigen preferentially detects aggressive prostate cancers in men with 2 to 4 ng/mL prostate specific antigen. J Urol 2004;171(6 Pt 1):2239–44.
41. Catalona WJ, et al. Serum pro prostate specific antigen improves cancer detection compared to free and complexed prostate specific antigen in men with prostate specific antigen 2 to 4 ng/mL. J Urol 2003;170(6 Pt 1):2181–5.
42. Finlay JA, et al. Development of monoclonal antibodies specific for human glandular kallikrein (hK2): development of a dual antibody immunoassay for hK2 with negligible prostate-specific antigen cross-reactivity. Urology 1998;51(5):804–9.
43. Magklara A, et al. The combination of human glandular kallikrein and free prostate-specific antigen (PSA) enhances discrimination between prostate cancer and benign prostatic hyperplasia in patients with moderately increased total PSA. Clin Chem 1999;45(11):1960–6.
44. Partin AW, et al. Use of human glandular kallikrein 2 for the detection of prostate cancer: preliminary analysis. Urology 1999;54(5):839–45.
45. National Cancer Institute. C.S.B. Surveillance, Epidemiology, and End Results (SEER) Program. www.seer.cancer.gov. Nov 2003 Sub (1973–2001).
46. Bartsch G, et al. Prostate cancer mortality after introduction of prostate-specific antigen mass screening in the Federal State of Tyrol, Austria. Urology 2001;58(3):417–24.

4

The Role of Complexed Prostate-Specific Antigen in Prostate Cancer Screening

Matthew E. Nielsen and Alan W. Partin

Abstract

Complexed prostate-specific antigen (cPSA) testing has been shown to have greater specificity in detecting prostate cancer than total PSA testing. Factors supporting the use of cPSA measurement in clinical screening include greater stability, longer half-life, less day-to-day variation, and less variation in the setting of confounding factors. Studies have found that cPSA offers comparable and perhaps superior performance to percent free PSA. cPSA may also have important predictive nomograms for pathologic staging of patients with localized prostate cancer. Investigation into the uses of cPSA testing has critical implications for the future of prostate cancer screening. The use of cPSA as a more specific method of detection for prostate cancer would reduce the number of biopsies performed and the overall cost of screening. To integrate cPSA testing into standard care, specific standards and guidelines are required.

Keywords: PSA isoforms, complexed PSA, percent free PSA, screening

With substantial application in the realm of prostate cancer screening, early diagnosis, risk stratification, and monitoring, prostate-specific antigen (PSA) testing has altered not only the management landscape, but in fact the natural history of prostate cancer over the past 25 years. More than any other solid malignancy, prostate cancer has seen a significant change resulting from the integration of molecular markers into standard clinical practice. After the widespread clinical application of this tumor marker, earlier diagnosis has led to a stage migration toward nonpalpable, clinically localized disease (stage T1c).[1] Two large randomized screening trials are

From: *Current Clinical Urology: Prostate Biopsy: Indications, Techniques, and Complications*
Edited by J.S. Jones © Humana Press, Totowa, NJ

underway in the United States and Europe to establish the degree to which concomitant observed improvements in prostate cancer-specific mortality trends have been directly attributable to the earlier diagnosis afforded by PSA screening.

Notwithstanding its tremendous impact on prostate cancer diagnosis and treatment, accumulated clinical experience points to the imperfect nature of PSA as a cancer screening test. Although the issues raised have been, to a certain extent, unique to prostate cancer and prostate disease, in a broader sense, they illuminate some fundamental practical issues generally relevant to the development of an effective cancer screening test. The basic performance features of any screening test are sensitivity (the ability of a test to identify correctly those who have the disease of interest) and specificity (the ability of the test to identify correctly those who do not have the disease).

The principal shortcoming of PSA as a serum marker for population-based prostate cancer screening is its relatively low specificity, reflecting the fact that PSA is organ-specific but not cancer-specific. The substantial overlap of PSA levels among men with and without cancer is particularly notable in the "diagnostic gray zone" of total serum PSA concentrations between 4 and 10 ng/mL, where up to 75% of men with PSA levels exceeding the most widely accepted threshold of elevated PSA will not have cancer detected on needle biopsy. The picture is further complicated by the finding in several studies of a substantial incidence, up to 20%, of prostate cancer in men with PSA levels of less than 4.0 ng/mL.[2-4] Even at the relatively conservative biopsy threshold of 4 ng/mL, PSA's relatively low specificity results in unnecessary biopsies, and any efforts to increase detection by simply lowering the PSA threshold run the risk of magnifying the diagnostic shortcoming of the test (unnecessary biopsies and diagnosis of insignificant tumors).

It is in this general context that further refinements of PSA testing were developed, categorized broadly in terms of new biochemical tests and new computational derivatives of serum PSA concentration. A complete discussion of PSA derivatives (PSA density, PSA velocity, age-adjusted PSA, etc.) is beyond the scope of this chapter and has been thoroughly covered in several excellent reviews.[5-7] We will focus on the field of serum testing based on the multiple circulating isoforms of the PSA molecule. Our review will proceed through relevant basic science and clinical chemistry of cPSA (complexed PSA), setting the backdrop for better understanding the literature describing the application of cPSA testing to clinical practice.

Molecular Forms of Prostate-Specific Antigen in Serum

PSA is a serine protease in the tissue kallikrein family, produced by prostate epithelial cells and secreted into prostatic ducts contributing to the proteolytic liquefaction of seminal fluid in the ejaculate. A small fraction of PSA enters the systemic circulation, where it exists in multiple forms that

TABLE 4.1. Prostate-specific antigen (PSA) type and percent in serum.

PSA type	Percent in serum
Complexed PSA	60–95
PSA-ACT	60–90
PSA-API	1–5
PSA-A2M	10–20
Free PSA	5–40

ACT = alpha-1-antichymotrypsin; API = alpha-protease inbibitor; A2M = alpha-2-macroglobulin.

for practical purposes are considered as two categories: unbound or "free" PSA (fPSA) and protein-bound or "complexed" PSA (cPSA) (Table 4.1). cPSA is the predominant molecular form found in the serum, with 65%–95% of circulating PSA existing in complexes with serum proteins. A number of serum proteins bind PSA, most notably alpha-1-antichymotrypsin (ACT), an abundant serum protease inhibitor that inhibits PSA's enzymatic activity.[8] To a lesser extent, PSA also forms stable covalent complexes in serum with other serum antiproteases, including alpha-2 macroglobulin, protein C inhibitor, and alpha-1-protease inhibitor.

Healthy patients without prostate disease or with benign prostatic disease have a greater proportion of their serum PSA existing in the unbound form (fPSA) than men with prostate cancer.[9] Although malignant prostate tissue does not produce a larger quantity of PSA than benign prostate epithelium, the proteolytic processing of PSA in cancer cells seems to be dysregulated, resulting in a greater fraction of cPSA in the serum of patients with prostate cancer.[10] These observations fueled studies of the different molecular forms of PSA in the serum as alternate approaches to enhance specificity for prostate cancer detection. In 1998, Catalona et al.[9] presented a landmark study in the field, demonstrating that a 25% fPSA cutoff in the total PSA (tPSA) range of 4–10 ng/mL could decrease unnecessary biopsies by 20% while maintaining 95% sensitivity in a large prospective clinical trial. There has been a groundswell of activity in the clinical research arena in the past 10 years toward the end of refining PSA testing with the application of the different molecular serum isoforms. Key studies with attention to the role of cPSA in prostate cancer screening will be reviewed below.

There are several theoretical advantages to cPSA relative to fPSA as a tumor marker. These include metabolic and kinetic issues germane to the relative in vivo stabilities of the two PSA isoforms. By virtue of interaction with serum proteins, cPSA has greater stability in serum than the unbound form. fPSA has a considerably shorter half-life than cPSA, reflecting the rapid exponential elimination of fPSA versus the slow, capacity-limited elimination of cPSA.[11] This may expose fPSA measurements to a greater degree of day-to-day variation.[12] Furthermore, cPSA levels seem to have less variation than fPSA in the setting of confounding factors such as

severe renal impairment or physical manipulation of the prostate gland, as
occurs with digital rectal examination, prostate biopsy, or cystoscopy.[12]
Finally, fPSA has been reported to suffer from significant in vitro instability
(Figure 4.1).[13,14]

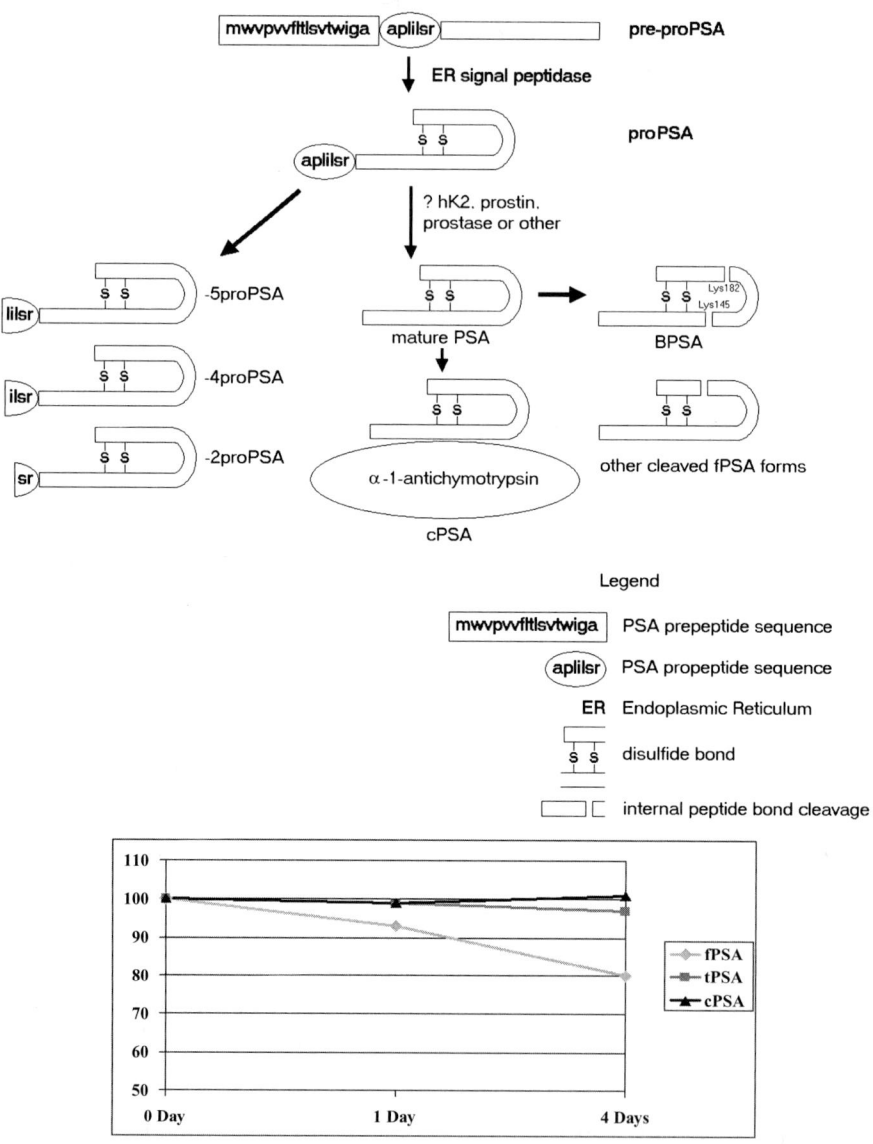

FIGURE 4.1. Stability of prostate-specific antigen (PSA) isoforms in serum at 4°C.
(Adapted from Jung K, Lein M, Brux B, Sinha P, Schnorr D, Loening SA. Different
stability of free and complexed prostate-specific antigen in serum in relation to
specimen handling and storage conditions. Clin Chem Lab Med 2000;38(12):
1271–75.)

Historical Background of Complexed Prostate-Specific Antigen Detection

PSA assays are based on monoclonal antibodies that measure the immunoreactive molecules circulating in serum. A substantial body of work has resulted in specific assays that permit the measurement of the relative fractions of free and complexed forms in a serum sample.

Early attempts to develop assays for cPSA in serum were hindered by nonspecific interference from other protease-ACT complexes, detrimental to the accuracy and reproducibility of cPSA measurements.[15] Initial immunoassays for fPSA were not similarly limited by nonspecific binding, resulting in its earlier widespread adoption into clinical practice. Continued efforts led to Bayer's development in 1998 of a commercially available immunoassay for cPSA that overcame the limitations of its predecessors, specifically by avoiding the use of antibodies to ACT. The basis of this test, the Bayer Immuno 1 cPSA (cPSA-BI) (Bayer Healthcare, Tarrytown, NY), involves preincubation with high concentrations of a "cold antibody" to the E epitope to effectively clear the sera of all fPSA, minimizing nonspecific binding.[16] This paved the way for the application of measurement of cPSA as a serum marker for prostate cancer detection.

Complexed Prostate-Specific Antigen Performance in Clinical Studies in Various Patient Subgroups

With rare exceptions, cPSA has been more specific than tPSA in a variety of patient populations across the clinically relevant range of PSA levels. More recently, additional evidence has accumulated suggesting that cPSA may have at least comparable and possibly superior performance to %fPSA for prostate cancer detection.

Several studies have indicated that cPSA may be a better initial test for prostate cancer detection than tPSA within the clinically relevant tPSA ranges of 2–20 and 4–10 ng/mL (Table 4.2). Brawer et al.[17] presented one of the initial clinical applications of the Bayer Immuno 1 assay in a retrospective study of archival sera from 300 men, 75 of whom had biopsy-proven prostate cancer. For the cohort as a whole, they found specificities for tPSA, %fPSA, and cPSA of 21.8%, 15.6%, and 26.7%, respectively, at cutoffs yielding 95% sensitivity. For the subgroup of patients in the tPSA range of 4–10 ng/mL, cPSA offered greater specificity than %fPSA, except at the 95% level of sensitivity.

In 2000, Brawer et al.[18] further evaluated the relative performance of tPSA, cPSA, and %fPSA in a larger group of patients, in which they found comparable specificity for cPSA and %fPSA in the group as a whole as well as patients with tPSA 4–10 ng/mL. Interestingly, they observed that the

TABLE 4.2. Complexed prostate-specific antigen (cPSA) in prostate cancer testing: diagnostic performance (AUC).

Author	N	cPSA AUC	Total PSA AUC
Miller (2001)	3000	0.539	0.522
Mitchell (2001)	160	0.706	0.671
Brawer (2000)	657	0.671	0.648
Okegawa (2000)	140	0.714	0.611
Jung (2000)	324	0.632	0.568
Filella (2000)	251	0.873	0.851
Stamey (2000)	170	0.568	0.519
Brawer (1998)	300	0.722	0.688
Tanguay (2002)	535	0.661	0.644

patient populations identified by cPSA and %fPSA in the tPSA range of 4–10 ng/mL were distinct from one another. Also in that year, Okegawa et al.[19] evaluated the performance of tPSA, %fPSA, and cPSA measured by the Bayer assay as well as the investigational Markit-M PSA-ACT assay in 182 Japanese patients with abnormal digital rectal examination or tPSA >4.0 ng/mL. Their results supported enhanced specificity for cPSA relative to tPSA for both cPSA immunoassay platforms. Subsequently, Mitchell et al.[20] and Miller et al.[21] confirmed the findings of enhanced specificity for cPSA relative to tPSA in 160 and 3368 men, respectively, with tPSA in the range of 2–20 ng/mL. It is notable that in all of these studies, cPSA seemed to have comparable performance to %fPSA, as measured by areas under the receiver-operator characteristics curves (ROC-AUCs).

   Partin et al.[22] confirmed the increased specificity of cPSA relative to tPSA in a large multiinstitutional prospective evaluation of 831 men undergoing initial prostate biopsy. This study demonstrated that the use of cPSA as a single test yielded enhanced specificity relative to tPSA across a range of relevant PSA strata, with negligible added value from %fPSA (Figure 4.2). Interestingly, in contrast to the earlier findings of Catalona et al.[9], they did not observe that %fPSA with a cutoff of 25% detected 95% of cancers and spared 20% of patients unnecessary biopsy. In this study, a %fPSA cutoff of 21% was required to achieve 95% detection, with a corresponding reduction in specificity to 11%. Similar findings were reported in a prospective multicenter European study by Djavan et al.[23], where the specificity of %fPSA at a 95% sensitivity threshold was <10%. Potential explanations for the discrepancy between the earlier report of Catalona et al. and these more recent prospective multicenter studies include a shift in contemporary practice toward automated assay platforms for measurement of fPSA and tPSA and/or extended core biopsy schemes, versus manual platforms and sextant biopsies, respectively. These potential confounding variables underscore the value of data from contemporary multicenter prospective trials with well-defined methodologies.

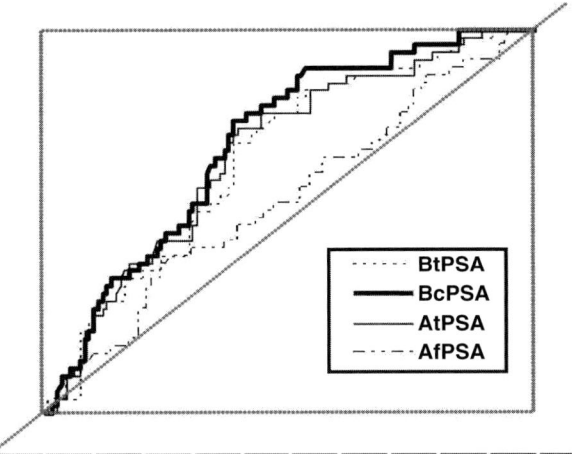

FIGURE 4.2. Diagnostic ROC (receiver-operator characteristics) curves for different prostate-specific antigen (PSA) isoforms [x-axis: 100-specificity (%), y-axis: sensitivity (%)]. BtPSA = Bayer total PSA, BcPSA = Bayer complexed PSA, AtPSA = Access/Beckman total PSA, AfPSA = Access/Beckman free PSA.

Other studies have specifically examined the performance of cPSA in the setting of tPSA values below the traditional threshold of 4.1 ng/mL, where the low specificity of tPSA raises the concern of increasing the number of unnecessary biopsies (Table 4.3). The importance of critical examination in this subgroup of patients has been underscored by data demonstrating a substantial number of younger men diagnosed with prostate cancer with tPSA levels of <4.1 ng/mL.[24] Parsons et al.[25] examined the relative performance of cPSA, tPSA, and %fPSA in the diagnosis of prostate cancer for

TABLE 4.3. Complexed prostate-specific antigen (cPSA) performance in low total PSA (tPSA) range.

Test (cutoff)	Sensitivity	Specificity	ROC-AUC
tPSA 2–6 ng/mL (n = 450)			
tPSA (2.5)	95	13.4	0.649
cPSA (2.1)	**95**	**21**	**0.680**
%fPSA (25%)	95	9	0.637
tPSA 2–4 ng/mL (n = 215)			
tPSA (2.5)	86	20.3	
cPSA (2.1)	**86**	**34.0**	
%fPSA (25%)	97	11.0	

Source: Adapted from Partin et al.[22]
ROC-AUC = areas under the receiver-operator characteristics curve, %fPSA = percent free PSA.

the tPSA range of 2.6–4.0 ng/mL in 316 men enrolled in two prospective multicenter studies. They found cPSA to have a significantly greater AUC than tPSA (0.63 vs. 0.58, respectively; p = 0.008) with respective specificities of 20.1% and 9.8% at threshold sensitivity values of 95%. In the 205 men who had %fPSA available, cPSA had a comparable AUC to %fPSA. These results confirmed previous reports in smaller groups of patients, both of cPSA performance improved relative to tPSA and at least comparable to %fPSA in the detection of clinically significant tumors in this important subpopulation of screened patients.[2,26,27]

The Role of Complexed Prostate-Specific Antigen in Nomograms Predicting Pathologic Stage

The publication of the Partin tables established the paradigm of predictive nomograms as a means of incorporating multiple prognostic elements to predict pathologic stage for patients with clinically localized prostate cancer.[28] Sokoll et al.[29] addressed the clinical utility of cPSA in this application in a prospective study of 420 men undergoing radical prostatectomy. They found a high degree of correlation (r = 0.985) between cPSA and tPSA, and on univariate analysis, the two assays were equivalent in predicting organ-confined disease and pathologic features. A multivariate logistic regression analysis including clinical stage, biopsy Gleason score, and cPSA predicted the likelihood of organ-confined disease as accurately as a model that replaced cPSA with tPSA. Additional studies incorporating cPSA into established nomograms may be useful to validate the concept that cPSA may be integrated into clinical practice without significantly affecting the predictive accuracy of these useful clinical tools.

Medical Economic Considerations Relevant to Complexed Prostate-Specific Antigen in Prostate Cancer Screening

Ellison et al.[30] presented an elegant analysis of cost-benefit relationships in prostate cancer screening comparing several thresholds of tPSA, cPSA, and %fPSA in conjunction with tPSA. The excellent performance features of cPSA among the various strategies studied were consistent with previously published reports, discussed above. Using decision-analysis techniques including estimates of cost for serum assays and prostate biopsies, their models predicted that cPSA with a positive threshold of 3.8 ng/mL would be the least costly strategy for population-based prostate cancer screening. Their analysis demonstrated that the primary determinant of cost in any prostate cancer screening strategy is the biopsy rate, underscoring the importance of balancing positive predictive value and test specificity. Their conclusions were based on the finding that the cPSA strategy would reduce the number of serum assays and, more importantly, biopsies needed without compromising diagnostic performance.

Measured Complexed Prostate-Specific Antigen Versus Calculated Complexed Prostate-Specific Antigen

Although the availability of a reliable and effective specific immunoassay enables the direct measurement of cPSA, serum cPSA levels may alternatively be indirectly ascertained via subtraction of the unbound fraction from the total serum PSA (tPSA − fPSA). This approach has several limitations. First, there are limited data to support that this computational approach yields comparable information to the direct measurement of the protein-bound PSA isoforms in the serum. Current commercially available immunoassays for cPSA detect the PSA-ACT complex, the predominant complexed form in serum. The calculation of cPSA, therefore, inaccurately reflects measured cPSA to the extent that there are small fractions of PSA bound to other serum proteins. Zhang et al.[31] developed an assay to detect complexes of PSA with alpha-1-protease inhibitor distinct from PSA-ACT complexes. This complex comprised up to 7.9% of immunoreactive PSA in serum from patients with prostate cancer and up to 12.2% in patients with benign prostatic hyperplasia. The clinical significance of this inherent discrepancy in calculated cPSA simply utilizing tPSA − fPSA is unknown. Additionally, discussed above, there are data suggesting that fPSA may have limitations with regard to its stability both in vivo and in vitro that may hamper the fidelity of calculations including fPSA to ascertain levels of cPSA.

Furthermore, the performance characteristics of calculated cPSA have received limited attention in the literature. Okihara et al.[26] specifically evaluated the performance of calculated cPSA for prostate cancer detection in 151 patients with a tPSA range of 2.5–4.0 ng/mL. Their results were comparable to those of other studies examining measured cPSA (AUC 0.718), and although one might argue that, conceptually, calculated cPSA is simply another expression of %fPSA, they found calculated cPSA to achieve superior cancer detection (AUC 0.729) in comparison to %fPSA (AUC 0.635) in their study population.

Because calculated cPSA relies on the difference of two separate assays, the cost disadvantages of this approach, discussed above in Ellison's analysis, argue in favor of measured cPSA versus calculated cPSA. Specifically, cPSA as a single diagnostic test offering comparable diagnostic accuracy to the combination of tPSA and fPSA may provide cost savings in healthcare delivery.

The Future of Complexed Prostate-Specific Antigen in Prostate Cancer Screening

cPSA has been targeted as a biomarker for prostate cancer screening with the potential of enhancing specificity of serum testing. The precise clinical niche for cPSA in the armamentarium of serum assays is in the process of being defined. The preponderance of clinical evidence suggests that cPSA offers enhanced specificity relative to tPSA and accumulating evidence suggests that cPSA offers at least comparable and perhaps superior performance to the application of %fPSA.

Critical future directions include further validation of cPSA in well-defined applications including nomograms predictive of pathologic stage as well as better characterization of the kinetic features of cPSA, as the importance of tPSA velocity as a prognostic marker has been reinforced in recent years.[32,33] Age- and race-specific performance features of tPSA are controversial and have been the subject of numerous investigations. Similar refinements of our understanding of more specific applications of cPSA have been investigated. As seen with tPSA, cPSA levels increase with age,[34,35] and early data suggest that higher cPSA cutoffs are required to preserve sensitivity.[36] The majority of patients in studies of cPSA have been Caucasian and the performance of cPSA in different racial groups is controversial. Initial data suggested comparable cPSA levels among African American and Caucasian men;[37] however, more recent data have called into question the robustness of cPSA in African American men.[38] Clearly, further race-stratified analyses of cPSA performance are indicated to guide recommendations for use of the test.

Additionally, clinically useful applications of the enhanced specificity afforded by the measurement of cPSA remain to be rigorously defined. Observations of the performance of %fPSA suggest some specific avenues of investigation. These may include identifying older patients with a less than 10-year age-adjusted life expectancy in whom a prostate biopsy may be deferred.[39] These tests may also add value in the identification of patients with a negative initial biopsy who may benefit from a repeated biopsy, a very real clinical dilemma in contemporary urologic practice.[40,41] Along these lines, the role of cPSA in active surveillance and expectant management protocols remains another potentially fruitful area for further investigation.

Fundamentally, the single greatest limitation to the use of cPSA in prostate cancer screening is the absence of accepted consensus guidelines for its application in clinical practice. The proliferation of rigorously designed and executed studies outlined above support the utility of cPSA in the field of prostate cancer detection. A critical next step in the application of cPSA to general use is the promulgation of specific standards and recommendations to facilitate its integration into standard care.

References

1. Stephenson RA. Prostate cancer trends in the era of prostate-specific antigen. An update of incidence, mortality, and clinical factors from the SEER database. Urol Clin North Am 2002;29:173–81.
2. Schroder FH, van der Cruijsen-Koeter I, de Koning HJ, Vis AN, Hoedemaeker RF, Kranse R. Prostate cancer detection at low prostate-specific antigen. J Urol 2000;163(3):806–12.
3. Catalona WJ, Smith DS, Ornstein DK. Prostate cancer detection in men with serum PSA concentrations of 2.6–4.0 ng/mL and benign prostate examination. Enhancement of specificity with free PSA measurements. JAMA 1998; 277(18):1452–5.
4. Colberg JW, Smith DS, Catalona WJ. Prevalence and pathological extent of prostate cancer in men with prostate specific antigen levels of 2.9 to 4.0 ng/mL. J Urol 1993;149(3):507–9.
5. Nishiya M, Miller GJ, Lookner DH, Crawford ED. Prostate-specific antigen density in patients with histologically proven prostate carcinoma. Cancer 1994;74(11):3002–9.
6. Carter HB, Morrell CH, Pearson JD, et al. Estimation of prostatic growth using serial prostate-specific antigen measurements in men with and without prostate disease. Cancer Res 1992;52(12):3323–8.
7. Oesterling JE, Jacobsen SJ, Chute CG, et al. Serum prostate-specific antigen in a community-based population of healthy men. Establishment of age-specific reference ranges. JAMA 1993;270(7):860–4.
8. Leinonen J, Zhang WM, Stenman UH. Complex formation between PSA iso-enzymes and protease inhibitors. J Urol 1996;155:1099–103.
9. Catalona WJ, Partin AW, Slawin KM, et al. Use of percentage of free prostate-specific antigen to enhance differentiation of prostate cancer from benign pros-tatic disease: a prospective multicenter clinical trial. JAMA 1998;279:1542.
10. Christensson A, Bjork T, Nilsson O, et al. Serum prostate specific antigen com-plexed to alpha 1-antichymotrypsin as an indicator of prostate cancer. J Urol 1993;150(1):100–5.
11. Bjork T, Ljungberg B, Piironen T, et al. Rapid exponential elimination of free prostate-specific antigen contrasts the slow, capacity-limited elimination of PSA complexed to alpha 1-antichymotrypsin from serum. Urology 1998;51: 57–62.
12. Lilja H, Haese A, Bjork T, et al. Significance and metabolism of complexed and noncomplexed prostate specific antigen forms, and human glandular kallikrein 2 in clinically localized prostate cancer before and after radical prostatectomy. J Urol 1999;162:2029–34; discussion 2034–5.
13. Piironen T, Pettersson K, Suonpaa M, et al. In vitro stability of free prostate-specific antigen (PSA) and prostate-specific antigen (PSA) complexed to alpha 1-antichymotrypsin in blood samples. Urology 1996;48:81–7.
14. Woodrum D, French C, Shamel LB. Stability of free prostate-specific antigen in serum samples under a variety of sample collection and sample storage condi-tions. Urology 1996;48:33–9.
15. Stenman UH, Leinonen J, Alfthan H, Rannikko S, Tuhkanen K, Alfthan O. A complex between prostate-specific antigen and alpha 1-antichymotrypsin is the major form of prostate-specific antigen in serum of patients with prostatic

cancer: assay of the complex improves clinical sensitivity for cancer. Cancer Res 1991;51:222–6.

16. Morris DL, Dillon PW, Very DL, et al. Bayer immuno 1 PSA assay: an automated, ultrasensitive method to quantitate total PSA in serum. J Clin Lab Anal 1998;12(1):65–74.

17. Brawer MK, Meyer GE, Letran JL, et al. Measurement of complexed PSA improves specificity for early detection of prostate cancer. Urology 1998;52(3): 372–8.

18. Brawer MK, Cheli CD, Neaman IE, et al. Complexed prostate-specific antigen provides significant enhancement of specificity compared with total prostate specific antigen for detecting prostate cancer. J Urol 2000;163(5):1476–80.

19. Okegawa T, Noda H, Nutahara K, Higashihara E. Comparison of two investigative assays for the complexed prostate-specific antigen in total prostate-specific antigen between 4.1 and 10.0 ng/mL. Urology 2000;55(5):700–4.

20. Mitchell ID, Croal BL, Dickie A, Cohen NP, Ross I. A prospective study to evaluate the role of complexed prostate-specific antigen and free/total prostate specific antigen ratio for the diagnosis of prostate cancer. J Urol 2001;165(5): 1549–53.

21. Miller MC, O'Dowd GJ, Partin AW, Veltri RW. Contemporary use of complexed PSA and calculated percent free PSA for early detection of prostate cancer: impact of changing disease demographics. Urology 2001;57(6): 1105–11.

22. Partin AW, Brawer MK, Bartsch G, et al. Complexed prostate specific antigen improves specificity for prostate cancer detection: results of a prospective multicenter clinical trial. J Urol 2003;170:1787–91.

23. Djavan B, Remzi M, Zlotta AR, et al. Complexed prostate-specific antigen, complexed prostate-specific antigen density of total and transition zone, complexed/total prostate-specific antigen ratio, free-to-total prostate-specific antigen ratio, density of total and transition zone prostate-specific antigen: results of the prospective multicenter European trial. Urology 2002;60(4 Suppl 1):4–9.

24. Punglia RS, D'Amico AV, Catalona WJ, et al. Effect of verification bias on screening for prostate cancer by measurement of prostate-specific antigen. N Engl J Med 2003;349:335–42.

25. Parsons JK, Brawer MK, Cheli CD, Partin AW, Djavan R. Complexed prostate specific antigen (PSA) reduces unnecessary biopsies in the 2.6–4.0 ng/mL range of total PSA. BJU Int 2004;94:47–50.

26. Okihara K, Fritsche H, Ayala A, Johnston DA, Allard WJ, Babaian RJ. Can complexed prostate-specific antigen enhance prostate cancer detection in men with total prostate specific antigen between 2.4 and 4 ng/mL. J Urol 2001;165: 1930–6.

27. Horninger W, Cheli CD, Babaian RJ, et al. Complexed prostate-specific antigen for early detection of prostate cancer in men with serum prostate-specific antigen levels of 2–4 ng/mL. Urology 2002;60(Suppl 1):31–5.

28. Partin AW, Kattan MW, Subong EN, et al. Combination of prostate-specific antigen, clinical stage, and Gleason score to predict pathologic stage of localized prostate cancer. A multi-institutional update. JAMA 1997;277(18):1445–51.

29. Sokoll LJ, Mangold LA, Partin AW, et al. Complexed prostate-specific antigen as a staging tool for prostate cancer: a prospective study in 420 men. Urology 2002;60:18–23.

30. Ellison L, Cheli CD, Bright S, Veltri RW, Partin AW. Cost-benefit analysis of total, free/total, and complexed prostate-specific antigen for prostate cancer screening. Urology 2002;60(Suppl 4A):42–6.
31. Zhang WM, Finne P, Leinonen J, Vesalainen S, Nordling S, Stenman UH. Measurement of the complex between prostate-specific antigen and alpha-1-protease inhibitor in serum. Clin Chem 1999;45:814–21.
32. D'Amico AV, Chen MH, Roehl KA, Catalona WJ. Preoperative PSA velocity and the risk of death from prostate cancer after radical prostatectomy. N Engl J Med 2004;351(2):125–35.
33. D'Amico AV, Renshaw AA, Sussman B, Chen MH. Pretreatment PSA velocity and risk of death from prostate cancer following external beam radiation therapy. JAMA 2005;294(4):440–7.
34. Cheli CD, Levine RL, Cambetas DR, et al. Age-related reference ranges for complexed prostate-specific antigen and complexed/total prostate-specific antigen ratio: results from East Texas Medical Center Cancer Institute screening campaign. Urology 2002;60:53–9.
35. Berger AP, Cheli CD, Levine RL, et al. Impact of age on complexed PSA levels in men with total PSA levels up to 20 ng/mL. Urology 2003;62:840–4.
36. Veltri RW, Miller MC, O'Dowd GH, et al. Impact of age on total and complexed prostate-specific antigen cutoffs in a contemporary referral series of men with prostate cancer. Urology 2002;60:47–52.
37. Martin B, Cheli C, Pollard S, et al. Similar age-specific PSA, complexed PSA, and percent cPSA levels among African-American and white men of southern Louisiana. Urology 2003;61(2):375–9.
38. Martin B, Cheli CD, Lifsey D, et al. Complexed PSA performance for prostate cancer detection in an African-American population. Urology 2003;62(5): 835–9.
39. Veltri RW, Miller MC. Free/total PSA ratios improve differentiation of benign and malignant disease of the prostate: critical analysis of two different test populations. Urology 1999;53:736–45.
40. O'Dowd GJ, Miller MC, Orozco R, et al. Analysis of repeat biopsy results within one year following a non-cancer diagnosis. Urology 2000;55:553–9.
41. Letran JL, Blasé AB, Loberiza FR, et al. Repeat ultrasound guided prostate needle biopsy: use of free-to-total prostate specific antigen ratio in predicting prostatic carcinoma. J Urol 1998;160:426–9.

5
Newly Recognized Forms of Prostate-Specific Antigen and Emerging Molecular Markers

Eduardo I. Canto and Kevin M. Slawin

Abstract

Total PSA has been the mainstay of diagnostic laboratory investigation for prostate cancer. However, a number of isoforms of this molecule and other emerging markers offer the promise of improved diagnostic strategies.

Keywords: prostate specific antigen (PSA), molecular forms of free PSA, prostate cancer screening, MALDI-TOF, SELDI-TOF

Prostate-specific antigen (PSA) is a member of the kallikrein family of serine proteases. Prostate luminal epithelial cells are the primary producers of PSA. These cells secrete PSA into the seminal fluid, where it degrades the major gel-forming proteins of human ejaculate, semenogelin I and II, and fibronectin. Even in the absence of any pathology, a small amount of PSA enters the circulation. Although reasonable theories abound, this process occurs through an unknown mechanism. In normal male serum, PSA reaches concentrations of only ng/mL, 10^6 times less concentrated than in the seminal plasma, where it reaches mg/mL concentrations.[1]

Although small amounts of PSA have been noted in endometrium, breast tissue, breast cancer, ileum, Skene's glands, and breast milk, only the prostate produces clinically significant quantities of PSA.[2,3] Both normal and hyperplastic or neoplastic prostate epithelial cells produce PSA. PSA is, therefore, an organ-specific rather than a hyperplasia- or cancer-specific marker. A large, and only partially characterized number of variables affect the serum PSA concentration of a given male. It has been well documented that neoplastic prostate tissue increases serum PSA concentrations more, on a per-gram basis, than hyperplastic prostate tissue. Benign prostatic

From: *Current Clinical Urology: Prostate Biopsy: Indications, Techniques, and Complications*
Edited by J.S. Jones © Humana Press, Totowa, NJ

hyperplasia (BPH), in turn, increases serum PSA concentration more than normal prostate on a per-gram basis.[4] Nevertheless, the amount of PSA that reaches the circulation per gram of cancerous, hyperplastic, or normal prostate varies from one individual to the other, and varies with time for a given individual.

The amount of PSA produced per gram of prostate tissue is influenced by many factors. Some of these include age, local androgen levels, the variable stroma-to-epithelium ratio of the prostate gland, and the presence or absence of inflammation.[5] Because of these and other inherent, biologically determined drawbacks to the clinical use of PSA as a prostate cancer screening tool, there is ample room for improvement to our current PSA-based prostate cancer screening methods. Much effort has been devoted to improving the performance of PSA by controlling for some of the factors that determine the serum PSA concentration in the absence cancer. Others have dedicated significant resources to discovering and testing distinct molecular forms of PSA or totally new non–PSA-based makers for prostate cancer screening.

Molecular Derivatives of Prostate-Specific Antigen in the Diagnosis of Prostate Cancer

PSA was isolated almost simultaneously from both seminal plasma and prostate tissue, by separate investigator groups for very different reasons. Forensic investigators first purified PSA from seminal plasma whereas investigators interested in prostate pathology first purified it from prostate tissue. Because almost all of the PSA found in seminal plasma and prostate tissue is free PSA (fPSA), PSA was first purified in its free, noncomplexed form. The first report documenting the isolation of PSA was published in 1971 by a group of forensic investigators in Japan. The newly discovered semen-specific antigen was named gamma-seminoprotein.[6] At the same time, a separate group of investigators were able to document the presence of prostate tissue–specific antigens by probing prostate tissue lysates with anti-prostate serum.[7] However, it was not until almost a decade later that a method for the purification of fPSA from prostate tissue was described by investigators interested in developing diagnostics for prostate disease.[8]

Because complexed PSA (cPSA) is found at relatively low concentrations in serum, it was not discovered until the 1990s. Interestingly, Papsidero et al.,[9] one of the first groups to purify PSA from the serum of cancer patients, noted in 1980 that serum PSA is found in a molecular complex of 90–100 kDa. Mistakenly, they believed this to represent polymerized PSA rather than PSA complexed with a protease inhibitor. The now well-known PSA complexes consisting of PSA complexed with α-1-antichymo-trypsin (PSA-ACT) and PSA complexed with α-2-macroglobulin (PSA-AMG) were not discovered until 1990, when in vitro studies consisting of mixing purified fPSA from semen with female serum revealed their existence.[10] Soon after, Stenman et al.[11] purified cPSA from the serum of cancer patients and showed that the fraction of PSA-ACT increased with increasing PSA and the presence of prostate cancer.

The process by which PSA complexes with protease inhibitors is not completely understood. One theory suggests that the loss of tissue architecture that results from disorganized cancer growth facilitates the binding of protease inhibitors to PSA and results in an increased release of cPSA into the bloodstream. PSA produced by BPH, however, is thought to follow the normal secretory pathway into the seminal spaces and, only after it reaches these, to leak back through the intercellular space into the circulation. This process is thought to expose BPH-produced PSA to proteases found in both BPH tissue and seminal plasma. Because cleaved, inactive forms of PSA are not able to bind to protease inhibitors, the higher proportion of internally cleaved PSA that arises from BPH tissue results in a lower proportion of cPSA in the presence of BPH. A second theory suggests that complex formation between PSA produced by prostate cancer and ACT is facilitated by the production of ACT by prostate cancer cells. Unlike neoplastic prostate epithelial cells, the epithelial cells found in BPH tissue do not produce ACT. PSA produced by BPH is, therefore, susceptible to protease degradation within the prostate and/or seminal spaces before it reaches the circulation. Although there is excess ACT available for binding in the circulation, enzymatically inactive, cleaved forms of PSA cannot bind ACT.[12]

It is now well established that about 75% of measurable serum PSA is irreversibly bound to the protease inhibitor ACT (PSA-ACT). The interaction of PSA with ACT results in the cleavage of ACT carboxy-terminal to the Leu residue at position 358. In the process, ACT covalently binds PSA and inactivates it. A lesser fraction of serum PSA is bound to either AMG (PSA-AMG) or α-1-protease inhibitor (PSA-API).[10] Up to 50% of serum PSA is in the free form. As with ACT, the interaction between PSA and API involves cleavage and inactivation of the protease. Complexes between PSA and API have been replicated in vitro. The process is not only slow but also inefficient. When complexed to PSA, API is cleaved between Met 358 and Ser 359.[10,13] Unlike ACT and API, AMG binds PSA by encapsulating it rather than by interacting with the active site. For this reason, PSA-AMG retains its enzymatic activity to small substrates that can penetrate the complex. PSA-AMG is less abundant than PSA-ACT because it is rapidly cleared from the circulation. Clearance rates for PSA-ACT are less than 1 ng/mL/day. PSA-ACT is not excreted by the kidneys because of the relatively large size of the complex.[11]

PSA has at least five epitopes. All five PSA epitopes are hidden in PSA-AMG whereas only two are hidden when it is bound to ACT. This allows commercial immunoassays to differentiate between PSA-ACT and fPSA. It also means that conventional total PSA assays detect only PSA-ACT and fPSA, but not PSA-AMG.[11] The only cPSA assay approved by the U.S. Food and Drug Administration is based on monoclonal antibody–mediated elimination of all fPSA followed by measurement of the remaining PSA with a polyclonal antibody (Bayer Immuno1 cPSA Assay, Bayer Diagnostics, Tarrytown, NY).[14] At least three fPSA assay systems are approved as adjuncts to PSA-based prostate cancer screening. The performance of the assays varies and, therefore, care should be taken to use the fPSA cutoffs established for each specific assay.[15,16]

Complexed Versus Free Prostate-Specific Antigen in Prostate Cancer Screening

Although PSA-ACT or cPSA was the first PSA molecular form to be associated with improved prostate cancer screening performance, the first large-scale trial of a molecular form of PSA in prostate cancer screening was performed using %fPSA (100 × fPSA/PSA) not cPSA. By 1998, many retrospective studies had suggested that use of %fPSA could reduce the number of unnecessary prostate biopsies in men with PSA between 4 and 10 ng/mL. However, it was a large, prospective trial involving 773 men that proved that %fPSA could enhance the specificity of PSA-based prostate cancer screening in men with a benign rectal examination and serum PSA concentration between 4 and 10 ng/mL. Using the Hybritech Tandem-E fPSA assay, this study demonstrated that, if men with a %fPSA greater than 25% did not undergo a prostate biopsy, the number of unnecessary biopsies could be reduced by 20% while 95% of all cancers that could be detected on an initial sextant biopsy would still be detected.[17] On the basis of this and other data, the U.S. Food and Drug Administration approved the use of %fPSA for prostate cancer screening in men with PSA between 4 and 10 ng/mL.

The use of %fPSA was later extended to PSA concentrations below 4 ng/mL. Of men with a PSA between 2.6 and 4 ng/mL, 25%–30% can be expected to have prostate cancer.[18] Catalona et al.,[19] using the Tandem-E PSA assay, showed that a %fPSA cutoff of ≤27% in patients with a PSA between 2.6 and 4 ng/mL detected 90% of cancers while avoiding 18% of unnecessary biopsies. In this study, 83% of the cancers diagnosed were considered clinically significant, yet 81% of patients who underwent surgery had organ-confined disease. Vashi et al.,[20] using the AxSYM PSA assay (Abbott Laboratories, Abbott Park, IL), found that by biopsying patients with a %fPSA below 19%, and PSA between 3 and 4 ng/mL, they detected

90% of cancers that would have been found if all men with a PSA within this range had undergone a biopsy. Using this %fPSA cutoff, they detected 1 cancer per 1.7 biopsies.

Because total PSA measurements include only PSA-ACT and fPSA, and the available cPSA assay measures the PSA remaining after immunologically removing all fPSA forms, the relationship between cPSA and fPSA is a straightforward equation: cPSA + fPSA = total PSA, and fPSA/PSA = 1 − cPSA/PSA. Despite the suggestion by early studies that cPSA by itself (not in a ratio to PSA) could outperform PSA, one would expect that if fPSA by itself does not outperform total PSA and the difference between fPSA/PSA and cPSA/PSA is a constant, then cPSA/PSA, and not cPSA alone should outperform total PSA. Contrary to the early studies and in accordance with the mathematical rationale, in the largest multicenter study of cPSA, cPSA/PSA, but not cPSA, performed as well as %fPSA. In this study, cPSA by itself performed as well as %fPSA only in patients with a PSA below 6 ng/mL. However, for the entire 2–10 ng/mL PSA range, the performance of cPSA/PSA was comparable to that of %fPSA, and both %fPSA and cPSA/PSA outperformed cPSA.[21] The fact that cPSA performed as well as %fPSA when the cohort was limited to patients with a PSA below 6 ng/mL is explained by the fact that as the PSA range narrows, for both %fPSA and cPSA/PSA, the contribution by the value of PSA to the discriminatory power of the marker diminishes.

Interestingly, in the previously mentioned cPSA study, as in other recent studies comparing prostate cancer markers, the performance of %fPSA was significantly less than that reported in the original Catalona study.[17,21–23] Our own data confirm this trend. This might be attributable to any or a combination of the following: differences in the fPSA testing methods, changes in patient population, or the bias toward the detection of smaller cancers caused by extended biopsy schemes involving more than 10 cores. The effect of extended biopsy schemes as compared with the traditional sextant biopsy used in the original Catalona study on the performance of %fPSA has been evaluated. At least one study showed a trend toward a decrease in the sensitivity of %fPSA at each biopsy threshold value without affecting specificity.[24] Nevertheless, others have reported that this trend toward a diminished %fPSA performance seems to be unrelated to the increase in the number of core taken at the time of prostate biopsy.[25]

If the diagnostic utility of cPSA/PSA and %fPSA is comparable, how does one decide which one to use? Although currently more widely used, %fPSA is not without drawbacks. The performance of %fPSA has been shown to decrease as prostate size increases. In men with prostates larger than 40 cc, %fPSA increases even in the presence of a small cancer. This results in a lower sensitivity for prostate cancer detection. Although not proven for cPSA/PSA, given the fact that cPSA = PSA − fPSA, the sensitivity of cPSA/PSA should be similarly negatively affected by prostate size.[26] There are practical matters that could favor the use of a direct assay for cPSA. cPSA is more stable than fPSA. Under common temporary storage conditions of 4 to −20°C, fPSA immunoreactivity is affected more than either total PSA or cPSA. It is recommended, therefore, that specimens that will not be processed within 8 hours of harvest be frozen at −70°C for fPSA testing. In contrast, loss of immunoreactivity of PSA and cPSA can be prevented by storage at −20°C.[27] Finally, cPSA has been shown to be less affected by prostate manipulation, such as digital rectal examination or cystoscopy, than fPSA.[28]

Free Prostate-Specific Antigen More Complex Than Once Thought

PSA is produced as a pre-pro-peptide. This means that the amino acid sequence of the protein includes both a hydrophobic endoplasmic reticulum–targeting sequence, the "pre" amino acids, and an additional amino acid sequence that maintains the protease in an inactive, "pro" or zymogen form. The endoplasmic reticulum–targeting sequence (amino acids −24 to −8) is clipped as soon as the N-terminus of the nascent protein enters the endoplasmic reticulum. The "pro" peptide (amino acids −7 to −1) is not removed until the protein is secreted into the target anatomic location. Here, another enzyme activates the protein by removing the "pro" peptide sequence (Ala-Pro-Leu-Ile-Leu-Ser-Arg).[1] Unlike pro-hK2 (human glandular kallikrein), which can activate itself by autoprocessing, proPSA activation requires the action of another enzyme.[29] A number of proteases with trypsin-like activity found in prostate tissue have been shown to be capable of activating proPSA. Among these are hK2, prostin, and prostase.[30–32] Whether one of these is the enzyme responsible for physiologic activation of PSA in seminal plasma remains to be determined.

Studies examining the actual amino terminal sequence of the various inactive forms of fPSA found in serum, seminal plasma, and normal, hyperplastic, and cancerous prostate tissue have demonstrated the existence of various alternatively processed forms that have retained some or all of the "pro" sequence or have internal cleavages. The study of these various newly recognized molecular forms of PSA has the potential to yield new markers or a combination of markers capable of improving not only our ability to screen for, stage, and predict prostate cancer outcomes, but also to diagnose and predict the outcomes of patients with BPH.

Internally Cleaved Free Prostate-Specific Antigen Forms

The discovery of cPSA raised the question of why not all the PSA in serum is found in complexed form. It was soon realized that only active PSA can complex with ACT and that only a fraction of the PSA found in either seminal plasma or prostate tissue is in an active form. In the mid-1990s, investigators focused their attention on deciphering how it is that PSA is inactivated in seminal plasma and prostate tissue. In 1995, Zhang et al.[33] showed that the PSA found in seminal plasma is inactivated by internal peptide bond cleavages. It was the ability to purify PSA, rather than the use of any novel analytic technique, that allowed this group to analyze the molecular forms of fPSA. Using an old biochemical technique, protein electrophoresis under reducing and nonreducing conditions, they showed that the inactive PSA in seminal plasma has internal cleavages, and that the resulting fragments are held together by disulfide bonds.

Two years later, in 1997, Chen et al.[34] showed that cleaved forms of fPSA were also found in fresh prostate tissue. These authors, however, did not compare BPH tissue to normal tissue. Furthermore, their purification method resulted in persistent contamination by one or more enzymes, likely hK2, with trypsin-like activity. Pure PSA exhibits only chymotrypsin-like enzymatic activity. It was Mikolajczyk et al.[35] who demonstrated, using a more specific purification method, namely, affinity purification with an anti-pan-fPSA–specific antibody followed by size exclusion chromatography, that most of the internally cleaved PSA in BPH tissue is cleaved at both Lys 145 and Lys 182. This mature, enzymatically inactive form of fPSA, found at highest concentration in BPH tissue, has been dubbed "BPSA."

Taking advantage of the change in conformation that this single internal cleavage at Lys 182 creates, the group at Hybritech created a sensitive immunoassay that detects BPSA. Because of the immunologic similarity between BPSA and fPSA cleaved only at Lys 182, this assay measures both true BPSA (cleaved at both Lys 145 and Lys 182) and fPSA cleaved only at Lys 182. Because PSA cleaved only at Lys 182 has been shown to compose a relatively fixed proportion (~30%) of fPSA in BPH tissues, it is unlikely that the performance of the assay will be negatively affected.[36]

Although biologically intriguing, the mere fact that there is more BPSA in BPH tissue than in normal transition zone tissue or peripheral zone tissue does not mean that this assay will be of clinical utility. Many factors other than tissue levels, such as rate of release into the circulation, clearance rate, and stability in serum, affect the final concentration of a given protein. Therefore, it was not guaranteed by any means, that serum BPSA levels would correlate with either prostate volume or other parameters of BPH. Nevertheless, the first study to carefully evaluate the correlation between serum BPSA concentration and prostate volume showed that BPSA does, indeed, correlate with prostate and transition zone volume in an age-independent manner. Total PSA, however, had a weaker and age-dependent correlation with transition zone volume. Serum

BPSA concentration outperformed both PSA and fPSA in its ability to predict transition zone enlargement.[37] Of note, this was also the second study to evaluate the correlation of fPSA, not in a ratio to PSA, with prostate volume. As demonstrated by the only other study to evaluate this correlation, fPSA displayed an age-independent correlation with transition zone volume.[38] When BPSA was subtracted from the absolute fPSA concentration, the correlation of fPSA with prostate volume decreased to below that of total PSA.[37,39] This suggests that the correlation between prostate volume and fPSA is primarily attributable to the contribution of BPSA.

Whether BPSA will be a clinically useful predictor of BPH pathology, progression, or outcomes remains to be determined. Studies are underway that should answer this question. Preliminary data generated by measuring BPSA levels in the stored serum from the MTOPS (Medical Therapy of Prostatic Symptoms) trial suggest that a threshold amount of BPH must be present to increase serum BPSA above background levels. These data show that BPSA correlates with baseline transition zone volume only in patients with a total PSA above 2.5 ng/mL. Furthermore, as the total PSA increases, the correlation between BPSA and transition zone volume also increases.[40] Data from the Glaxo ARIA 3001–3003 phase III trials suggest that BPSA may, indeed, predict BPH progression and together with fPSA more accurately identify prostate enlargement than PSA. Receiver operating characteristic curve analysis for prediction of baseline prostate volume >30 cc, >40 cc, and >50 cc revealed that a model including both fPSA and BPSA outperformed total PSA, and either BPSA or fPSA alone.[41] Addition of BPSA to a nomogram that included each patient's AUA SI, BPH impact index, maximum flow rate, history of alpha-blocker use, and dutasteride treatment improved its concordance index from 0.724 to 0.738. This improvement could not be matched or improved by the addition of baseline prostate volume.[42] This suggests that serum BPSA concentration may provide additional predictive value beyond that of prostate volume measurement.

Noncleaved Free Prostate-Specific Antigen Forms

The existence of an inactive zymogen form of PSA was initially noted when the cDNA coding for PSA was expressed in *Spodoptera frugiperda* Sf9 insect cells. Although made possible 8 years earlier by the cloning of PSA, this experiment was not reported until 1995. The investigators noted that half of the PSA purified from the culture medium of the transfected cells was in an inactive zymogen form containing two extra amino-terminal amino acids (−2proPSA). These two amino acids correspond to those at positions −1 and −2 of the pro-peptide form of PSA. However, the investigators make no mention in their report of the possible significance of this finding.[43] Two years later, a similar experiment consisting of expressing PSA cDNA in the Syrian hamster tumor cell line AV12–664 demonstrated the existence of two additional zymogen forms of PSA, –5, and –7proPSA. –5proPSA contains five of the seven pro-peptide PSA amino acids, whereas –7proPSA contains all seven pro-peptide amino acids. Unlike the Sf9 insect cells, the AV12–664 cells expressed only the zymogen forms. The investigators also showed that these zymogen forms could be converted to active mature PSA by hK2's trypsin-like protease activity. The group at Hybritech that conducted the experiment realized that their findings suggested that PSA may be expressed in an inactive form in human prostate and later activated in the seminal spaces.[44] Because the microstructural anomalies found in prostate cancer may result in spilling of zymogen forms of PSA into the circulation, the Hybritech investigators searched for these forms in the serum of prostate cancer patients and found them.[45] Three years later, the same group showed that an additional inactive form of PSA was produced by LNCaP cells. Unlike the other inactive forms described previously, that had either internal cleavages or consisted of zymogen forms, this inactive PSA was mature (no extra amino-terminal amino acids) and had no internal cleavages.[46]

The Hybritech group was not the first to study fPSA from the serum of prostate cancer patients. Noldus et al.[47] had already purified fPSA from prostate cancer serum and found only inactive mature PSA and cleaved forms of mature PSA. The difference between the two reports can be explained by the difference in purification methods used by the two groups. Mikolajczyk et al.[45] used immunoadsorption as the purification method, whereas Noldus et al.[47] used gel filtration. The product of the gel filtration purification contained contaminants because it displayed trypsin-like activity. PSA displays only chymotrypsin-like activity. It is likely that the trypsin-like activity (probably hK2 contamination) converted any zymogen PSA forms to the mature PSA form, explaining the lack of any zymogen forms in the study by Noldus et al. Multiple subsequent studies have confirmed that zymogen forms of PSA including 2, 4, 5, or all 7 of the pro amino acids exist in the serum of prostate cancer patients.[48–50]

By examining the molecular forms of PSA from normal peripheral zone tissue, prostate cancer, and both normal and hyperplastic transition zone tissue, Mikolajczyk et al.[35,49] later showed that production of zymogen forms of PSA was restricted to peripheral zone tissue and prostate cancer, whereas cleaved forms of mature PSA were produced primarily by transition zone tissue. This further suggested that the zymogen forms of PSA found in the serum of prostate cancer patients likely originated in neoplastic prostate cells.

fPSA has been conclusively shown by multiple independent groups to contain the following forms: a) mature yet inactive noncleaved PSA, b) inactive zymogen forms including –2, –4, –5, and –7proPSA, and c) cleaved, thereby inactive, forms of otherwise mature PSA, including cleavages at Ile 1, Hist 54, Phen 157, Lys 145, and Lys 182. The fPSA that can be isolated from BPH tissue (transition zone nodular tissue) is devoid of zymogen forms and demonstrates a number of internal cleavages that render the enzyme inactive.[34,35,49] Likewise, PSA isolated from seminal plasma does not contain any of the zymogen forms associated with prostate cancer, but contains a different proportion of internally cleaved forms.[34] PSA isolated from BPH tissue has been shown to have more internal cleavages than PSA isolated from either normal peripheral- or transition zone tissue or seminal plasma. The internal cleavage sites include Ile 1, Hist 54, Phen 157, Lys 145, and Lys 182.[33–35,49]

At least three different methods of measuring the concentration of the various molecular forms of fPSA have been developed. The first consists of a traditional enzyme-linked immunosorbent assay (ELISA), in which all fPSA forms are captured by an anti-pan-fPSA monoclonal antibody followed by labeling of one or more zymogen forms with specific antibodies coupled to a fluorofor.[23] The second is also an ELISA-type fluorogenic assay (fSPA-I assay), but differs from the first in that it uses antibodies raised against LNCaP-produced fPSA to directly measure the concentration of all noncleaved forms of fPSA, including both the zymogen and the mature inactive molecules.[51] Although this assay is said to detect "intact" PSA, it detects both zymogen (–2, –4, –5, –7proPSA) and mature forms of noncleaved PSA. There is currently no ELISA for the detection of *only* the mature, enzymatically inactive, noncleaved form of fPSA. The concentration of this mature enzymatically inactive form of fPSA can only be calculated indirectly. The third approach is a functional assay that detects all zymogen forms of PSA by first capturing all fPSA forms and then activating the zymogen forms exclusively by exposing the captured fPSA to hK2. The concentration of proPSA is determined by adding a PSA-specific substrate.[52]

Because both zymogen forms of PSA and mature noncleaved PSA were initially identified in serum of patients with very high total PSA concentrations and in prostate tissue extracts, it was not expected that they would necessarily be of diagnostic value in men with PSA levels less than 10 ng/mL. Nevertheless, clinical testing of these three assays has shown significant potential. The first studies to be performed not only demonstrated that these PSA isoforms were detectable in patients with PSA less than 10 ng/mL, but they also demonstrated that the ratio of noncleaved forms of fPSA to all forms of fPSA (not necessarily the absolute concentration of noncleaved forms of fPSA) was higher in patients with prostate cancer than in patients with BPH.[48] Using fluorogenic assays for the various proPSA forms (–2proPSA, –4proPSA, and combined –5 and –7proPSA), Catalona et al.[23] demonstrated, in a retrospective study of 1091 patients, that either –2proPSA or panproPSA (sum of –2, –4, –5 and –7proPSA) in a ratio with fPSA both outperformed either %fPSA or cPSA in patients with a serum PSA in the 2–10 ng/mL range. In this PSA range, panproPSA/fPSA spared 21% of unnecessary biopsies, whereas %fPSA spared only 13%, and cPSA spared 9% of unnecessary biopsies (p < 0.0001).

The fPSA-I assay that measures noncleaved forms of fPSA has not performed as well as the direct assays or the various proPSA forms. The most extensive study (282 patients) of the utility of measuring noncleaved forms of fPSA in patients with a PSA between 2 and 10 ng/mL demonstrated that the ratio of noncleaved PSA/fPSA [area under the receiver-operator characteristics curve (AUC) = 0.620] performed marginally worse than %fPSA.[51] Because it measures all noncleaved fPSA forms, the fPSA-I assay can be used to measure all cleaved forms of fPSA by subtracting the value of fPSA-I from that of fPSA. In a study of 282 patients with total PSA between 2 and 10 ng/mL, the ratio of cleaved to total PSA outperformed the ratio of fPSA-I to fPSA (AUC 0.704 vs. 0.620).[51] By subtracting fPSA-I from fPSA, one indirectly calculates the sum of BPSA and fPSA cleaved only at Lys 145. Whether this assay detects fPSA that is cleaved only at Lys 182 is unclear.

A number of important biologic questions relating to the various fPSA forms remain to be answered: a) Why does the ratio of proPSA/fPSA rather than the absolute concentration of proPSA correlate with the presence of prostate cancer? b) What enzyme cleaves off the pro-peptide from PSA? c) Does cleavage of the pro-peptide normally occur within the intercellular spaces of the prostate or within the seminal spaces? d) Why does prostate cancer and, to a lesser extent, normal peripheral zone produce the various zymogen forms of fPSA? e) What enzyme cleaves the zymogen form of PSA to generate −2, −4, −5proPSA? f) What enzyme cleaves fPSA at Lys 145 and/or Lys 182?

Novel Prostate Cancer Markers and Mass Spectrometry

The prostate cancer markers mentioned up to this point have all been discovered and studied using classic biochemical techniques that are both laborious and inefficient. Recently, a high-throughput method for small protein biomarker discovery has gained significant momentum. Surface-enhanced laser desorption and ionization time-of-flight mass spectrometry (SELDI-TOF) combines two simple, yet powerful, techniques: on-chip separation of complex protein mixtures by adsorption on a stationary-phase and mass spectrometry of proteins ionized by laser energy. A typical experiment consists of: 1) directly applying the fluid to be studied onto the treated surface of a protein chip (specialized surfaces include: hydrophobic, ionic, metal binding, and cationic) so as to allow a subset of proteins or fragments thereof to bind to the surface; 2) the surface of the chip is treated with acid in order to ionize the adhered proteins; 3) under vacuum conditions, the chip is exposed to a laser that causes desorption and ionization of the bound proteins; 4) the detached ionized proteins travel toward an oppositely charged electrode; and 5) the mass-to-charge (m/z) ratio of each ionized protein is calculated from the time it takes the ion to travel from the chip's surface to the electrode.

The described experiment yields a spectrum consisting of the m/z ratios of the proteins bound to the chip's surface that subsequently desorbed in the form of ions when excited by the laser's energy. This spectrum pattern or fingerprint is the discriminator. When SELDI-TOF is used as a diagnostic tool, no attempt is made to identify the proteins or protein fragments that make up each peak. Interestingly, although the height of each peak in the m/z spectrum represents the number of ionized proteins of a given m/z ratio that successfully bound to the chip's surface and subsequently desorbed, it does not necessarily correlate with the abundance of that peptide in the original sample. In fact, the minimum concentration of a given peptide in a sample required for detection by SELDI-TOF has not been determined.

Because of the complexity of each sample's m/z spectrum, specialized data mining systems have evolved. Rather than identifying a multiplex list of biomarkers or m/z peaks, these bioinformatics systems create one or more patterns in N-dimensional space from the combined relative amplitudes of ions at each m/z ratio. If a supervised system is being used, the patterns of disease samples are compared with those of known normal samples in order to define a classification algorithm. In unsupervised bioinformatics systems, the SELDI-TOF spectra are first grouped, without prior knowledge of the disease classification, and later the groups are scored as disease or normal. Because a typical SELDI-TOF profile may have between 10,000 and 400,000 data points, the computational power needed to evaluate the most discriminatory patterns is far from trivial. Fortunately, algorithms that shorten the time to determination of near-optimal solutions to a few days have been developed. A detailed discussion of these artificial intelligence algorithms is beyond the scope of this review, and has been reviewed elsewhere.[53]

With respect to prostate cancer, SELDI-TOF has been used to identify both prostate cancer–specific serum patterns and tissue-derived cancer-specific proteins. Three recent reports highlight the impressive potential of SELDI-TOF as a tool in the molecular diagnosis of prostate cancer. These three studies were able to obtain 95%–100% sensitivity at 78%–100% specificity.[54-56] Although the studies were conducted on relatively small sets of selected serum samples, clearly the potential for this technology is impressive. Nevertheless, a closer examination of these three reports reveals that the major problem with SELDI-TOF is its lack of reproducibility. Two of the studies were from the same group and used the same type of chip (IMAC-3; Ciphergen Biosystems, Fremont, CA), serum extraction method, and mass spectrometer, and focused on the same range of molecular weight proteins, 2–40 kDa. Nevertheless, of the 12 major peaks selected by Qu et al.[54] and the 9 peaks selected by Adam et al.,[55] only 2 shared peaks in their algorithms at m/z ratios of 704 and 9656. A third peak at m/z ratio of 7820 was used by Adam et al. to distinguish cancer from noncancer and by Qu et al. to distinguish normal from BPH.

SELDI-TOF has also been used as a method of screening for new prostate cancer markers. Investigators at Harvard have applied SELDI-TOF to prostate tissue rather than the serum of prostate cancer patients. They were able to identify a prostate cancer–specific peak at an m/z = 24,730.1. They then showed by laser capture microdissection that this peak corresponds to a prostate cancer–specific protein produced by cancerous, but not BPH-associated or normal, epithelium.[57] Although this study showed the potential of SELDI-TOF technology to identify tissue in addition to serum biomarkers, it also highlighted the difficulty in identifying the actual protein or peptide that generates a peak in the mass spectrometer.

SELDI-TOF–based prostate cancer screening faces two fundamental challenges. The first is that the technique itself is difficult to reproduce. Each step of the process, from sample handling and preparation to the calibration and performance of the mass spectrometer, may affect the final results and reproducibility. Because it is an empiric science, large numbers of patients must be tested to both define diagnostic patterns and evaluate their accuracy. This is the second fundamental challenge. Because SELDI-TOF likely recognizes the most abundant peptide in serum only, it is likely that these are not produced by the prostate or prostate cancer, but rather, are epiphenomena and as such are more likely to be affected by comorbidities, differences in the host response to cancer, or many not yet recognized factors that might vary with time and geographic location, to name only two variables. For this reason, some investigators have suggested that SELDI-TOF should be standardized across the country with data stored and analyzed by a centralized laboratory with constant modification of the scoring algorithm based on real-time data gathered from prostate biopsies on patients being tested so as to continually update and improve the scoring algorithms as the population of tested individuals changes over time.

Conclusion

The knowledge gained over the last 15 years through the study of the molecular biology of PSA has the potential to change the markers that we use for prostate cancer screening. The first major step toward improving the performance of PSA assays resulted from the discovery, in the 1990s, that PSA exists in bound and unbound form. This newly gained knowledge led to the development of both %fPSA and cPSA measures as new assays meant to complement total PSA in the 4–10 ng/mL gray zone. It would take almost a decade for investigators to discover that fPSA is actually a mixture of various internally cleaved and zymogen forms of PSA. These newly discovered molecular forms of fPSA have the potential to improve our ability to detect and stage prostate cancer, and to diagnose BPH and predict its outcomes. Although it is almost certain that non–PSA-based molecular markers of prostate cancer will reach the clinic, it is unlikely that any one new non–PSA-based marker will replace all PSA-based markers. Rather, with time, combinations of markers, whether PSA or non–PSA-based, will prove most useful in prostate cancer screening and staging.

Acknowledgments. Carolyn Schum provided indispensable editorial assistance of the manuscript.

References

1. Lilja H. Biology of prostate-specific antigen. Urology 2003;62(5 Suppl 1):27–33.
2. Diamandis EP. Prostate specific antigen—new applications in breast and other cancers. Anticancer Res 1996;16(6C):3983–4.
3. Olsson AY, Bjartell A, Lilja H, Lundwall A. Expression of prostate-specific antigen (PSA) and human glandular kallikrein 2 (hK2) in ileum and other extraprostatic tissues. Int J Cancer 2005;113(2):290–7.
4. Stamey TA, Yang N, Hay AR, McNeal JE, Freiha FS, Redwine E. Prostate-specific antigen as a serum marker for adenocarcinoma of the prostate. N Engl J Med 1987;317(15):909–16.
5. Bunting PS. A guide to the interpretation of serum prostate specific antigen levels. Clin Biochem 1995;28(3):221–41.
6. Hara M, Inorre T, Fukuama T. Some physico-chemical characteristics of gamma-seminoprotein, an antigenic component specific for human seminal plasma. Jpn J Leg Med 1971;25:322.
7. Ablin RJ, Soanes WA, Bronson P, Witebsky E. Precipitating antigens of the normal human prostate. J Reprod Fertil 1970;22(3):573–4.
8. Wang MC, Valenzuela LA, Murphy GP, Chu TM. Purification of a human prostate specific antigen. Invest Urol 1979;17(2):159–63.
9. Papsidero LD, Wang MC, Valenzuela LA, Murphy GP, Chu TM. A prostate antigen in sera of prostatic cancer patients. Cancer Res 1980;40(7):2428–32.
10. Christensson A, Laurell CB, Lilja H. Enzymatic activity of prostate-specific antigen and its reactions with extracellular serine proteinase inhibitors. Eur J Biochem 1990;194(3):755–63.
11. Stenman UH, Leinonen J, Alfthan H, Rannikko S, Tuhkanen K, Alfthan O. A complex between prostate-specific antigen and alpha 1-antichymotrypsin is the major form of prostate-specific antigen in serum of patients with prostatic cancer: assay of the complex improves clinical sensitivity for cancer. Cancer Res 1991;51(1):222–6.

12. Lilja H. Regulation of the enzymatic activity of prostate-specific antigen and its reactions with extracellular protease inhibitors in prostate cancer. Scand J Clin Lab Invest Suppl 1995;220:47–56.
13. Zhang WM, Leinonen J, Kalkkinen N, Stenman UH. Prostate-specific antigen forms a complex with and cleaves alpha 1-protease inhibitor in vitro. Prostate 1997;33(2):87–96.
14. Zhou Z, Armstrong EG, Belenky A, Freeman JV, Yeung KK. Equivalent recognition of free and ACT-complexed PSA in a monoclonal-polyclonal sandwich assay is conferred by binding specificity of the monoclonal antibody. J Clin Lab Anal 1998;12(4):242–9.
15. Junker R, Brandt B, Zechel C, Assmann G. Comparison of prostate-specific antigen (PSA) measured by four combinations of free PSA and total PSA assays. Clin Chem 1997;43(9):1588–94.
16. Nixon RG, Meyer GE, Blase AB, Gold MH, Brawer MK. Comparison of 3 investigational assays for the free form of prostate specific antigen. J Urol 1998;160(2):420–5.
17. Catalona WJ, Partin AW, Slawin KM, et al. Use of the percentage of free prostate-specific antigen to enhance differentiation of prostate cancer from benign prostatic disease: a prospective multicenter clinical trial. JAMA 1998; 279(19):1542–7.
18. Gann PH, Hennekens CH, Stampfer MJ. A prospective evaluation of plasma prostate-specific antigen for detection of prostatic cancer. JAMA 1995;273(4): 289–94.
19. Catalona WJ, Smith DS, Ornstein DK. Prostate cancer detection in men with serum PSA concentrations of 2.6 to 4.0 ng/mL and benign prostate examination. Enhancement of specificity with free PSA measurements. JAMA 1997;277(18): 1452–5.
20. Vashi AR, Wojno KJ, Henricks W, et al. Determination of the "reflex range" and appropriate cutpoints for percent free prostate-specific antigen in 413 men referred for prostatic evaluation using the AxSYM system. Urology 1997;49(1): 19–27.
21. Partin AW, Brawer MK, Bartsch G, et al. Complexed prostate specific antigen improves specificity for prostate cancer detection: results of a prospective multicenter clinical trial. J Urol 2003;170(5):1787–91.
22. Djavan B, Remzi M, Zlotta AR, et al. Complexed prostate-specific antigen, complexed prostate-specific antigen density of total and transition zone, complexed/total prostate-specific antigen ratio, free-to-total prostate-specific antigen ratio, density of total and transition zone prostate-specific antigen: results of the prospective multicenter European trial. Urology 2002;60(4 Suppl 1):4–9.
23. Catalona WJ, Bartsch G, Rittenhouse HG, et al. Serum pro prostate specific antigen improves cancer detection compared to free and complexed prostate specific antigen in men with prostate specific antigen 2 to 4 ng/ml. J Urol 2003;170(6 Pt 1):2181–5.
24. Canto EI, Singh H, Shariat SF, et al. Effects of systematic 12-core biopsy on the performance of percent free prostate specific antigen for prostate cancer detection. J Urol 2004;172(3):900–4.
25. Roddam AW, Duffy MJ, Hamdy FC, et al. Use of prostate-specific antigen (PSA) isoforms for the detection of prostate cancer in men with a PSA level of 2–10 ng/ml: systematic review and meta-analysis. Eur Urol 2005;48(3):386–99; discussion 98–9.

26. Meyer A, Jung K, Lein M, Rudolph B, Schnorr D, Loening SA. Factors influencing the ratio of free to total prostate-specific antigen in serum. Int J Cancer 1997;74(6):630–6.
27. Arcangeli CG, Smith DS, Ratliff TL, Catalona WJ. Stability of serum total and free prostate specific antigen under varying storage intervals and temperatures. J Urol 1997;158(6):2182–7.
28. Lynn NN, Collins GN, O'Reilly PH. Prostatic manipulation has a minimal effect on complexed prostate-specific antigen levels. BJU Int 2000;86(1):65–7.
29. Denmeade SR, Lovgren J, Khan SR, Lilja H, Isaacs JT. Activation of latent protease function of pro-hK2, but not pro-PSA, involves autoprocessing. Prostate 2001;48(2):122–6.
30. Takayama TK, Carter CA, Deng T. Activation of prostate-specific antigen precursor (pro-PSA) by prostin, a novel human prostatic serine protease identified by degenerate PCR. Biochemistry 2001;40(6):1679–87.
31. Nelson PS, Gan L, Ferguson C, et al. Molecular cloning and characterization of prostase, an androgen-regulated serine protease with prostate-restricted expression. Proc Natl Acad Sci USA 1999;96(6):3114–19.
32. Lovgren J, Rajakoski K, Karp M, Lundwall A, Lilja H. Activation of the zymogen form of prostate-specific antigen by human glandular kallikrein 2. Biochem Biophys Res Commun 1997;238(2):549–55.
33. Zhang WM, Leinonen J, Kalkkinen N, Dowell B, Stenman UH. Purification and characterization of different molecular forms of prostate-specific antigen in human seminal fluid. Clin Chem 1995;41(11):1567–73.
34. Chen Z, Chen H, Stamey TA. Prostate specific antigen in benign prostatic hyperplasia: purification and characterization. J Urol 1997;157(6):2166–70.
35. Mikolajczyk SD, Millar LS, Wang TJ, et al. "BPSA," a specific molecular form of free prostate-specific antigen, is found predominantly in the transition zone of patients with nodular benign prostatic hyperplasia. Urology 2000;55(1):41–5.
36. Wang TJ, Slawin KM, Rittenhouse HG, Millar LS, Mikolajczyk SD. Benign prostatic hyperplasia-associated prostate-specific antigen (BPSA) shows unique immunoreactivity with anti-PSA monoclonal antibodies. Eur J Biochem 2000;267(13):4040–5.
37. Canto EI, Singh H, Shariat SF, et al. Serum BPSA outperforms both total PSA and free PSA as a predictor of prostatic enlargement in men without prostate cancer. Urology 2004;63(5):905–10; discussion 10–11.
38. Morote J, Encabo G, Lopez M, de Torres IM. Prediction of prostate volume based on total and free serum prostate-specific antigen: is it reliable? Eur Urol 2000;38(1):91–5.
39. Linton HJ, Marks LS, Millar LS, Knott CL, Rittenhouse HG, Mikolajczyk SD. Benign prostate-specific antigen (BPSA) in serum is increased in benign prostate disease. Clin Chem 2003;49(2):253–9.
40. Slawin KM, Levitt JM, Roehrborn CG, et al. The relationship between PSA isoforms and BPH-related prostate volume at baseline in the MTOPS trial. Presented at the 101st American Urological Association Annual Meeting, 2006.
41. Slawin KM, Levitt JM, Lamb DJ, et al. Prediction of prostate volume using molecular forms of PSA in men with BPH enrolled on the GSK phase III dutasteride trials. Presented at the 101st American Urological Association Annual Meeting, 2006.

42. Slawin KM, Levitt JM, Lamb DJ, et al. Baseline serum BPH-A level enhances the accuracy of a nomogram to predict BPH progression in men enrolled on the GSK phase III dutasteride trials. Presented at the 101st American Urological Association Annual Meeting, 2006.

43. Kurkela R, Herrala A, Henttu P, Nai H, Vihko P. Expression of active, secreted human prostate-specific antigen by recombinant baculovirus-infected insect cells on a pilot-scale. Biotechnology (NY) 1995;13(11):1230–4.

44. Kumar A, Mikolajczyk SD, Goel AS, Millar LS, Saedi MS. Expression of pro form of prostate-specific antigen by mammalian cells and its conversion to mature, active form by human kallikrein 2. Cancer Res 1997;57(15): 3111–4.

45. Mikolajczyk SD, Grauer LS, Millar LS, et al. A precursor form of PSA (pPSA) is a component of the free PSA in prostate cancer serum. Urology 1997;50(5): 710–4.

46. Kumar A, Mikolajczyk SD, Hill TM, Millar LS, Saedi MS. Different proportions of various prostate-specific antigen (PSA) and human kallikrein 2 (hK2) forms are present in noninduced and androgen-induced LNCaP cells. Prostate 2000;44(3):248–54.

47. Noldus J, Chen Z, Stamey TA. Isolation and characterization of free form prostate specific antigen (f-PSA) in sera of men with prostate cancer. J Urol 1997;158(4):1606–9.

48. Mikolajczyk SD, Marker KM, Millar LS, et al. A truncated precursor form of prostate-specific antigen is a more specific serum marker of prostate cancer. Cancer Res 2001;61(18):6958–63.

49. Mikolajczyk SD, Millar LS, Wang TJ, et al. A precursor form of prostate-specific antigen is more highly elevated in prostate cancer compared with benign transition zone prostate tissue. Cancer Res 2000;60(3):756–9.

50. Mikolajczyk SD, Catalona WJ, Evans CL, et al. Proenzyme forms of prostate-specific antigen in serum improve the detection of prostate cancer. Clin Chem 2004;50(6):1017–25.

51. Steuber T, Nurmikko P, Haese A, et al. Discrimination of benign from malignant prostatic disease by selective measurements of single chain, intact free prostate specific antigen. J Urol 2002;168(5):1917–22.

52. Niemela P, Lovgren J, Karp M, Lilja H, Pettersson K. Sensitive and specific enzymatic assay for the determination of precursor forms of prostate-specific antigen after an activation step. Clin Chem 2002;48(8):1257–64.

53. Petricoin EE, Paweletz CP, Liotta LA. Clinical applications of proteomics: proteomic pattern diagnostics. J Mammary Gland Biol Neoplasia 2002;7(4): 433–40.

54. Qu Y, Adam BL, Yasui Y, et al. Boosted decision tree analysis of surface-enhanced laser desorption/ionization mass spectral serum profiles discriminates prostate cancer from noncancer patients. Clin Chem 2002;48(10):1835–43.

55. Adam BL, Qu Y, Davis JW, et al. Serum protein fingerprinting coupled with a pattern-matching algorithm distinguishes prostate cancer from benign prostate hyperplasia and healthy men. Cancer Res 2002;62(13):3609–14.

56. Petricoin EF 3rd, Ornstein DK, Paweletz CP, et al. Serum proteomic patterns for detection of prostate cancer. J Natl Cancer Inst 2002;94(20):1576–8.

57. Zheng Y, Xu Y, Ye B, et al. Prostate carcinoma tissue proteomics for biomarker discovery. Cancer 2003;98(12):2576–82.

6

The Role of Prostate-Specific Antigen Velocity in the Diagnosis and Management of Prostate Cancer

H. Ballentine Carter

Abstract

Interpretation of absolute PSA values can be confusing both when used for diagnosis and management. Clinicians are beginning to appreciate that PSA changes (kinetics) may provide important information beyond an absolute PSA value for assessing the risk of cancer presence, cancer significance, and risk of death from prostate cancer after curative intervention. Because PSAV correlates with the likelihood that life threatening disease is present, use of PSAV may help reduce the over diagnosis and over treatment of prostate cancer that has occurred with PSA screening. In addition, after curative intervention for prostate cancer, PSADT is a surrogate for survival and can be used to help identify those men with biochemical failure who are most likely to benefit from salvage treatments.

Keywords: screening, PSA velocity, PSA doubling time, PSA kinetics

Prostate-specific antigen (PSA) screening is widely used today for the diagnosis and management of men with prostate cancer. Although PSA screening has not been proven to reduce prostate cancer mortality, many experts believe that widespread use of this marker for diagnosis has been—in part—responsible for the decrease in prostate cancer deaths observed in the last decade. Prostate cancer mortality rates are lowest in areas where the rates of distant-stage disease are lowest, and distant-stage disease is lowest in areas with the highest PSA utilization[1]—findings that suggest a PSA effect on mortality. PSA is also widely used for assessing disease extent after diagnosis of prostate cancer, and for monitoring patients who have undergone treatment for the disease. Even though PSA has been widely used for 2 decades, interpretation of PSA values can be confusing

From: *Current Clinical Urology: Prostate Biopsy: Indications, Techniques, and Complications*
Edited by J.S. Jones © Humana Press, Totowa, NJ

when used for both diagnosis and management. Clinicians are beginning to appreciate that PSA changes (kinetics) may provide important information beyond an absolute PSA value for assessing the risk of cancer presence, cancer significance, and death from prostate cancer after curative intervention. This chapter reviews the role of PSA kinetics in the diagnosis and management of men with prostate cancer with an emphasis on diagnosis and assessment of disease significance.

What Is Prostate-Specific Antigen Kinetics?

The changes in a physical or chemical system are broadly referred to as kinetics. Two PSA kinetic terms have been coined to describe changes in PSA: PSA velocity (PSAV) and PSA doubling time (PSADT). PSAV is the rate of change in PSA or the change corrected for the elapsed time usually expressed in nanograms/milliliter per year (i.e., annualized), whereas PSADT reflects "growth" of PSA and is the time to double the marker, usually expressed in months or years. PSADT is calculated from the slope of the regression of the log-transformed PSA on time, and thus assumes an exponential relationship between PSA and time. PSADT could be constant while PSA is increasing exponentially (see Figure 6.1).

The slope of the line of the regression of PSA on time is the rate of change in PSA or PSAV. The equation that describes a straight line is $y = mx + b$ where m is the slope and b is the intercept. This approach assumes a linear relationship between PSA and time as shown in Figure 6.1. The slope (PSAV) in this example is 3.6 ng/mL per year over 4 years. Another method for calculating PSAV is the running average or the simple PSAV

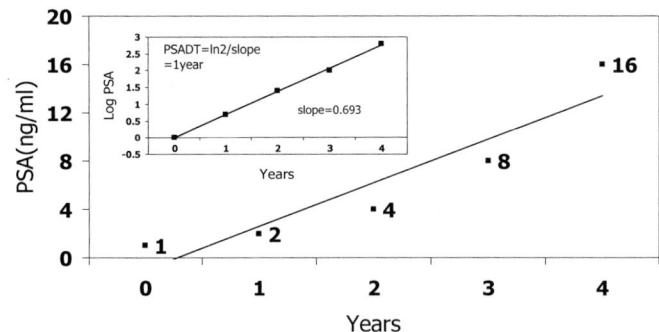

FIGURE 6.1. Prostate specific antigen (PSA) as a function of time (years). Line represents regression of PSA on time. Inset is log transformation of PSA as a function of time. PSADT = PSA doubling time, ln = natural logarithm.

(change divided by time) between 2 points, plus the PSAV between the next 2 points, all divided by 2.[2] For example, the average rate of change in Figure 6.1 for years 2–4 is ([8 – 4 ng/mL]/1 year) + ([16 – 8 ng/mL]/1 year)/2 = 6 ng/mL per year. If one plots the log-transformed PSA on time for the above example (see Figure 6.1 inset), then the PSADT is calculated from the formula: ln (2)/slope = PSADT. The ln2 = 0.693 and the slope = 0.693 giving a PSADT of 1 year.

Prostate-Specific Antigen Kinetics: Predicting the Presence of Prostate Cancer

There can be substantial changes or variability in serum PSA between measurements in the presence or absence of prostate cancer.[3–7] The short-term changes in PSA are primarily a result of physiologic variation.[6] A number of studies have shown that men who harbor prostate cancer have more rapid increases in PSA compared with those without the disease[2,3,8–13]—a finding that is useful for assessing the risk that prostate cancer is present.

Using frozen sera to measure PSA years before the diagnosis of prostate disease in men with and without prostate cancer, Carter and colleagues[2] found that at 5–10 years before clinical diagnosis, the median PSAV for men with localized prostate cancer (0.27 ng/mL per year) and metastatic disease (1.33 ng/mL per year) was significantly greater compared with those men with benign prostatic hyperplasia (BPH) (0.09 ng/mL per year) and controls (0.01 ng/mL per year) (see Figure 6.2). At 10–15 years before clinical diagnosis, the median PSAV for men with localized prostate cancer (0.14 ng/mL per year) and metastatic disease (0.30 ng/mL per year) was significantly greater compared with controls (0.02 ng/mL per year) but not those with BPH (0.09 ng/mL per year). In that study, 72% of men with cancer and 5% of men without cancer had a PSAV of more than 0.75 ng/mL per year. Specificity of PSAV using a cut point of 0.75 ng/mL per year remained high (more than 90%) when PSA levels were between 4 and 10 ng/mL or below 4 ng/mL, but sensitivity for cancer detection was 11% at levels below 4 ng/mL, compared with 79% for levels between 4 and 10 ng/mL.

Table 6.1 compares the PSAV findings in men with and without prostate cancer from studies with different designs (i.e., prospective and retrospective). In my opinion, differences in PSAV between studies is probably attributable to differences in cohort age, absolute PSA levels, and cancer grade and extent—all of which can influence PSAV. For example, PSAV increases directly with PSA and age,[3] and changes in PSA are greater for men with high-grade cancers compared with those with low-grade cancers.[14]

More recently, it has been shown that PSAV might be useful for prostate cancer detection among men with PSA levels below 4.0 ng/mL. In a longi-

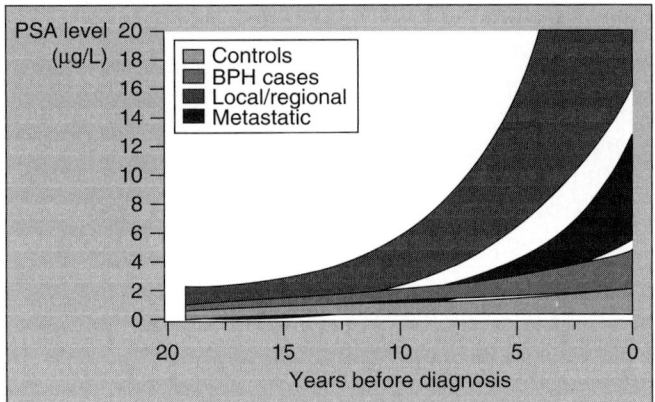

FIGURE 6.2. The curves represent the average prostate-specific antigen (PSA) levels and the 95% confidence limits of PSA among men without prostate disease (bottom curve), men with benign prostatic hyperplasia (BPH) who underwent simple prostatectomy (next to bottom), localized prostate cancer (third from bottom), and metastatic prostate cancer (top curve) as a function of years before diagnosis (prostate cancer), simple prostatectomy (BPH) or last visit to the Baltimore Longitudinal Study of Aging (BLSA) indicated by time 0. Men in this study were diagnosed before the PSA era and were more likely to have life-threatening disease compared with men diagnosed today. (Adapted from Carter et al.[2])

tudinal aging study, the cumulative probability of freedom from prostate cancer at 10 years after a baseline PSA between 2–4 ng/mL was 97.1% (range 91.4%–100%) and 35.2% (range 14.0%–56.4%) when the PSAV was less than and greater than 0.1 ng/mL per year, respectively.[15] However, Roobol et al.[16] did not find that PSAV was an independent predictor of a prostate cancer diagnosis at the second screening round of a randomized screening trial when PSA was less than 4.0 ng/mL. I believe that similar to PSA, PSAV has greater predictive value for cancer among men without

TABLE 6.1. Prostate-specific antigen velocity (PSAV) in men with and without prostate cancer.

Study	Study design	PSAV (ng/mL per year)*	
		No cancer	Cancer
Carter et al.[2,3]	Longitudinal aging study	0.04	0.75
Oesterling et al.[13]	Longitudinal BPH study	0.04	—
Berger et al.[12]	Invitational screening over 10 years	0.03	0.4
Raaijmakers et al.[11]	Randomized screening at 4-year intervals	0.09	0.62

* Average PSAV.
BPH = benign prostatic hyperplasia.

prostatic enlargement. Men without prostatic enlargement are more likely to have lower PSA values (below 4.0 ng/mL) and less likely to have PSA changes caused by noncancerous causes.

The minimal length of follow-up—time over which changes in PSA should be adjusted—for PSAV to be useful in cancer detection has been calculated in separate studies to be 18 months.[4,8,9] Furthermore, evaluation of three repeated PSA measurements, to determine an average rate of change in PSA, would seem to optimize the accuracy of PSAV for cancer detection.[2–4]

Prostate-Specific Antigen Kinetics: Prediction of Life-Threatening Disease

Before Curative Intervention

D'Amico et al.[17,18] demonstrated that PSAV in the year before treatment of presumed localized prostate cancer was associated with the probability of prostate cancer death after curative intervention. In a landmark study, the authors evaluated PSAV in the year before surgery for men who were thought to have localized prostate cancers.[17] They found that compared with a PSAV below 2 ng/mL per year in the year before diagnosis, a PSAV greater than 2 ng/mL per year was associated with a 10-fold greater risk of prostate cancer death in the 7 years after surgery. Thus, failure of local therapy among men with presumed localized disease was associated with a higher PSAV. This seminal observation suggested that PSAV could be useful in assessing the biologic behavior of prostate cancer before treatment. The authors have made the same observations after radiation therapy for prostate cancer.[18] In addition, Sengupta et al.[19] showed that both PSAV and PSADT were significant predictors of prostate cancer death at a median follow-up of 7 years after surgical treatment for prostate cancer.

It seems intuitive that PSA would increase faster in those men with high-grade cancer compared with those with lower-grade cancers if PSA gains access to the systemic circulation by alterations in prostatic architecture caused by cancer. In addition, PSA may have greater access to the circulation in men with micrometastatic deposits compared with those with organ-confined disease. Data from the Prostate Cancer Prevention Trial (PCPT) have shown that men with high-grade cancers have faster PSA increases (annual percent change in PSA) compared with those with lower-grade cancers.[14] In the end of study biopsies (biopsies done not for elevated PSA or abnormal digital rectal examination) in the PCPT, those men with high-grade cancers (Gleason score 7 and above) had an annual change in PSA of 11%–12% compared with those with low-grade cancers (Gleason score 6 or below) where annual changes were 5%–6% (i.e., twofold higher for high-grade cancers vs. low-grade cancers). For a man with a PSA of 2.5 ng/mL, this would translate into a PSAV of 0.3 ng/mL per year for high-grade cancer and 0.15 ng/mL per year for low-grade cancer.

The data from D'Amico et al.[17,18] demonstrated that a higher PSAV in the year before diagnosis was associated with a greater likelihood that presumed localized disease would not be cured with local therapy (radiation and surgery). An unanswered question is whether PSAV could help identify those men with life-threatening cancers at a time when cure might still be possible. We addressed this question by exploring PSAV among men enrolled in a longitudinal aging study (the Baltimore Longitudinal Study of Aging; National Institute on Aging).[20] We found that at 10–15 years before diagnosis when absolute PSA levels were below 4.0 ng/mL in most men, PSAV predicted cancer-specific survival 25 years later. Using a PSAV cutoff of 0.35 ng/mL per year, cancer-specific survival was 92% (84%–96%) for those with a PSAV of 0.35 ng/mL per year or less compared with 54% (15%–82%) for men with a PSAV more than 0.35 ng/mL per year (p = 0.0001). The relative risk of prostate cancer death was 4.7 (1.3–16.5) for those patients with a PSAV more than 0.35 ng/mL per year compared with those whose PSAV was 0.35 ng/mL per year or less (p = 0.02). These preliminary data suggest that even among men with PSA levels that are traditionally considered to be low (below 4.0 ng/mL), the rate of increase in PSA may be helpful in identifying those men who need further evaluation for the presence of life-threatening disease. The evaluation of the rate at which PSA increases to a given PSA level (PSAV), rather than using a dichotomous PSA cut point, to help determine the need for a prostate biopsy could greatly reduce the overdiagnosis and overtreatment of prostate cancer that has occurred today with PSA screening.

After Failed Curative Intervention

It has been estimated that 20%–40% of men who undergo curative intervention for presumed localized prostate cancer with radiotherapy or surgery will have evidence of biochemical failure over the 10 years after treatment.[21] Because a detectable or increasing PSA after treatment is not a valid surrogate for clinical relapse (radiographic or physical evidence of disease) or more importantly overall survival, it is difficult to identify the patients who will benefit from further treatment.[21–26] In a series of men with a detectable PSA after surgical treatment of prostate cancer followed without additional treatments, 34% developed metastatic disease at a median of 8 years after PSA failure, and of these 43% (or 15% of those with metastatic disease) died of prostate cancer at a median of 5 years after development of metastatic disease.[22] Ward et al.[23] found that 29% of men who experienced biochemical failure progressed to clinical failure, and that 8% of those with biochemical failure died of prostate cancer at a median of 10 years after clinical failure was documented. Thus, biochemical failure after curative intervention is not synonymous with death from prostate cancer, but instead represents a heterogeneous state that is a continuum from insignificant disease to development of metastatic disease and death.

The clinical dilemma of biochemical failure after curative intervention is difficult because of uncertainty regarding future progression to clinically apparent disease, and the inability to accurately determine by imaging if microscopic disease is localized or distant. Because most men with bio-chemical failure after definitive therapy will not develop metastatic disease and die from prostate cancer[22,23] within 10 years, it is important to identify those with life-threatening disease for whom further treatment may be most beneficial.

D'Amico et al.[24] have shown that the PSADT, in subjects with biochemi-cal failure, is a surrogate end point for prostate cancer mortality and overall mortality independent of curative treatment received (radiation or surgery). In their study, the posttreatment PSADT (but not treatment received) was statistically significantly associated with time to prostate cancer–specific mortality and with time to all-cause mortality. A PSADT of less than 3 months was associated with a median time to prostate cancer–specific mor-tality of 6 years and a hazard ratio of 19.6 for prostate cancer–specific mortality—values confirmed by Freedland et al.[25] who followed untreated men with biochemical failure after surgical intervention. The proportion of patients with biochemical failure postsurgery who have a PSADT less than 3 months is approximately 10% (Table 6.2). These men are more likely to benefit from "early" androgen deprivation therapy given the imminent development of metastatic disease predicted by a PSADT below 3 months.

PSADTs (specific values) above 3 months are also surrogate end points for prostate cancer–specific mortality after curative intervention in those

TABLE 6.2. Distributions of prostate-specific antigen doubling time (PSADT) after failure of local therapy.

Study (no. of subjects)	PSADT (months)	Distribution (%) of subjects
D'Amico et al.[24] (n = 8669)	<3	12
	3–5.9	16
	6–11.9	28
	≥12	44
Freedland et al.[25] (n = 379)	<3	6
	3–5.9	15
	6–11.9	29
	≥12	50
Stephenson et al.[26] (n = 501)	<7.4	50
	>7.4	50
Ward et al.[23] (n = 211)	<7.3	50
	>7.3	50

TABLE 6.3. Estimated risk of prostate cancer–specific survival 15 years after biochemical failure following surgery.

	Risk estimate, % (95% confidence interval)			
	Recurrence >3 years after surgery		Recurrence ≤3 years after surgery	
PSADT (months)	Gleason score <8	Gleason score ≥8	Gleason score <8	Gleason score ≥8
≥15	94 (87–100)	87 (79–92)	81 (57–93)	62 (32–85)
9–14.9	86 (57–97)	72 (35–92)	59 (24–87)	31 (7–72)
3–8.9	59 (32–81)	30 (10–63)	16 (4–49)	1 (<1–51)
<3	19 (5–51)	2 (<1–38)	<1 (<1–26)	<1 (<1–2)

Source: Adapted from Freedland et al.[25]
PSADT = prostate-specific antigen doubling time.

with biochemical failure.[24] Freedland et al.[25] found that PSADT, pathologic Gleason score, and time from surgery to biochemical recurrence were all significant risk factors for time to prostate cancer–specific mortality. However, a PSADT below 9 months was associated with a higher risk of prostate cancer death compared with time from surgery to recurrence (≤3 vs.>3 years) and pathologic Gleason score (≥8 vs.<8). Thus, PSADT should be used in the decision-making process when determining the need for salvage treatments in those with biochemical failure after curative intervention. Estimates of the risk of biochemical recurrence at 15 years after biochemical failure as a function of PSADT, grade, and time from surgery to recurrence were made by Freedland et al.[25] to help physicians and patients choose management options (Table 6.3).

Recently, D'Amico et al.[27] identified a subset of patients who seem to have clinically insignificant PSA failure and probably could safely forego salvage therapy. A PSADT of 12 months or more and a pretreatment PSAA that did not exceed 0.5 ng/mL per year in the year before surgery (12% of population) was associated with maintenance of a minimally detectable PSA, and associated with pathologic features at surgery that were not different from those who did not sustain PSA failure. Further follow-up may identify a larger proportion of patients with biochemical failure after curative intervention who should consider surveillance instead of salvage therapy.

Conclusions

Evaluation of PSA changes over time (PSA kinetics) is a method that can be used to help assess the risk that prostate cancer is present. Accumulating data suggest that there is no PSA level below which we can reassure a man that prostate cancer is not present. Therefore, instead of performing a biopsy on all men who reach a given PSA threshold, another approach would be to evaluate the rate at which the PSA increases to a given level and use this information as part of the decision-making process regarding the need for biopsy. Because PSAV correlates with the likelihood that life-threatening disease is present, this approach may help reduce the overdiagnosis and overtreatment of prostate cancer that has occurred with PSA screening. In addition, after curative intervention for prostate cancer, PSADT is a surrogate for survival and can be used to help identify those men with biochemical failure who are most likely to benefit from salvage treatments.

References

1. Jemal A, Ward E, Wu X, Martin HJ, McLaughlin CC, Thun MJ. Geographic patterns of prostate cancer mortality and variations in access to medical care in the United States. Cancer Epidemiol Biomarkers Prev 2005;14:590–5.
2. Carter HB, Pearson JD, Metter JE, et al. Longitudinal evaluation of prostate specific antigen levels in men with and without prostate disease. JAMA 1992;267:2215–20.
3. Carter HB, Morrell CH, Pearson JD, et al. Estimation of prostatic growth using serial prostate-specific antigen measurements in men with and without prostate disease. Cancer Res 1992;52:3323–8.
4. Carter HB, Pearson JD, Waclawiw Z, et al. Prostate-specific antigen variability in men without prostate cancer: the effect of sampling interval and number of repeat measurements on prostate-specific antigen velocity. Urology 1995;45: 591–6.
5. Riehmann M, Rhodes PR, Cook TD, et al. Analysis of variation in prostate-specific antigen values. Urology 1993;42:390–7.
6. Prestigiacomo AF, Stamey TA. Physiological variation of serum prostate specific antigen in the 4.0 to 10.0 ng/mL range in male volunteers. J Urol 1996;155: 1977–80.
7. Eastham JA, Riedel E, Scardino PT, et al.; Polyp Prevention Trial Study Group. Variation of serum prostate-specific antigen levels: an evaluation of year-to-year fluctuations. JAMA 2003;289:2695–700.
8. Smith DS, Catalona WJ. Rate of change in serum prostate specific antigen levels as a method for prostate cancer detection. J Urol 1994;152:1163–7.
9. Kadmon D, Weinberg AD, Williams RH, et al. Pitfalls in interpreting prostate specific antigen velocity. J Urol 1996;155:1655–7.
10. Lujan M, Paez A, Sanchez E, et al. Prostate specific antigen variation in patients without clinically evident prostate cancer. J Urol 1999;162:1311–13.
11. Raaijmakers R, Wildhagen MF, Ito K, et al. Prostate-specific antigen change in the European Randomized Study of Screening for Prostate Cancer, section Rotterdam. Urology 2004;63:316–20.
12. Berger AP, Deibl M, Steiner H, et al. Longitudinal PSA changes in men with and without prostate cancer: assessment of prostate cancer risk. Prostate 2005; 64:240–5.
13. Oesterling JE, Jacobsen SJ, Chute CG, et al. Serum prostate-specific antigen in a community-based population of healthy men: establishment of age-specific reference ranges. JAMA 1993;270:860–4.

14. Etzioni RD, Howlader N, Shaw PA, et al. Long-term effects of finasteride on prostate specific antigen levels: results from the prostate cancer prevention trial. J Urol 2005;174:877–81.
15. Fang J, Metter EJ, Landis P, Carter HB. PSA velocity for assessing prostate cancer risk in men with PSA levels between 2.0 and 4.0 ng/mL. Urology 2002;59:889–93.
16. Roobol MJ, Kranse R, de Koning HJ, Schroder FH. Prostate-specific antigen velocity at low prostate-specific antigen levels as screening tool for prostate cancer: results of second screening round of ERSPC (ROTTERDAM). Urology 2004;63:309–13.
17. D'Amico AV, Chen MH, Roehl KA, Catalona WJ. Preoperative PSA velocity and the risk of death from prostate cancer after radical prostatectomy. N Engl J Med 2004;351:125–35.
18. D'Amico AV, Renshaw AA, Sussman B, Chen MH. Pretreatment PSA velocity and risk of death from prostate cancer following external beam radiation therapy. JAMA 2005;294:440–7.
19. Sengupta S, Myers RP, Slezak JM, Bergstralh EJ, Zincke H, Blute ML. Preoperative prostate specific antigen doubling time and velocity are strong and independent predictors of outcomes following radical prostatectomy. J Urol 2005;174:2191–6.
20. Carter HB, Ferrucci L, Metter EJ. PSA velocity and risk of prostate cancer death in the Baltimore Longitudinal Study of Aging. J Urol 2005;173:257. Abstract 951.
21. Ward JF, Moul JW. Treating the biochemical recurrence of prostate cancer after definitive primary therapy. Clin Prostate Cancer 2005;4:38–44.
22. Pound CR, Partin AW, Eisenberger MA. Natural history of progression after PSA elevation following radical prostatectomy. JAMA 1999;281:1591–7.
23. Ward JF, Blute ML, Slezak J, Bergstralh EJ, Zincke H. The long-term clinical impact of biochemical recurrence of prostate cancer 5 or more years after radical prostatectomy. J Urol 2003;170:1872–6.
24. D'Amico AV, Moul JW, Carroll PR, Sun L, Lubeck D, Chen MH. Surrogate end point for prostate cancer-specific mortality after radical prostatectomy or radiation therapy. J Natl Cancer Inst 2003;95:1376–83.
25. Freedland SJ, Humphreys EB, Mangold LA, et al. Risk of prostate cancer-specific mortality following biochemical recurrence after radical prostatectomy. JAMA 2005;294:433–9.
26. Stephenson AJ, Shariat SF, Zelefsky MJ, et al. Salvage radiotherapy for recurrent prostate cancer after radical prostatectomy. JAMA 2004;291:1325–32.
27. D'Amico AV, Chen MH, Roehl KA, Catalona WJ. Identifying patients at risk for significant versus clinically insignificant postoperative prostate-specific antigen failure. J Clin Oncol 2005;23:4975–9.

7
Prostate Cancer Screening: Navigating the Controversy

Timothy C. Brand and Ian M. Thompson

Abstract

National medical societies are diverse in their recommendations for prostate cancer screening. Digital rectal examination and prostate-specific antigen level continue to be the accepted practice, with transrectal ultrasound–guided biopsy recommended for patients with abnormal findings. Although there has been a dramatic increase in the rate of prostate cancer detection, prostate cancer mortality has decreased only marginally. The benefit of screening hinges upon the efficacy of prevention and treatment for which there currently exist few options. An ideal screening test for prostate cancer would have both high sensitivity and specificity and also be indicative of prognosis. The ability to differentiate between latent, low-risk and more clinically significant, high-risk prostate cancer represents an enormous factor in the risks and benefits of digital rectal examination, prostate-specific antigen level testing, and biopsy as screening modalities.

Keywords: screening, prostate cancer, prostate-specific antigen, prevention

Since the early 1900s, prostate cancer screening consisted of a digital rectal examination (DRE). The DRE, examined as a "biomarker" for early detection of prostate cancer, has relatively poor sensitivity and specificity. In a study of 2005 men undergoing screening, only 65 men were noted to have an abnormal DRE and of these 65, biopsy proved only 17 men to have prostate cancer.[1] Another large study published in 1986 demonstrated that prostate cancer was initially detected by DRE in only 45% of patients.[2] Other studies have shown similar unreliability of the DRE in detecting cancer.[3]

From: *Current Clinical Urology: Prostate Biopsy: Indications, Techniques, and Complications*
Edited by J.S. Jones © Humana Press, Totowa, NJ

The identification of prostate-specific antigen (PSA) as a biomarker for prostate cancer forever altered prostate cancer screening. PSA was first described by Ablin and colleagues in 1970 with confirmation by other investigators in later years.[4–6] Public interest increased in PSA screening as several series found a positive predictive value of approximately 25% in men with a PSA value >4 ng/mL, and a positive predictive value of approximately 50% for values >10 ng/mL.[7–12] It is unclear to the authors exactly how the cutoff value of 4 ng/mL was selected and became the de facto upper limit of normal, but it may be because approximately 8% of the population had a PSA value >4 ng/mL and that was the same lifetime risk of prostate cancer in the mid-1980s in the United States.

After the widespread implementation of PSA for prostate cancer screening, the reported results with the utilization of the test began to change. This might be partly attributable to the way the procedure of prostate biopsy was changing in the same era. Prostate biopsies were routinely initially performed with digital guidance, and the spring-loaded biopsy device entered clinical practice shortly after the initiation of PSA screening, replacing the Tru-Cut large-core biopsy needle. In 1989, Huggins and Hodges[13] published recommendations for using transrectal ultrasound imaging to perform a sextant biopsy of the prostate to include sampling from different regions of the prostate. Currently, most urologists obtain between 10 and 12 core biopsies to minimize risk of missing cancer.[14,15]

With a combination of the use of PSA for screening, and improved biopsy technique, there was a steep increase in the number of prostate cancer cases diagnosed in the United States[16] (see Figure 7.1).

This spike in cases may be described as a "harvest effect" and is often seen when a new screening test is introduced in a screening-naïve population. The rate of prostate cancers detected eventually decreased to a level somewhat above that of the late 1980s.

The stage of the tumors that were diagnosed was substantially altered by the ability of PSA to detect clinically localized disease. There was a sub-

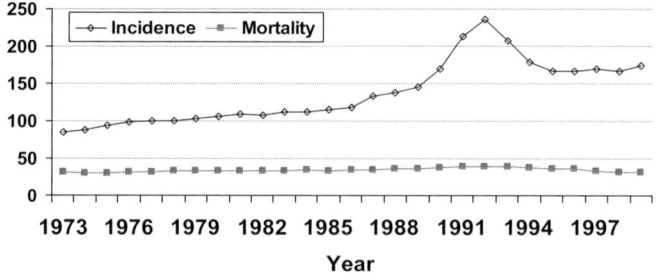

FIGURE 7.1. Prostate cancer trends in incidence and mortality, 1973–1999. (From CDC online resources at: http://www.cdc.gov/cancer/prostate/resourcematerials. htm.)

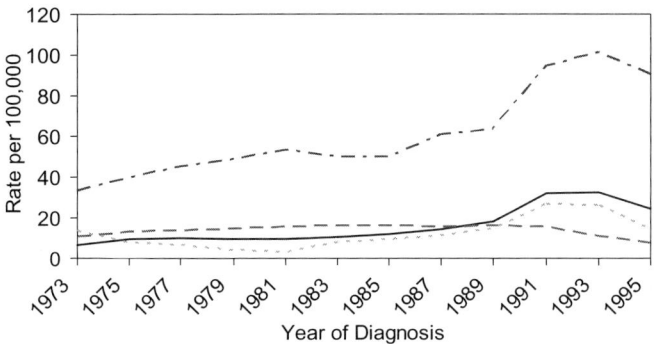

FIGURE 7.2. Prostate cancer incidence rates by stage, 1973–1995. (From CDC online resources at: http://www.cdc.gov/cancer/prostate/resourcematerials.htm.)

stantial increase in the rate of cancers that were identified as localized to the prostate, and a corresponding decrease in the rate of distant-stage prostate cancer during the same era[17] (see Figure 7.2).

There was an increase in the diagnosis of prostate cancers of every tumor grade during the early 1990s, but proportionally, the greatest increase in detection occurred for those cancers of moderate grade (Gleason 5–7)[18,19] (see Figure 7.3).

Unfortunately, although there has been a dramatic increase in the rate of prostate cancer diagnosis, prostate cancer mortality has changed only marginally. It has been reported that the U.S. mortality from the disease has decreased by 27% since 1994.[16,20] However, it is important to recognize that shortly after the onset of screening, prostate cancer mortality actually *increased*. As such, the degree of decrease in mortality, if based on the rate before the outset of screening, has been smaller. Additionally, when one compares the rates of increase of prostate cancer detection between the United States and the United Kingdom, where there is little PSA screening,

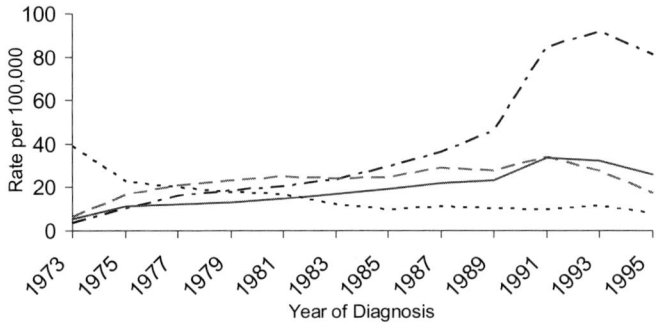

FIGURE 7.3. Tumor rates by grade. (From CDC online resources at: http://www.cdc.gov/cancer/prostate/resourcematerials.htm.)

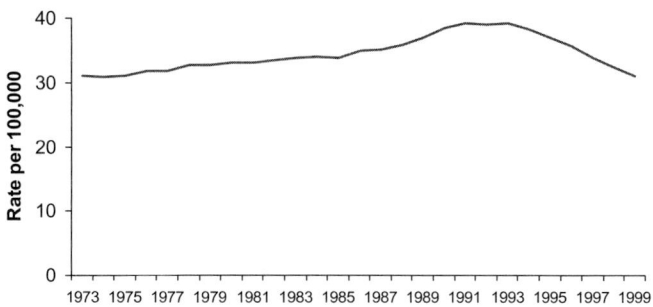

FIGURE 7.4. Top: Prostate cancer mortality in the United States, in an era of increased screening. Bottom: Prostate cancer mortality in the United Kingdom, where screening was seldom used. (From CDC online resources at: http://www.cdc. gov/cancer/prostate/resourcematerials.htm.)

whereas a corresponding enormous increase in incidence was not seen in the United Kingdom, a similar decrease in mortality was seen in both countries[21] (Figure 7.4).

It has been unclear how the positive predictive value of PSA has changed since the introduction of PSA testing. In 2004, the results of the Prostate Cancer Prevention Trial (PCPT) dramatically changed our understanding of the performance of PSA, and it is now recognized that there is a high prevalence of prostate cancer at levels below 4.0 ng/mL.[22] Although it had been known that prostate cancer incidence rates in the aging male population were quite high, it was assumed that these generally small tumors detected at autopsy were generally not found with prostate biopsies using 6–12 cores.[23] In the PCPT, for the first time, a group of men all underwent prostate biopsy regardless of PSA level. In this study, 2950 men in the placebo group that had a normal DRE and PSA, who had never had an abnormal DRE or PSA over the 7 years of the study, underwent an end of study biopsy, and 24.4% of men were found to have cancer on biopsy.[22] Further analysis demonstrated a 24.5% sensitivity for PSA using an upper limit of normal of 4 ng/mL. Additionally, to achieve a 90% sensitivity for cancer detection, a PSA of approximately 1 ng/mL would be necessary.[24] The performance of PSA was found to be better for higher-grade tumors, but a cut point of 4.0 ng/mL would still miss 60% of Gleason 7 or higher tumors.[24] Other recent studies have had similar findings.[20]

Prevention

Because of the modest reduction in mortality seen after implementation of prostate cancer screening in the United States, and while considering the side effects associated with therapy including erectile dysfunction, urinary incontinence or retention, bowel toxicity, emotional consequences, and the anxiety and stigma associated with the diagnosis of the disease, the opportunity to *prevent* prostate cancer is extremely attractive. The evidence is now clear that this is a proven option for some patients.

To date, the only agent that has been definitively proven in a randomized, placebo-controlled, prospective clinical trial to prevent prostate cancer is finasteride. The PCPT was activated in 1993 shortly after Food and Drug Administration approval of finasteride, a selective inhibitor of type II five-alpha reductase (5αR), previously shown to lower intraprostatic dihydrotestosterone levels. Because of overwhelming evidence that the trial was positive, an independent Data and Safety Monitoring Committee recommended study closure 15 months before the anticipated date of completion. In 2003, the results of PCPT were published. It was found that the prevalence of prostate cancer was reduced from 24.4% in the placebo group to 18.4% in the group taking finasteride (a 24.8% reduction). Balanced against the significant reduction in prostate cancers was a greater number and proportion of high-grade tumors in the finasteride group. The prevalence of Gleason 7–10 cancers was 6.4% in the finasteride group compared with 5.1% with placebo.

There are several possible reasons for the detection of higher-grade tumors in the finasteride group. The finasteride could have resulted in a hormonal pathologic effect because of an alteration of the appearance of tumors that were detected with finasteride. Another bias could have been related to disease ascertainment. Because finasteride acts to reduce the size of the prostate gland (22% size reduction in this study), it is possible that the "sampling density" at the time of prostate biopsy favored the detection of higher-grade disease. Arguing against the concept that finasteride induced high-grade disease were two observations: 1) The increased rate of high-grade disease was seen at year 1 of the study and did not change over the 7 years, and 2) the increased risk of high-grade disease was seen in those biopsies performed for elevated PSA or abnormal DRE whereas those performed at the end of the study—after the greatest length of exposure to the medication—showed no increased detection.

Several authors have examined the impact of finasteride for chemoprevention in the population on life expectancy or death from prostate cancer.[25,26] Unger et al.[27] modeled the results of finasteride use on the general U.S. population using the metric of person-years of life saved. In this analysis, they predicted more than 300,000 person-years of life saved over 10 years in the United States with generalized finasteride use.

For patients considering finasteride for cancer prevention, it is important to consider potential other risks and benefits of this drug. The primary side effect that was noted was a group of sexual symptoms including erectile dysfunction, decreased libido, and decreased volume of ejaculate but, in general, the rates were only slightly greater in finasteride than in the placebo group. Additionally, other studies have demonstrated that discontinuation of the drug resolves this symptom. An additional benefit of finasteride use was related to urinary symptoms and included a reduced risk of complaints of benign prostatic hyperplasia, lower rate of transurethral resection of the prostate, and a lower risk of prostatitis.

Arguments in Favor of Prostate Cancer Screening

No one should have to die of prostate cancer if it's detected and treated early enough. But avoidance of the subject is simply a matter of playing a losing game of Russian roulette.

—General Norman Schwarzkopf

An often-used argument for prostate cancer screening is the number of men that fall victim to the disease each year. It is the most common nondermatologic malignancy in men, and more than 30,000 men die of prostate cancer each year.[16] It is the sixth most common cause of death for men after age 40 (National Center for Health Statistics U.S. mortality data 1995–1999), and the lifetime risk of prostate cancer death is 3% (or 4% if African American).[28]

By the time symptoms develop, prostate cancer is usually advanced. With regular screening, prostate cancer is usually detected while clinically confined to the prostate. This is evidenced by Figure 7.2. Treatment for clinically localized prostate cancer results in very high survival rates. Cancer-specific survival at 5 years after treatment is 100% for localized prostate cancer, versus 34% for patients with distant disease.[29]

Data do exist that demonstrate that intervention for early prostate cancer does reduce mortality. Bill-Axelson et al.[30] published results of a trial in which 695 men with localized prostate cancer were randomized to radical prostatectomy or observation only. After a median of 8.2 years of follow-up, there were 83 deaths (of 347 men) from the surgery group, and 106 deaths (of 348 men) from the watchful waiting group (p = 0.04); 8.6% of men assigned to surgery died as a result of prostate cancer compared with 14.4% of men in the watchful waiting group. The risk of metastasis and local progression was also diminished in the prostatectomy group.

Studies that have been designed to evaluate the impact of prostate cancer screening on mortality are frequently limited by the duration of study that is necessary to demonstrate change. A recent case-control study suggested that screening with DRE decreased mortality from prostate cancer.[31] Several data limitations precluded this study's estimation of the impact of PSA screening compared with DRE. Although from a public health standpoint, broad-based PSA screening may be perceived as expensive, it was recently shown that prostate cancer screening would probably be perceived as cost-effective if potentially curable patients gained on average just one additional year of survival.[32]

The treatment of cancer has advanced significantly, with improvement in quality-of-life outcomes. Technical advances in radical retropubic prosta-tectomy to include the nerve-sparing technique,[33] the introduction of brachytherapy, as well as increasingly targeted external beam techniques have significantly reduced patient morbidity. A recent study evaluating self-reported quality of life after retropubic radical prostatectomy using the Rand 36-Item Health Survey demonstrated no statistically significant change in health-related quality of life in >80% of patients at 1 year of follow-up.[34] Similar findings hold true in brachytherapy, with return to baseline for a majority of patients at measurement of quality of life after 1 year. Outcomes do correlate with radiotherapy dose.[35]

Arguments Against Prostate Cancer Screening

At the present time "non-treatment" is what most individuals with stage 1 (prostate) cancer receive, if for no other reason than lack of detection. When one considers the tremendous number of latent prostatic cancers, the death rate from prostatic cancer in this country becomes relatively less impressive. This is another way of saying that "non-treatment" has been a relatively effective method of management of latent cancer.

—Willet F. Whitmore Jr., M.D., 1956

No randomized clinical trials have confirmed that prostate cancer screening significantly reduces the risk of prostate cancer death in the population. There are currently several studies underway (described further below) but an advantage to screening has never been demonstrated in a prospective, randomized study. In the interpretation of smaller, nonrandomized studies, it is important to avoid giving screening an undeserved benefit because of the presence of lead-time bias, which may be seen in the interpretation of studies that compare disease progression for tumors detected early and later. If a cancer is *found* earlier, there may be an illusion of delayed pro-gression or improved survival for those patients with early detection even when attempts are made at standardization for tumor stage, etc. In other words, the treatments must be effective for there to be a true benefit with earlier detection.

Given population statistics, 96%–97% of men who undergo screening for prostate cancer would not die of prostate cancer without screening, whereas at least 8% of men who undergo screening for prostate cancer are found to have an elevated PSA level (>4 ng/mL) and are advised to have a biopsy of the prostate. With current evidence of the prevalence of cancer at lower PSA values, this percentage may increase substantially, increasing the risk of detection of indolent disease. As such, if prostate cancer is found, it is possible that the cancer is not of clinical significance. Age of the patient and grade of tumor may be useful in assessing the patient's risk from that tumor, but for a 65- to 69-year-old man with a Gleason 7 tumor, about half the men who have passed will have died of prostate cancer and half the men will have died of something else in 15 years after diagnosis with conservative management of the prostate cancer.[36] So far, we have not been able to reliably predict the clinically significant cancers with accuracy.

Despite the two previous citations that report minimal effect of prostate cancer treatments on quality of life,[34,35] there are many other studies that reveal significant consequences for treating prostate cancer for the patient. These quality-of-life issues include incontinence, urinary obstruction, urinary frequency, loss of ejaculation, loss of sexual desire, loss of erections, irritable bowels, and blood in the stool. These, of course, vary with the type of treatment administered.[37] Finally, even with screening, some tumors are incurable, and treatment may not affect the outcome in these patients.

Conclusions

The recommendations of national medical organizations are diverse regarding prostate cancer screening. The American Cancer Society advocates that PSA and DRE be offered yearly, beginning at age 50, to men who have at least a 10-year life expectancy, with some additional recommendations for men at a younger age who are at increased risk. The recommendation of the American Urological Association is very similar to that of the American Cancer Society. The U.S. Preventative Service Task Force summary of recommendations regarding prostate cancer screening reports that the evidence is insufficient to recommend for or against routine screening for prostate cancer using PSA and DRE. The American College of Preventive Medicine recommends against routine population screening with DRE and PSA with the caveat that men 50 or older with a life expectancy greater than 10 years should be given information regarding benefits and harms of screening and limits of current evidence and be allowed to make their own choice regarding screening.

We advocate that prostate cancer screening with PSA and DRE be offered to the patient after counseling, similar to what most national organizations are currently recommending. Most men expect to have a PSA. Currently, more than half of men older than 50 years have annual screening, and approximately 75% of men have had a PSA determination at some point.[16,23]

It is expected that the results of the Prostate, Lung, Colorectal, and Ovarian (PLCO) Cancer Screening Trial will provide definitive evidence regarding the impact of prostate cancer screening on population mortality. This very large study is sponsored by the National Cancer Institute's Division of Cancer Prevention, in collaboration with the Division of Cancer Epidemiology and Genetics. The study opened in 1992, and enrollment ended in 2001. A total of 76,705 men between the ages of 55 and 74 enrolled in the study. The PLCO randomized patients to either routine healthcare from their provider or a series of examinations to screen for prostate and the other cancers. Trigger for biopsy in this study is PSA > 4.0 ng/mL or abnormal DRE. Screening will continue until 2007 and follow-up will continue for up to 10 years.[38] Another large, ongoing study designed to assess benefit in prostate cancer screening is the European Randomized Study of Screening for Prostate Cancer. This study began in 1993 and includes patients from eight countries. Results are anticipated in the next few years.[39]

Future Directions

The ideal screening test would be very sensitive and specific for prostate cancer, and not only specific, but specific for the tumor with a poor prognosis. The Early Detection Research Network of the National Cancer Institute is currently conducting a three-phase validation study to evaluate the role of surface-enhanced laser desorption/ionization time-of-flight (SELDI-TOF) in the detection of prostate cancer.[40] The goals of this study are to determine the portability and reproducibility of the assay, refine the predictive algorithm in a case-control study design across a multiinstitutional study patient population, and eventually, to prospectively validate SELDI for the detection of prostate cancer. This study is unique in that it is incorporating prognosis in addition to cancer detection by analyzing two groups of cancer cases: those with high-risk disease (Gleason score ≥7) versus those with low-risk disease (Gleason ≤6).

Another opportunity for improvement for gaining information of prostate cancer prognosis would be at the time of biopsy. In addition to grade and volume of tumor, there is active investigation to determine which molecular markers would be useful in predicting whether the cancer is predictably latent or one that will become clinically significant. Limitations in this area include the scant amount of tissue that is available after prostate biopsy for additional testing, and the fact that an ideal scenario would avoid biopsy all together for those latent cancers.

References

1. Thompson IM, Ernst JJ, Gangai MP, et al. Adenocarcinoma of the prostate: results of routine urological screening. J Urol 1984;132:690.
2. Schmidt JD, Mettlin CJ, Natarajan N, et al. Trends in patterns of care for prostatic cancer, 1974–1983: results of surveys by the American College of Surgeons. J Urol 1986;136:416.
3. Chodak GW, Schoenberg HW. Early detection of prostate cancer by routine screening. JAMA 1984;252:3261.

4. Ablin RJ, Bronson P, Soanes WA, et al. Tissue- and species-specific antigens of normal human prostatic tissue. J Immunol 1970;104:1329.
5. Hara M, Koyanagi Y, Inoue T, et al. Some physico-chemical characteristics of "-seminoprotein," an antigenic component specific for human seminal plasma. Forensic immunological study of body fluids and secretion. VII. Nippon Hoigaku Zasshi 1971;25:322.
6. Li TS, Beling CG. Isolation and characterization of two specific antigens of human seminal plasma. Fertil Steril 1973;24:134.
7. Catalona WJ, Smith DS, Ratliff TL, et al. Measurement of prostate-specific antigen in serum as a screening test for prostate cancer. [Erratum appears in N Engl J Med 1991;325(18):1324]. N Engl J Med 1991;324:1156.
8. Brawer MK, Chetner MP, Beatie J, et al. Screening for prostatic carcinoma with prostate specific antigen. J Urol 1992;147:841.
9. Brawer MK, Beatie J, Wener MH, et al. Screening for prostatic carcinoma with prostate specific antigen: results of the second year. J Urol 1993;150:106.
10. Wang TY, Kawaguchi TP. Preliminary evaluation of measurement of serum prostate-specific antigen level in detection of prostate cancer. Ann Clin Lab Sci 1986;16:461.
11. Cooner WH, Mosley BR, Rutherford CL Jr, et al. Prostate cancer detection in a clinical urological practice by ultrasonography, digital rectal examination and prostate specific antigen. J Urol 1990;143:1146.
12. Terris MK, Stamey TA. Utilization of polyclonal serum prostate specific antigen levels in screening for prostate cancer: a comparison with corresponding monoclonal values. Br J Urol 1994;73:61.
13. Huggins C, Hodges CV. Studies on prostatic cancer: I. The effect of castration, of estrogen and of androgen injection on serum phosphatases in metastatic carcinoma of the prostate. 1941. J Urol 2002;168:9.
14. Presti JC Jr, Chang JJ, Bhargava V, et al. The optimal systematic prostate biopsy scheme should include 8 rather than 6 biopsies: results of a prospective clinical trial. J Urol 2000;163:163.
15. Presti JC Jr, O'Dowd GJ, Miller MC, et al. Extended peripheral zone biopsy schemes increase cancer detection rates and minimize variance in prostate specific antigen and age related cancer rates: results of a community multi-practice study. J Urol 2003;169:125.
16. Weir HK, Thun MJ, Hankey BF, et al. Annual report to the nation on the status of cancer, 1975–2000, featuring the uses of surveillance data for cancer prevention and control. [Erratum appears in J Natl Cancer Inst 2003;95(21):1641]. J Natl Cancer Inst 2003;95:1276.
17. Screening for prostate cancer: sharing the decision slide set. In: Cancer Prevention and Control. Centers for Disease Control (CDC).
18. Humphrey PA, Keetch DW, Smith DS, et al. Prospective characterization of pathological features of prostatic carcinomas detected via serum prostate specific antigen based screening. J Urol 1996;155:816.
19. Gilliland FD, Gleason DF, Hunt WC, et al. Trends in Gleason score for prostate cancer diagnosed between 1983 and 1993. J Urol 2001;165:846.
20. Pelzer AE, Tewari A, Bektic J, et al. Detection rates and biologic significance of prostate cancer with PSA less than 4.0 ng/mL: observation and clinical implications from Tyrol screening project. Urology 2005;66:1029.

21. Oliver SE, Gunnell D, Donovan JL. Comparison of trends in prostate-cancer mortality in England and Wales and the USA. [Erratum appears in Lancet 2000;356(9237):1278]. Lancet 2000;355:1788.
22. Thompson IM, Pauler DK, Goodman PJ, et al. Prevalence of prostate cancer among men with a prostate-specific antigen level ≤4.0 ng per milliliter. [Erratum appears in N Engl J Med 2004;351(14):1470]. N Engl J Med 2004;350:2239.
23. Sirovich BE, Schwartz LM, Woloshin S. Screening men for prostate and colorectal cancer in the United States: does practice reflect the evidence? JAMA 2003;289:1414.
24. Thompson IM, Ankerst DP, Chi C, et al. Operating characteristics of prostate-specific antigen in men with an initial PSA level of 3.0 ng/ml or lower. JAMA 2005;294:66.
25. Zeliadt SB, Etzioni RD, Penson DF, et al. Lifetime implications and cost-effectiveness of using finasteride to prevent prostate cancer. Am J Med 2005;118:850.
26. Lotan Y, Cadeddu JA, Lee JJ, et al. Implications of the prostate cancer prevention trial: a decision analysis model of survival outcomes. J Clin Oncol 2005;23:1911.
27. Unger JM, LeBlanc M, Thompson IM, et al. The person-years saved model and other methodologies for assessing the population impact of cancer-prevention strategies. Urol Oncol 2004;22:362.
28. Surveillance epidemiology and end results: U.S. National Institute of Health. Available at: www.seer.cancer.gov. 2005.
29. Wingo PA, Tong T, Bolden S. Cancer statistics, 1995. [Erratum appears in CA Cancer J Clin 1995;45(2):127–8]. CA Cancer J Clin 1995;45:8.
30. Bill-Axelson A, Holmberg L, Ruutu M, et al. Radical prostatectomy versus watchful waiting in early prostate cancer. N Engl J Med 2005;352:1977.
31. Weinmann S, Richert-Boe KE, Van Den Eeden SK, et al. Screening by prostate-specific antigen and digital rectal examination in relation to prostate cancer mortality: a case-control study. [Erratum appears in Epidemiology 2005;16(4):515]. Epidemiology 2005;16:367.
32. Sennfalt K, Sandblom G, Carlsson P, et al. Costs and effects of prostate cancer screening in Sweden—a 15-year follow-up of a randomized trial. Scand J Urol Nephrol 2004;38:291.
33. Walsh PC, Mostwin JL. Radical prostatectomy and cystoprostatectomy with preservation of potency. Results using a new nerve-sparing technique. Br J Urol 1984;56:694.
34. Ficarra V, Novara G, Galfano A, et al. Twelve-month self-reported quality of life after retropubic radical prostatectomy: a prospective study with Rand 36-Item Health Survey (Short Form-36). BJU Int 2006;97:274.
35. Van Gellekom MPR, Moerland MA, Van Vulpen M, et al. Quality of life of patients after permanent prostate brachytherapy in relation to dosimetry. Int J Radiat Oncology, Biol Phys 2005;63:772.
36. Albertsen PC, Hanley JA, Gleason DF, et al. Competing risk analysis of men aged 55 to 74 years at diagnosis managed conservatively for clinically localized prostate cancer. JAMA 1998;280:975.
37. Quek ML, Penson DF. Quality of life in patients with localized prostate cancer. Urol Oncol 2005;23:208.

38. Andriole GL, Levin DL, Crawford ED, et al. Prostate Cancer Screening in the Prostate, Lung, Colorectal and Ovarian (PLCO) Cancer Screening Trial: findings from the initial screening round of a randomized trial. J Natl Cancer Inst 2005;97:433.
39. Roobol MJ, Schroder FH. European Randomized Study of Screening for Prostate Cancer: achievements and presentation. BJU Int 2003;92(Suppl 2):117.
40. Fabian CJ, Kimler BF, Elledge RM, et al. Models for early chemoprevention trials in breast cancer. Hematol Oncol Clin North Am 1998;12:993.

8
Prostate Cancer Nomograms and How They Measure Up to Neural Networks

Pierre I. Karakiewicz and Michael W. Kattan

Abstract

Nomograms and neural networks represent two distinct methodologic approaches toward prediction of prostate cancer outcomes. The authors of this chapter recommend nomograms because of advantages including increased accuracy and graphic display of input variables and their relative importance. Accuracy, level of complexity, performance characteristics, model generalizability, and advantages relative to available alternatives are important considerations in selecting a predictive tool. Benefiting from continued improvement, prostate cancer nomograms have become accepted in clinical practice worldwide.

Keywords: nomograms, prediction models, neural networks, screening

The field of prognostics has exploded in the last decade, and clinicians have been provided with numerous tools to assist with medical decision-making in the most evidence-based manner. Most of these tools consist of nomograms, look-up tables, and neural network models.[1–16] They address numerous prostate cancer (PCa) outcomes, which range from prediction of biopsy outcome[1] in men considered at risk of PCa to prediction of death from hormone-refractory PCa.[2]

Choice of Decision Aids

The presence of several decision aids requires a careful selection of tools that should be used for prediction of the outcomes of interest. The following criteria provide an objective and systematic approach in that complex process:

From: *Current Clinical Urology: Prostate Biopsy: Indications, Techniques, and Complications*
Edited by J.S. Jones © Humana Press, Totowa, NJ

1. Accuracy represents the first consideration. Current statistical methods offer the possibility of assessing a model's predictive accuracy. Usually, it is quantified using the area under the receiver operating characteristic curve and is expressed as a percentage. Values range from 0.5 to 1.0, where 0.5 is equivalent to a flip of a coin and 1.0 represents perfect prediction. No model is perfect, and generally acceptable accuracy ranges from 70% to 80%.[1–16] Accuracy should be confirmed in either an external cohort or internally, using statistical methods such as bootstrapping.[17,18]

2. Level of complexity represents an important consideration. Excessively complex models are difficult to integrate in a busy clinical practice. For example, lengthy logistic regression equations require the use of multiple functions and access to scientific calculators. These are clearly impractical in busy clinical practice. Neural networks can accurately predict several outcomes of interest.[3–11] Despite high reported accuracy, the use of these models is frequently restricted to centers with adequate computer infrastructure, because predictions require access to and expertise with specific software. Look-up tables, such as the Partin Tables[12] or nomograms represent user-friendly alternatives. In either paper-based format or within palm digital assistants, they are ideally suited for busy clinical practice.[12–16]

3. Performance characteristics represent another important consideration. Accuracy indicates the overall ability of the model to predict the outcome of interest. However, the overall predictive accuracy does not inform the user on how good or how bad the predictions may be in specific patient subgroups. Some models may be ideally suited to predict in high-risk patients, but may predict poorly in low-risk patients. Other models may predict well throughout the range of predictions.

4. Model generalizability is important, because patient characteristics can vary. For example, PCa characteristics may not be the same in Europe as in the United States.[14] Before using a tool, the clinician should ideally ensure that it was validated in patients with similar disease characteristics.

5. Finally, when judging a new tool,[19,20] one should examine its accuracy, validity, and performance characteristics relative to established models, with the intent of determining whether the new model offers advantages relative to available alternatives.

Availability of several high-quality predictive models should encourage the clinician to adopt these tools into everyday clinical practice. Arguments favoring such behavior include standardization of care and of decision-making. Moreover, nomograms predict more accurately than clinicians.[15] For example, Specht and colleagues[15] addressed the ability to predict presence of axillary nodal metastases in women with invasive breast cancer. Nomogram predictions were compared with 17 breast cancer specialists from the Memorial Sloan-Kettering Cancer Center. The nomogram predictions were 18% (p = 0.01) more accurate than those of the expert clinicians. This implies that if predictions were made for 100 consecutive women, 18 would have been staged incorrectly if expert clinician predictions were used instead of nomogram predictions. Thus, it seems that nomograms have better ability to predict the outcomes of interest than even expert clinicians. It is conceivable that the advantage related to the use of nomogram predictions may be even more important if clinical ratings were obtained from less expert clinicians.

Besides the methodologic and practical considerations, patient perspective also deserves a mention when considering the use of unbiased decision tools. Patients are becoming increasingly aware of the existence of predictive tools. This trend is likely to increase in future years. Patients are also increasingly demanding to actively participate in decision-making, which might in part be explained by the following observations:

1. Advances in therapeutics have offered numerous treatment options, and men no longer accept paternalistic physician-centered treatment decision-making. Instead, they demand to know the efficacy and detailed side-effect profiles of treatment alternatives.

2. The patient is increasingly recognized as a pivotal player in medical decision-making. Decisions can no longer be made by the physician alone. For example, the American Urological Association suggests a detailed informed consent before prostate-specific antigen (PSA) testing.

3. Healthcare "consumerism" is a growing phenomenon in North America and Europe. Patients select what option of healthcare to purchase, rather than passively receiving a given treatment modality.

4. Attention to bioethical considerations has greatly increased over the past decade and has promoted autonomous decision-making.

Thus, it may be postulated that increasingly greater emphasis will be placed on standardized predictions, which will further promote the development of new tools and/or the improvement of existing predictive tools. These considerations may motivate clinicians to adopt the use of decision tools. Their motivation may also stem from the wealth of clinical data that are used for the development and validation of each model. Most decision tools are based on thousands of observations and it is virtually impossible to achieve that level of clinical exposure and expertise on an individual level. Moreover, most clinicians do not have the capacity to systematically record or remember the risk characteristics of several thousands of patients. Additionally, unlike computers, clinicians are incapable of systematically and cumulatively processing the recorded risk characteristics and outcomes of historic cases, to derive an estimated probability of outcome for a new case at hand. Thus, it may be expected that the majority of physician-derived estimates are not as accurate as computer-derived decision models.[15] Despite this advantage, these tools are not meant to replace clinical judgment. Their input needs to be weighed against the pros and cons of several other considerations, such as comorbidity, cost, or social, religious, or emotional considerations.

Prostate Cancer Detection Nomograms

Several authors have developed nomograms for prediction of PCa on needle biopsy. One is limited to men with serum PSA values less than 4 ng/mL.[21] This restriction precludes inclusion of many men with PSA values in excess of 4, in whom a biopsy may not always be indicated because of age and/or comorbidity. However, in these men, it might be desirable to quantify the probability of finding cancer. Another nomogram relies on ultrasound findings to determine the probability of finding PCa.[22] This requirement also undermines the practical application of this tool. Clinicians decide whether to perform a biopsy well ahead of the ultrasonic assessment of the gland. These findings emphasize the importance of inclusion of readily and routinely available predictor variables, which represent a sine qua non of any predictive tool developed for broad use.

To circumvent the limitations of previously developed models, we recently developed a nomogram predicting the probability of PCa on needle biopsy in men undergoing an initial biopsy.[1] This tool only requires the input of variables that are routinely available at the time of a prostatic evaluation, namely age, digital rectal examination (DRE) findings, serum PSA, and percent free PSA (%fPSA). The combined predictive accuracy of this model is 78% in the development cohort and 77% in the external validation cohort (Figure 8.1). The benefit related to the use of this tool is its ability to consider the simultaneous contribution of four variables. Its multivariate performance is appreciably higher than that of PSA (64%), age (52%), DRE (62.9%), or %fPSA (73%) alone. These substantially lower predictive accuracy estimates clearly demonstrate the benefit related to consideration of all four variables.

Besides the combined contribution of the four variables, the nomogram users can ascertain the relative importance of each predictor variable, because all risk factors are graphically depicted in the form of "risk axes." For example, assessment of the nomogram axes indicates that the effect of a suspicious DRE, as well as the effect of serum PSA in excess of 50 ng/mL, has a limited effect on the probability of diagnosing PCa on needle biopsy. Suspicious DRE contributes 20 risk points. Similarly, PSA of 50 ng/mL contributes approximately the same number of risk points. Conversely, %fPSA can contribute as many as 100 risk points. Thus, the potential effect of %fPSA is fivefold stronger than that of the other predictors. Such information cannot readily be derived from look-up tables or from neural networks.

Moreover, assessment of nomogram axes can situate the user with regard to the magnitude of the effect associated with each predictor. For example,

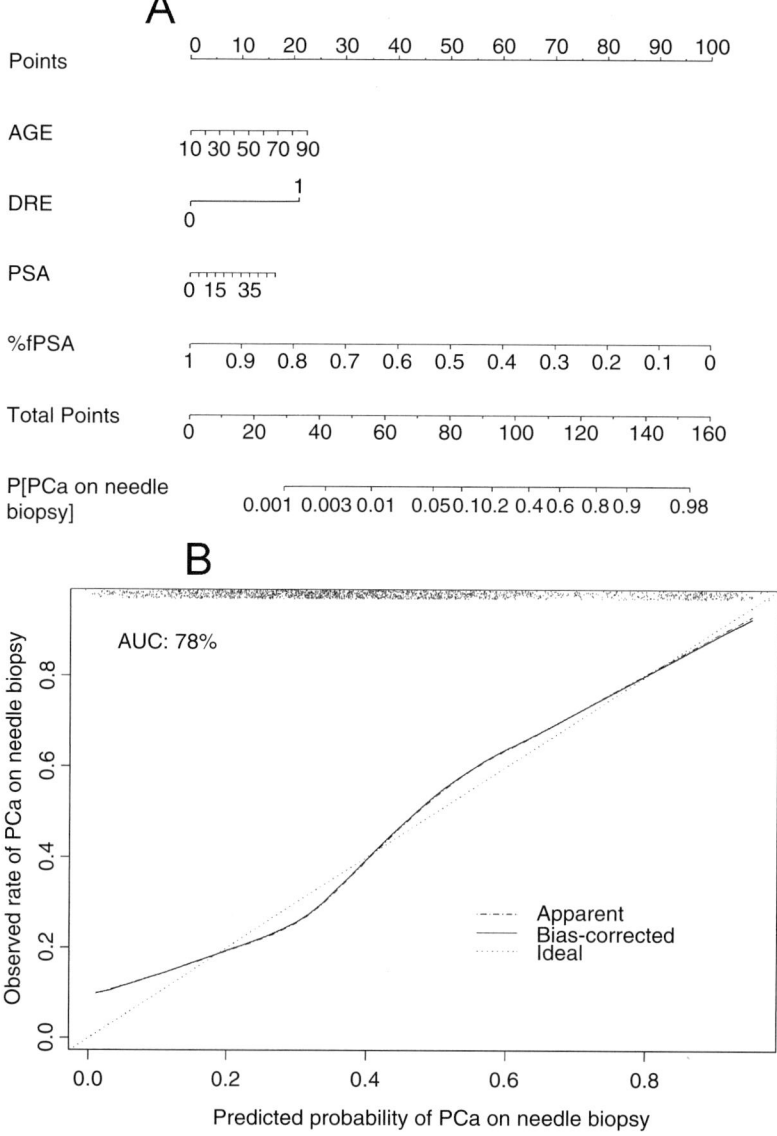

FIGURE 8.1. **A**: Initial biopsy nomogram based on four variables [age, digital rectal examination (DRE), prostate-specific antigen (PSA), and percent free PSA (%fPSA)]. Instructions for physicians: To obtain nomogram-predicted probability of biopsy outcome, locate patient values at each axis. Draw a vertical line to the "Point" axis to determine how many points are attributed for each variable value. Sum the points for all variables. Locate the sum on the "Total Points" line. Draw a vertical line toward the "P(PCa on needle biopsy)"—axis to determine the patient's probability of presence of prostate cancer on initial prostate biopsy. **B**: Calibration plot of the initial biopsy nomogram. Instructions for readers: Perfect prediction would correspond to the 45° line. Points estimated below the 45° line correspond to nomogram overprediction, whereas points situated above 45° line correspond to nomogram underprediction. DRE: 1 = suspicious, 0 = normal; %fPSA = percent free PSA.

the PSA risk axis indicates a limited magnitude of the effect of PSA. Men with PSA values between 10 and 15 ng/mL are given 10 risk points. Suspicious DRE and age of 75 years both contribute approximately 20 risk points. These contributions are modest at best, in the light of %fPSA, for which a value of 10% contributes 90 risk points. The above example illustrates how useful the graphical display of nomogram axes can be with regard to familiarizing the clinician with differential contribution of key risk factors.

Neural Networks

The graphical display of risk factors, which allows a clear and user-friendly depiction of the risk variables, distinguishes nomograms from neural networks, for which graphical display cannot be provided in paper format. Although the structure of neural networks can be presented in schematic form (Figure 8.2), the actual effect of the input variables on the output cannot. This is attributable to the numerous interactions that are allowed, when data are processed from the input units toward hidden neuron layers and then eventually to one or several output units. Neural networks predicting the outcome of needle biopsy have been generally limited to one layer of hidden neurons. Two investigators relied on "several" layers of hidden neurons.[3,4]

Use of several layers of hidden neurons renders the computational data manipulations highly complex and lacks transparence. Multiple interactions are allowed between input variables at each level. These are weighed to promote the most accurate prediction of the outcome of interest, for example presence of cancer on needle biopsy. At each hidden neuron, outputs are transmitted to the next level of hidden neurons. These resemble

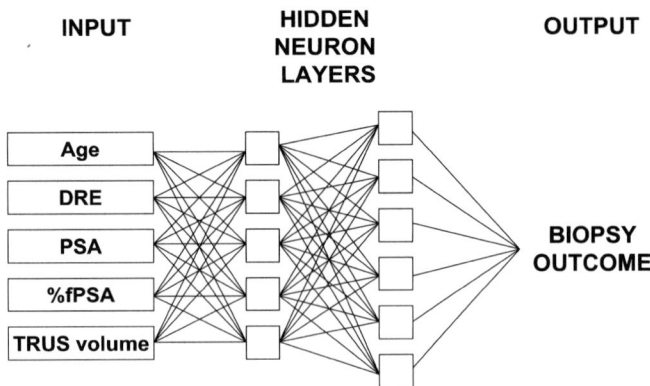

FIGURE 8.2. Schematic architecture of an artificial neural network to predict prostate cancer on initial biopsy.

multiple outputs within a logistic regression model. Interactions between these outputs, which again can be weighed to further promote accuracy, increase the complexity of the model. The process contributes to highly accurate prediction of the outcome of interest, which in several reported neural network models closely approximates the 85%–95% range. Although accuracy is of key importance, models that underlie predictions need to be tested before their discriminant ability can be taken at face value. Unfortunately, lack of familiarity with biostatistical considerations frequently severely undermines the validity of reported predicted accuracy estimates, which are exaggerated and reported in a biased and methodologically incorrect way.[23,24] Thus, despite good intentions, many investigators report spuriously high ability to predict the outcome of interest.

Head-to-Head Comparison of a Neural Network and a Nomogram

To substantiate the claim that neural network predictions are less accurate when they are subjected to strict external validity tests, we compared the ability to predict presence of cancer on biopsy between our nomogram and a neural network model that was made available by investigators at the Charité Hospital in Berlin, Germany.[5] The nomogram is based on four input variables, namely, age, DRE findings, serum PSA, and %fPSA, and its maximum predictive accuracy was estimated at 78%.[1] The neural network additionally includes prostate volume as a risk variable, and its predictive accuracy has been estimated at 84%. Prostate volume represents an important predictor of PCa risk on needle biopsy in several contemporary analyses.[25-28] Thus, its inclusion should bias the ability of the network to predict more accurately than the nomogram, where this variable is not considered. Moreover, unlike the neural network, the nomogram variables are not allowed to interact with one another, which should further undermine the predictive ability of the nomogram.

Both models were tested on a cohort of 4093 patients subjected to at least 8-core initial biopsy. Despite these a priori disadvantages, our results have indicated that the nomogram (70.6%) was 3.6% more accurate than the neural network (67.0%). Both models predicted less accurately than in the original studies, where they were described.[1,5] The decrease in predictive accuracy relative to original data was related to development of both tools on populations subjected to virtually exclusive sextant biopsies, whereas their head-to-head comparison was performed on a cohort exposed to extended biopsy schemes.

Besides overall model accuracy, we explored the performance characteristics of the nomogram and then of the neural network, because these are instrumental in the decision to adopt one tool versus another. As shown in Figure 8.3A, the performance characteristics of the nomogram virtually

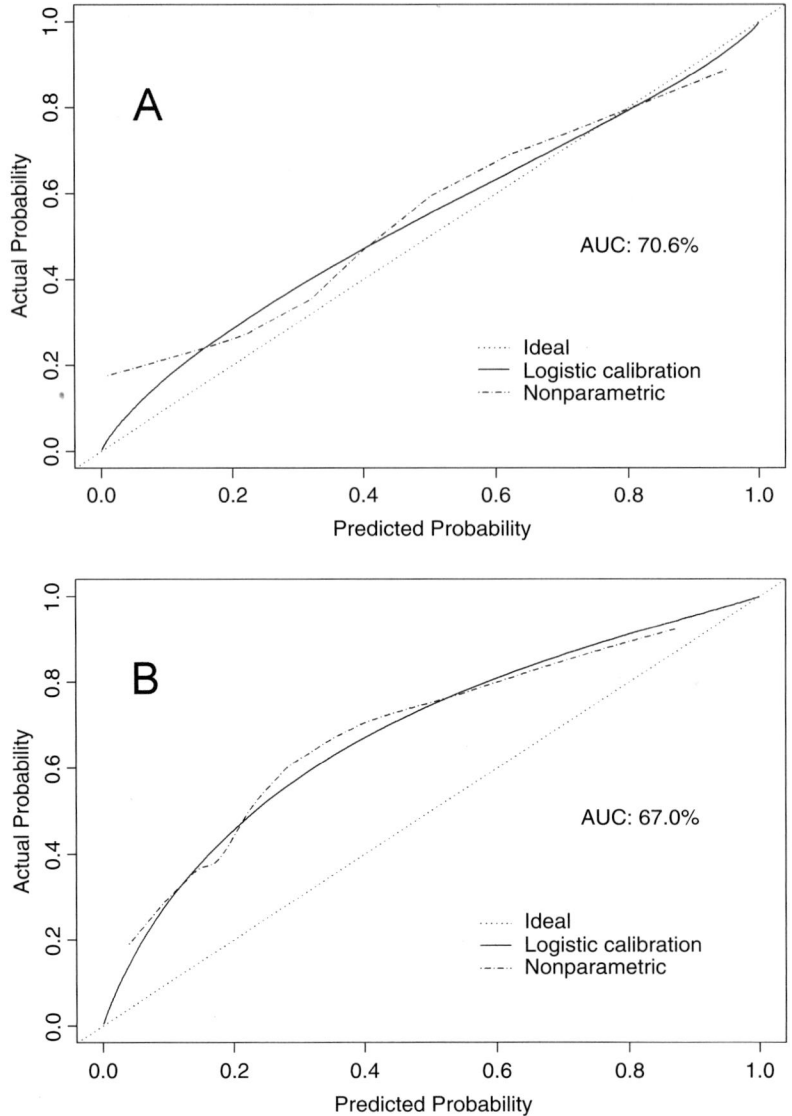

FIGURE 8.3. Local regression nonparametric smoothing plots that demonstrate performance of external validations of a previously published initial biopsy nomogram1 **(A)** and of a previously published artificial neural network5 **(B)** to predict initial biopsy outcome. **A**: External validation (n = 4093) of the previously published four variables [age, digital rectal examination (DRE), prostate-specific antigen (PSA), and percent free PSA (%fPSA)] sextant nomogram1 for prediction of prostate cancer in men exposed to initial biopsy, in which the x-axis represents predicted probability and the y-axis represents observed fraction with evidence of prostate cancer. **B**: External validation (n = 4093) of the previously published artificial neural network5 (age, DRE, PSA, %fPSA, prostate volume) for prediction of prostate cancer in men exposed to initial biopsy in which the x-axis represents predicted probability and the y-axis represents observed fraction with evidence of prostate cancer. Perfect predictions correspond to the 45° line. Points estimated below the 45° line correspond to nomogram overprediction, whereas points situated above the 45° line correspond to nomogram underprediction.

paralleled the ideal 45° prediction line. Conversely, the neural network demonstrated important departures from ideal predictions (Figure 8.3B), which were manifested by severe underestimation throughout the range of predicted probabilities. The most important departures were recorded for predicted probabilities between 20% and 80%.

Taken together, our comparison demonstrated that neural networks do not exceed the ability of logistic regression models to predict the outcome of interest. Moreover, we have shown that the performance characteristics of the nomogram, which consist of a comparison between predicted and observed rate of PCa on needle biopsy, were far superior to the neural network. This example of a head-to-head comparison between a nomogram and a neural network shows that nomograms seem to be more accurate and are associated with better performance characteristics. This directly contradicts several urologic publications, in which the accuracy of neural networks was substantially higher than that of nomograms. Moreover, this example illustrates some of the concerns that experts in prognostics have voiced about the true predictive ability of neural networks.[29]

Our findings and their interpretation are not meant to suggest that the neural network methodology should be abandoned. Instead, they indicate the need for methodologically sound application and critical appraisal of this approach.[30]

Concerns with Current Neural Network Applications

Several important problems have been identified with the methodology of contributions addressing neural network models. The potential for the emergence of these problems has been signaled as early as 1977, when statistical packages, such as SPSS, SAS, and others became widely available for nonspecialists.[31] Despite these early warnings, a recent review of existing neural networks for prediction and diagnostic classification in oncology found numerous crucial methodologic mistakes in 43 identified articles.[32] These were summarized as: 1. biased and/or inefficient estimation, 2. overfitting and fitting of implausible functions, 3. incorrect or missing description of the complexity of the network, 4. use of inadequate statistical competitors or insufficient statistical comparisons, and 5. naive and inappropriate application to survival data.

1. Mistakes in the estimation of predictive accuracy represent without doubt the most dangerous flaw of many neural networks in oncology. These relate to inappropriate use of data sets to estimate the predictive ability of these models. For example, most reports divide the data sets into learning and validation sets. Such methodology is appropriate when the accuracy of a regression model is tested. Neural networks behave differently.

Therefore, validation sets demonstrate excessively optimistic predicted accuracy, relative to regression models. The degree of optimism has been estimated at between 9% and 13%.[32] Thus, a model may be reported to predict accurately 90% of the time, whereas in reality only 80% of predictions are correct.

Appropriate assessment of predictive accuracy requires the use of test sets. These can be derived from the original cohort. However, such approach results in fewer observations that can be used for learning and validation. Alternatively, cross-validation techniques can be used, in which the test set is generated from a randomly drawn proportion of the population. Another test set can then be randomly identified and the process may be repeated several times. Each time, the predictive accuracy of the neural network is determined. Once all repetitions have been completed, an average predictive accuracy is determined. This method is more sophisticated than simple splitting of the data set among learning, validation, and test sets. It allows testing of the unbiasedness of the model on substantially larger test sets, relative to when the cohort is split into three subsets. The most efficient validation may be provided by a computer-intensive resampling technique called bootstrapping.[18] This methodology replicates the process of test set generation from an underlying validation set by drawing samples with replacement from the original validation data set. Each sample is of the same size as the original validation set. Use of resampling maximizes the efficiency of predictive accuracy testing. Thus, instead of dividing the population among three subsets, only the learning and validation sets are required. Use of cross-validation or bootstrapping techniques may allow fewer instances of overfitting, in which neural network's learning sets rely on a few dozen observations and numerous input nodes. It is of note, that regression models do not require a test set. Instead, their validation may be achieved either using the split sample or cross-validation methodologies. Finally, resampling with replacement represents a frequently used and efficient validation approach of regression models.

2. Overfitting may undermine the validity of neural networks, which have the ability to closely reflect the underlying data. For example, neural networks, which are based on numerous hidden units, have a tendency to result in implausible functions to describe the relation between the input nodes and the output node. Such models may be associated with spuriously high accuracy, which may be difficult to confirm in a test set. Despite great ability to replicate the relations between input and output nodes, the neural networks, similar to regression models, do require between 5 and 10 observations for each parameter to be estimated. Thus, readers are cautioned about taking at face value the predictive ability of neural networks that bypass that key consideration.

3. Incorrect or incomplete description of the neural network represents a common limitation in the ability of the reader to independently assess the properties of the network at hand as well as those of the learning, valida-

tion, and testing steps. For example, it is not uncommon that multiple hidden layers are mentioned, without specifying how many.

4. Excessively optimistic performance of neural networks may be attributable to comparisons with inappropriate, insufficient, or inadequate statistical competitors. For example, neural networks are frequently compared with logistic regression models. Although we have demonstrated that logistic regression models can favorably outcompete neural networks, this is not invariably the case. The advantage of neural networks is their complexity relative to straightforward regression models, which rely on linear relations between predictors and the outcome of interest. To provide comparable conditions, regression models should be fitted with multiple interaction terms and with cubic as well as quadratic predictor terms. Such methodology would result in comparable ability of the predictors to interact with one another in a nonlinear manner, as in neural networks.

5. The above methodologic problems are compounded by inappropriate applications of neural networks. For example, the statistical assumptions governing neural networks generally do not allow the use of censored data. Thus, neural networks are not amenable to modeling of survival data. Many investigators have attempted to circumvent this methodologic limitation by ignoring censored cases, omitting censored cases, imputing censored cases, or finally by using time to event data as an additional input. All these approaches are methodologically flawed and are known to result in biased estimate of the outcome of interest.

Finally, neural networks have been popularized in the medical literature by overinflated praises, such as "ability to learn . . . makes them formidable tools in the fight against cancer,"[33] and "neural computation may be as beneficial to medicine and urology in the twenty-first century as molecular biology has been in the twentieth."[34] Despite these praises, neural networks have made little difference in the diagnosis or management of localized PCa, despite their introduction in the early 1990s.[35] Besides severely limited availability, practical considerations related to the misuses of neural network methodology have without doubt contributed to the observed marginal use of these tools in clinical practice.

Conclusion

Prediction of several PCa-related outcomes can be achieved with nomograms, look-up tables, or neural networks. Whereas look-up tables represent a simplification of logistic regression, nomograms and neural networks represent two distinct methodologic approaches toward prediction of clinical outcomes. Nomograms offer several advantages. They allow users to understand the underlying effect of risk factors on the outcome of interest. Their predictive accuracy and performance characteristics can be easily tested and graphically displayed. Finally, their accuracy and performance characteristics tend to be at least as good as those of neural networks. These properties have resulted in the use of nomograms in clinical practice across several continents.[36,37] Conversely, neural networks are less popular. Despite numerous methodologic flaws in existing neural network models, this approach represents a valid alternative to nomograms, providing that its methodology is used with equal scrutiny to that used in nomogram applications.

References

1. Karakiewicz PI, Benayoun S, Kattan MW, et al. Development and validation of a nomogram predicting the outcome of prostate biopsy based on patient age, digital rectal examination and serum prostate specific antigen. J Urol 2005;173(6):1930–4.
2. Svatek R, Karakiewicz PI, Shulman M, Karam J, Perrotte P, Benaim E. Pretreatment nomogram for disease-specific survival of patients with chemotherapy-naive androgen independent prostate cancer. Eur Urol 2006;49(4): 666–74.
3. Djavan B, Remzi M, Zlotta A, Seitz C, Snow P, Marberger M. Novel artificial neural network for early detection of prostate cancer. J Clin Oncol 2002;20(4):921–9.
4. Remzi M, Anagnostou T, Ravery V, Zlotta A, Stephan C, Marberger M, Djavan B. An artificial neural network to predict the outcome of repeat prostate biopsies. Urology 2003;62(3):456–60.
5. Stephan C, Cammann H, Semjonow A, et al. Multicenter evaluation of an artificial neural network to increase the prostate cancer detection rate and reduce unnecessary biopsies. Clin Chem 2002;48(8):1279–87.
6. Matsui Y, Utsunomiya N, Ichioka K, et al. The use of artificial neural network analysis to improve the predictive accuracy of prostate biopsy in the Japanese population. Jpn J Clin Oncol 2004;34(10):602–7.
7. Babaian RJ, Fritsche H, Ayala A, et al. Performance of a neural network in detecting prostate cancer in the prostate-specific antigen reflex range of 2.5 to 4.0 ng/mL. Urology 2000;56(6):1000–6.
8. Porter CR, Gamito EJ, Crawford ED, et al. Model to predict prostate biopsy outcome in large screening population with independent validation in referral setting. Urology 2005;65(5):937–41.
9. Poulakis V, Witzsch U, de Vries R, et al. Preoperative neural network using combined magnetic resonance imaging variables, prostate specific antigen, and Gleason score to predict prostate cancer recurrence after radical prostatectomy. Eur Urol 2004;46(5):571–8.
10. Poulakis V, Witzsch U, De Vries R, et al. Preoperative neural network using combined magnetic resonance imaging variables, prostate specific antigen and Gleason score to predict prostate cancer stage. J Urol 2004;172(4 Pt 1): 1306–10.
11. Han M, Snow PB, Epstein JI, et al. A neural network predicts progression for men with Gleason score 3 + 4 versus 4 + 3 tumors after radical prostatectomy. Urology 2000;56(6):994–9.

12. Partin AW, Kattan MW, Subong EN, et al. Combination of prostate-specific antigen, clinical stage, and Gleason score to predict pathological stage of localized prostate cancer. A multi-institutional update. JAMA 1997;277(18): 1445–51.

13. Finne P, Auvinen A, Aro J, et al. Estimation of prostate cancer risk on the basis of total and free prostate-specific antigen, prostate volume and digital rectal examination. Eur Urol 2002;41(6):619–26.

14. Steuber T, Graefen M, Haese A, et al. Validation of a nomogram for prediction of side specific extracapsular extension at radical prostatectomy. J Urol 2006; 175(3 Pt 1):939–44.

15. Specht MC, Kattan MW, Gonen M, Fey J, Van Zee KJ. Predicting nonsentinel node status after positive sentinel lymph biopsy for breast cancer: clinicians versus nomogram. Ann Surg Oncol 2005;12(8):654–9.

16. Chun FK, Steuber T, Erbersdobler A, et al. Development and Internal validation of a nomogram predicting the probability of prostate cancer Gleason sum upgrading between biopsy and radical prostatectomy pathology. Eur Urol 2006;49(5):820–6.

17. Bradley E, Tibshirani RJ. Monographs on Statistics and Applied Probability: An Introduction to the Bootstrap. Boca Raton: Chapman & Hall/CRC; 1993:275.

18. Steyerberg EW, Harrell FE Jr, Borsboom GJ, Eijkemans MJ, Vergouwe Y, Habbema JD. Internal validation of predictive models: efficiency of some procedures for logistic regression analysis. J Clin Epidemiol 2001;54(8):774–81.

19. Katz EM, Kattan MW. How to judge a tumor marker. Natl Clin Pract Oncol 2005;2:482–3.

20. Kattan MW. Statistical prediction models, artificial neural networks, and the sophism "I am a patient, not a statistic." J Clin Oncol 2002;20(4):885–7.

21. Eastham JA, May R, Robertson JL, Sartor O, Kattan MW. Development of a nomogram that predicts the probability of a positive prostate biopsy in men with an abnormal digital rectal examination and a prostate-specific antigen between 0 and 4 ng/mL. Urology 1999;54:709.

22. Garzotto M, Hudson RG, Peters L, et al. Predictive modeling for the presence of prostate carcinoma using clinical, laboratory, and ultrasound parameters in patients with prostate specific antigen levels ≤10 ng/mL. Cancer 2003;98:1417.

23. Moul JW, Snow PB, Fernandez EB, Maher PD, Sesterhenn IA. Neural network analysis of quantitative histological factors to predict pathological stage in clinical stage I nonseminomatous testicular cancer. J Urol 1995;153:1674–7.

24. Truong H, Morimoto R, Walts AE, Erler B, Marchevsky A. Neural networks as an aid in the diagnosis of lymphocyte-rich effusions. Anal Quant Cytol Histol 1995;17:48–54.

25. Karakiewicz PI, Bazinet M, Aprikian AG, et al. Outcome of sextant biopsy according to gland volume. Urology 1997;49(1):55–9.

26. Uzzo RG, Wei JT, Waldbaum RS, Perlmutter AP, Byrne JC, Vaughan ED Jr. The influence of prostate size on cancer detection. Urology 1995;46(6):831–6.

27. Eskicorapci SY, Guliyev F, Akdogan B, Dogan HS, Ergen A, Ozen H. Individualization of the biopsy protocol according to the prostate gland volume for prostate cancer detection. J Urol 2005;173(5):1536–40.

28. Schwarzer G, Schumacher M. Artificial neural networks for diagnosis and prognosis in prostate cancer. Semin Urol Oncol 2002;20(2):89–95.

29. Freedland SJ, Isaacs WB, Platz EA, et al. Prostate size and risk of high-grade, advanced prostate cancer and biochemical progression after radical prostatectomy: a search database study. J Clin Oncol 2005;23(30):7546–54.
30. Sargent DJ. Comparison of artificial neural networks with other statistical approaches: results from medical data sets. Cancer 2001;91:1636–42.
31. Lachenbruch PA. Some misuses of discriminant analysis. Methods Inf Med 1977;16(4):255–8.
32. Schwarzer G, Vach W, Schumacher M. On the misuses of artificial neural networks for prognostic and diagnostic classification in oncology. Stat Med 2000;19(4):541–61.
33. Burke HB. Artificial neural networks for cancer research: outcome prediction. Semin Surg Oncol 1994;10(1):73–9.
34. Niederberger CS. This month in Investigative Urology. Commentary on the use of neural networks in clinical urology. J Urol 1995;153(5):1362.
35. Snow PB, Smith DS, Catalona WJ. Artificial neural networks in the diagnosis and prognosis of prostate cancer: a pilot study. J Urol 1994;152(5 Pt 2):1923–6.
36. Graefen M, Karakiewicz PI, Cagiannos I, et al. International validation of a preoperative nomogram for prostate cancer recurrence after radical prostatectomy. J Clin Oncol 2002;20(15):3206–12.
37. Graefen M, Karakiewicz PI, Cagiannos I, et al. Validation study of the accuracy of a postoperative nomogram for recurrence after radical prostatectomy for localized prostate cancer. J Clin Oncol 2002;20(4):951–6.

9
Preparation for Prostate Biopsy

Alan M. Nieder and Mark S. Soloway

Abstract

Although a very routine procedure, transrectal ultrasound biopsy lacks accepted guidelines for technique and patient preparation. This chapter explains the preparation protocol at the University of Miami, including the administration of prophylactic antibiotics, the lack of necessity for the use of enemas, and the need for obtaining a detailed consent describing the procedure and possible complications. All patients undergoing transrectal ultrasound biopsy receive periprostatic lidocaine injection to minimize discomfort during the procedure.

Keywords: prostate biopsy, antibiotics, enema, patient preparation

It is estimated that more than 230,000 American men will be diagnosed with prostate cancer in 2007.[1] Transrectal ultrasound-guided biopsy of the prostate (TRUS-Bx) is the most common method for diagnosing prostate cancer and has been frequently performed by urologists since the 1970s. Although a relatively safe procedure, significant complications such as sepsis can occur.[2,3] More common side effects such as hematuria and hematospermia are nearly universal. Rodriguez and Terris[4] prospectively recorded all complications related to TRUS-Bx in 128 patients. Moderate to severe hematuria and rectal bleeding occurred in 71% and 8%, respectively. Chills, fever, and dysuria were reported in 3%, 2%, and 9%, respectively. Although TRUS-Bx is one of the most frequent procedures performed in the outpatient setting, there are few guidelines addressing the performance of the biopsy, including the preparation of the patient, the use of anesthetic agents, and the number of biopsy cores. Furthermore, despite the proven efficacy of periprostatic local lidocaine to reduce pain during

From: *Current Clinical Urology: Prostate Biopsy: Indications, Techniques, and Complications*
Edited by J.S. Jones © Humana Press, Totowa, NJ

TRUS-Bx,[5,6] many do not use this to minimize the patient's discomfort during the procedure.

Practice Patterns

Although the American Urological Association has created guidelines for the management of a variety of urologic conditions, such as benign prostatic hyperplasia, staghorn calculi, and priapism,[7–9] no guidelines have been created for the technique and patient preparation related to TRUS-Bx. Shandera et al.[10] surveyed 900 practicing United States urologists and reported a wide discordance among prostate biopsy preparation. Eighty-one percent of the survey respondents asked their patients to have an enema before biopsy. Although nearly all urologists (98.6%) provided their patients with antibiotics, there was no consensus regarding a specific antibiotic or dose. Furthermore, the cost of the various antibiotic preparations (in 1998) ranged from $8.79 to $160.54, with a mean of $27.06. Davis et al.[11] published similar results of a survey of urologists in 2002. Seventy-nine percent of survey respondents requested that their patients have an enema before biopsy, although there was a discordance regarding the timing of the enema. Ninety-nine percent of urologists prescribed their patients with an antibiotic, usually an oral fluoroquinolone.

Use of Antibiotics

Despite the fact that nearly all patients receive prophylactic antibiotics before TRUS-Bx, Enlund and Varenhorst[12] prospectively evaluated 426 men undergoing prostate biopsy without antibiotic prophylaxis. Patients who absolutely required antibiotics [i.e., those with a history of recurrent urinary tract infections (UTIs) or cardiac valvular disease] were excluded. The only preparation consisted of an enema which patients received 1 hour before the biopsy. A questionnaire regarding any complications was completed by 97.4% of patients. Twelve patients (2.9%) reported fever; three required hospitalization. The authors concluded that routine antibiotic prophylaxis is unwarranted in most patients if an enema is used.

Conversely, two prospective, placebo-controlled studies have compared prophylactic antibiotics with placebo and reported significantly less infections in those who received prophylaxis. Aron et al.[13] performed a prospective, placebo-controlled, randomized study evaluating 231 patients who underwent prostate biopsy. Patients were randomized to placebo, a single dose of ciprofloxacin 500 mg and tinidazole 600 mg (for anaerobic coverage), or ciprofloxacin 500 mg and tinidazole 600 mg twice daily for 3 days. All patients received an enema. The incidence of infectious complications was significantly greater in the placebo group than the antibiotic groups: 25.3%, 7.6%, and 10.4%, respectively. The authors concluded that a single dose of an antibiotic provides adequate prophylaxis and continuing the prophylaxis for 3 days provides no further benefit. Kapoor et al.[14] similarly performed a prospective, double-blind, placebo-controlled, randomized, multicenter trial comparing single-dose ciprofloxacin 500 mg with placebo in 537 men. All patients received an enema before biopsy. Follow-up urinalysis and urine cultures at 9–15 days after the biopsy were used as the primary determinant. Of the 457 patients available for analysis, there was a significant increased risk of bacteriuria in the placebo group compared with the antibiotic group—8% and 3%, respectively. Furthermore, whereas no patient in the antibiotic group required hospitalization, four in the placebo group developed urosepsis. In an economic analysis, the authors demonstrated that despite the cost of the antibiotic, there was an overall cost savings for antibiotic use.

Most urologists use and believe in prophylactic antibiotics and investigators have thus sought to evaluate the most effective and necessary number of antibiotic doses. Aus et al.[15] performed a prospective, randomized study evaluating twice-daily norfloxacin 400 mg for either 1 day or 1 week in 491 patients who underwent prostate biopsy. Patients were recommended to use an enema before biopsy. For those patients at increased risk of UTI (e.g., indwelling catheter, a history of UTI, diabetes, or prostatitis), 1 week of antibiotics significantly decreased the risk of UTI from 17.9% to 3.3%. The authors concluded that for low-risk patients, a single day of antibiotics is adequate; however, for those at risk of UTI, 1 week of prophylaxis is preferable.

Griffith et al.[16] also agreed that for low-risk patients, a single dose of an oral fluoroquinolone was adequate prophylaxis. These authors performed a prospective study evaluating the risk of UTI after prostate biopsy in men receiving a single dose of Levaquin 500 mg. All patients received a single dose 30–60 minutes before biopsy. Importantly, no patient received an enema before biopsy. If the patients were at increased risk for infectious complications (i.e., diabetics, prostates larger than 75 cc, recent steroid use, severe lower urinary tract symptoms, or immune compromised), they then received two subsequent doses of Levaquin. Only 1 of 377 (0.27%) low-risk patients developed a symptomatic UTI. None of the 23 patients at increased risk experienced a complication. The authors concluded that a single dose of Levaquin 500 mg was adequate prophylaxis for low-risk patients undergoing prostate biopsy. Shandera et al.[17] performed a similar prospective study evaluating the risk of UTI in 150 men undergoing prostate biopsy who received an enema and a single dose of ofloxacin 300 mg 1 hour before biopsy. Only one patient (0.67%) developed a UTI, and the authors thus concluded that a single dose of an oral fluoroquinolone combined with an enema is adequate and effective prophylaxis before prostate biopsy.

At the University of Miami, we typically prophylaxis all patients with a 3-day regimen of an oral fluoroquinolone and we do not ask our patients to perform an enema the morning prior. Although a single dose is likely adequate for most patients, we believe that the extra doses allow us to safely biopsy those patients who may be at increased risk for complications, such as those with larger glands, diabetics, and those with significant voiding symptoms. We have found this 3-day regimen to be efficacious as well as simple for improved patient compliance. For those who have had a recent, documented episode of a urinary tract infection, we typically ensure a negative urinalysis or culture before biopsy.

Use of Antibiotics in Patients at Risk for Endocarditis

Patients at increased risk for endocarditis after invasive procedures require prophylactic antibiotics before TRUS-Bx because the genitourinary tract is second only to the oral cavity as a portal of entry for organisms that cause endocarditis. Although most cases of postbiopsy bacteremia are caused by gram-negative bacilli, it is the gram-positive bacilli (e.g., enterococcus) that are the most likely culprit in cases of endocarditis.[18,19] High-risk patients are those with prosthetic heart valves, a history of endocarditis, complex cyanotic congenital heart defects, and surgically constructed pulmonary shunts.[18,20] Moderate-risk patients include those with mitral valve prolapse with regurgitation, acquired valvular disease (e.g., rheumatic fever), and those with cardiomyopathy and other congenital malformations.

The American Heart Association recommends that prophylaxis for patients at increased risk of endocarditis includes coverage for both gram-positive and gram-negative bacilli. Patients should be given gentamicin and either ampicillin or amoxicillin 1 hour before TRUS-Bx.[18,20,21] Patients with penicillin allergies should be given vancomycin instead of ampicillin or amoxicillin. Patients at high risk should be given a second dose of oral amoxicillin 6 hours after biopsy.

Use of Enemas

Many urologists empirically prescribe an enema to their patients before TRUS-Bx in an attempt to reduce the bacteria level in the rectum.[10] Carey and Korman[22] retrospectively reviewed 410 patients who underwent prostate biopsy and compared those who received enemas with those who did not. Patients had received the enemas based on their treating physician's protocol: one physician provided his patients with enemas and two did not. All patients received ciprofloxacin 500 mg twice daily for 3 days starting the evening before the biopsy. There was no significant difference in clinical complications between those who received enemas and those who did not: 4.4% versus 3.2%, respectively. The authors concluded that enemas do not provide a clinically significant improvement in outcome and are therefore unnecessary.

Jeon et al.[23] also published a retrospective review of 879 prostate biopsies and compared those who received bisacodyl suppositories with those who did not. Patients also received levofloxacin or a third-generation cephalo-sporin (cefixime) for a total of 7 days. Decision to give rectal preparation was determined by individual physician choice. Complications were recorded at follow-up within 2 weeks. Infectious complications occurred significantly less frequently in those patients who received an enema com-pared with those who did not: 1.3% versus 9.5%, respectively. The authors also found that an increased number of biopsy cores were a significant risk factor for infectious complications. The authors acknowledged that their results are discordant with the findings of Carey and Korman; however, they comment that this discordance may be related to the fact that both studies were retrospective and prevalence bias may have existed.

Lindert et al.[19] performed a prospective, randomized study evaluating 50 men undergoing prostate biopsy. Twenty-five men received an enema and 25 did not. Furthermore, all patients had prebiopsy urine culture and post-biopsy blood and urine cultures. As a departure from the authors' normal protocol, all patients received ciprofloxacin 500 mg and metronidazole 500 mg only *after* the biopsy and cultures were performed. All patients received a repeat dose of an antibiotic the evening of the biopsy. Seven (25%) of the patients who did not receive an enema had postbiopsy bacte-remia compared with only one (4%) patient who had an enema. However, only one patient with bacteremia developed a fever, which was treated with further oral ciprofloxacin. The authors concluded that enemas decrease the risk of bacteremia. Furthermore, despite recommending prebiopsy antibi-otics, the authors noted that postbiopsy antibiotics were effective in pre-venting any significant clinical complications of bacteremia. In a follow-up letter to the editor, Carey and Korman addressed Lindert et al.'s high rate of bacteremia subsequent to prostate biopsy and argued that the risk was increased because patients were not provided with appropriate prophylaxis *before* biopsy.[24] In a similarly designed follow-up study by the authors, Lai et al.[25] reported that uncircumcised men have a greater risk of postbiopsy bacteremia compared with circumcised men. Based on these studies, at the University of Miami, we do not ask our patients to use an enema before TRUS-Bx.

Consent for Prostate Biopsy

Before performing a prostate biopsy, the physician and the nurse discuss the risks of the biopsy with the patient. We specifically discuss the risks of hematuria, urinary retention, infection, rectal bleeding, and hematosper-mia. We provide the patient with a detailed consent form specifically addressing these risks (Appendix I). It is the policy of the University of Miami that all patients sign the consent form and a copy is filed in the chart. Whereas many practices may simply discuss the risks and benefits of the procedure with the patient, we believe that a signed consent is more appropriate. We also provide the patient with a detailed postbiopsy instruction form (Appendix II).

Conclusion

Although a very routine procedure, there is no general consensus or guidelines regarding the preparation for patients undergoing TRUS-Bx. Further prospective, randomized, multicenter trials will provide physicians with the optimal protocol for their patients. At the University of Miami, our protocol is as below:

- No enemas are required.
- No cardiac monitoring is typically required.
- All low-risk patients receive a single dose of an oral fluoroquinolone antibiotic 1 hour before biopsy. Patients are instructed to take additional doses on the following 2 days.
- Patients at high risk for endocarditis receive oral amoxicillin and intramuscular gentamicin 1 hour before biopsy and a second oral dose of amoxicillin the evening of the biopsy.
- All patients sign a detailed consent form describing the procedure and possible complications. Patients also receive a form describing typical postbiopsy signs and symptoms and are instructed to call the office immediately if there are any problems.
- All patients receive a periprostatic lidocaine injection.[6]

References

1. Jemal A, Siegel R, Ward E, Murray T, Xu J, Thun MJ. Cancer statistics, 2007. CA Cancer J Clin 2007;57:43–66.
2. Raaijmakers R, Kirkels WJ, Roobol MJ, Wildhagen MF, Schrder FH. Complication rates and risk factors of 5802 transrectal ultrasound-guided sextant biopsies of the prostate within a population-based screening program. Urology 2002;60:826–30.
3. Borer A, Gilad J, Sikuler E, Riesenberg K, Schlaeffer F, Buskila D: Fatal *Clostridium sordellii* ischio-rectal abscess with septicaemia complicating ultrasound-guided transrectal prostate biopsy. J Infect 1999;38:128–9.
4. Rodriguez LV, Terris MK. Risks and complications of transrectal ultrasound guided prostate needle biopsy: a prospective study and review of the literature. J Urol 1998;160:2115–20.
5. Soloway MS. Do unto others—why I would want anesthesia for my prostate biopsy. Urology 2003;62:973–5.
6. Alavi AS, Soloway MS, Vaidya A, Lynne CM, Gheiler EL. Local anesthesia for ultrasound guided prostate biopsy: a prospective randomized trial comparing 2 methods. J Urol 2001;166:1343–5.
7. Montague DK, Jarow J, Broderick GA, et al. American Urological Association guideline on the management of priapism. J Urol 2003;170:1318–24.

8. Preminger GM, Assimos DG, Lingeman JE, Nakada SY, Pearle MS, Wolf JS Jr. Chapter 1: AUA guideline on management of staghorn calculi: diagnosis and treatment recommendations. J Urol 2005;173:1991–2000.
9. AUA guideline on management of benign prostatic hyperplasia (2003). Chapter 1: Diagnosis and treatment recommendations. J Urol 2003;170:530–47.
10. Shandera KC, Thibault GP, Deshon GE Jr. Variability in patient preparation for prostate biopsy among American urologists. Urology 1998;52:644–6.
11. Davis M, Sofer M, Kim SS, Soloway MS. The procedure of transrectal ultrasound guided biopsy of the prostate: a survey of patient preparation and biopsy technique. J Urol 2002;167:566–70.
12. Enlund AL, Varenhorst E. Morbidity of ultrasound-guided transrectal core biopsy of the prostate without prophylactic antibiotic therapy. A prospective study in 415 cases. Br J Urol 1997;79:777–80.
13. Aron M, Rajeev TP, Gupta NP. Antibiotic prophylaxis for transrectal needle biopsy of the prostate: a randomized controlled study. BJU Int 2000;85:682–5.
14. Kapoor DA, Klimberg IW, Malek GH, et al. Single-dose oral ciprofloxacin versus placebo for prophylaxis during transrectal prostate biopsy. Urology 1998;52:552–8.
15. Aus G, Ahlgren G, Bergdahl S, Hugosson J. Infection after transrectal core biopsies of the prostate—risk factors and antibiotic prophylaxis. Br J Urol 1996;77:851–5.
16. Griffith BC, Morey AF, Ali-Khan MM, Canby-Hagino E, Foley JP, Rozanski TA. Single dose levofloxacin prophylaxis for prostate biopsy in patients at low risk. J Urol 2002;168:1021–3.
17. Shandera KC, Thibault GP, Deshon GE Jr. Efficacy of one dose fluoroquinolone before prostate biopsy. Urology 1998;52:641–3.
18. Dajani AS, Taubert KA, Wilson W, et al. Prevention of bacterial endocarditis. Recommendations by the American Heart Association. JAMA 1997;277:1794–801.
19. Lindert KA, Kabalin JN, Terris MK. Bacteremia and bacteriuria after transrectal ultrasound guided prostate biopsy. J Urol 2000;164:76–80.
20. Steckelberg JM, Wilson WR. Risk factors for infective endocarditis. Infect Dis Clin North Am 1993;7:9–19.
21. Leport C, Horstkotte D, Burckhardt D. Antibiotic prophylaxis for infective endocarditis from an international group of experts towards a European consensus. Group of Experts of the International Society for Chemotherapy. Eur Heart J 1995;16(Suppl B):126–31.
22. Carey JM, Korman HJ. Transrectal ultrasound guided biopsy of the prostate. Do enemas decrease clinically significant complications? J Urol 2001;166:82–5.
23. Jeon SS, Woo SH, Hyun JH, Choi HY, Chai SE. Bisacodyl rectal preparation can decrease infectious complications of transrectal ultrasound-guided prostate biopsy. Urology 2003;62:461–6.
24. Terris MK. Re: Transrectal ultrasound guided biopsy of the prostate. Do enemas decrease clinically significant complications? J Urol 2002;167:2145–6; author reply 2146.
25. Lai FC, Kennedy WA 2nd, Lindert KA, Terris MK. Effect of circumcision on prostatic bacterial colonization and subsequent bacterial seeding following transrectal ultrasound-guided prostate biopsies. Tech Urol 2001;7:305–9.

Appendix I: Prostate Biopsy Consent Form

Your physician has determined that you may have an abnormality of the prostate gland that requires a biopsy. A needle biopsy of the prostate is a procedure in which the physician inserts a special needle through the rectal wall into the prostate and cuts off a small sample of tissue, which is analyzed. This procedure is not a treatment for any disease but rather a more complete examination to assist your physician in formulating a diagnosis and treatment plan specific to your needs.

Although complications from this procedure are very uncommon, they do occasionally occur. No guarantee can be made as to the results that might be obtained from this procedure. Some of the complications that do occur occasionally include rectal or urinary bleeding and infection. Very rarely, an allergic or other adverse reaction occurs to one of the antibiotics or anesthetic agents used during the procedure, and a prolonged illness or permanent deformity could result.

There may be alternatives to this procedure available to you such as other types of diagnostic tests; however, these alternative methods have their own risks of complications and have a varying degree of success. Therefore, in those patients for whom the needle biopsy of the prostate is indicated, the procedure may provide the patient with best chance of successful diagnosis and treatment and the lowest risk of complications.

I certify that I have read or have had read to me the contents of this form and I understand the risks and alternatives associated with this procedure. I hereby authorize the physician named above who is a member of the University of Miami Department of Urology to perform the procedure described herein. I have been given the opportunity to ask questions about this procedure and all of my questions have been answered.

Appendix II: Instructions after a Prostate Biopsy

The procedure of transrectal ultrasound guided prostate biopsy is one that allows us to accurately guide a specially designed needle into the prostate and obtain tissue to determine whether there is an area of cancer or inflammation in the prostate gland. In addition, the procedure allows us to measure the size of your prostate.

After the biopsy, if you have fever or chills, it is important for you to call us immediately. It is very common to have small amounts of blood or blood clots in the urine and in the bowel movements after the procedure. It is unlikely that this bleeding would be sufficient to cause significant blood loss or obstruct the flow of urine. If you are concerned, however, please call us. It is not uncommon to have blood in the ejaculate (semen) for several days or weeks after the biopsy. You may resume your usual activities after the procedure.

10
Principles of Prostate Ultrasound

Martha K. Terris

Abstract

Although most urologists use transrectal ultrasound imaging of the prostate predominantly as a tool to accurately direct biopsies, identification of prostatic abnormalities on sonographic images can be critical in some patients.[1] To accurately decipher the pathology conveyed in the areas of shadow and brightness displayed in ultrasound images, an understanding of the physical principles generating these images is essential.[2]

Keywords: ultrasound, hypoechoic, imaging

Basic Concepts

Ultrasound is defined as sound with a frequency too high for the human ear to hear.[3,4] Frequency, or the number of sound waves per second, is measured in hertz (Hz). Sound with a frequency over 20 kilohertz (kHz) is outside human hearing range. Transrectal prostate ultrasound is generally performed at very high frequencies of 5–10 megahertz (mHz). By comparison, adult renal imaging is performed at frequencies of 2–3 mHz.

Wavelength is the distance between the onset of one sound wave to the next. In general, as wavelength increases, frequency decreases. The relationship of the wavelength to the frequency defines the velocity. Velocity

From: *Current Clinical Urology: Prostate Biopsy: Indications, Techniques, and Complications*
Edited by J.S. Jones © Humana Press, Totowa, NJ

is the speed at which sound waves travel through a particular medium or tissue, and is equal to the frequency multiplied by the wavelength. This becomes clinically important when interpreting ultrasound because velocity depends upon the medium through which the ultrasound wave is traveling. The velocity through human soft tissues is approximately 1540 meters per second, very similar to the velocity through water. The change in velocity when ultrasound waves encounter air, bone, and other structures accounts for many of the artifacts and landmarks encountered during ultrasound imaging. For example, air has a velocity of 330 meters per second, dramatically lower than soft tissue. Therefore, when air is present between the ultrasound probe and the tissue of interest, the image can be distorted or completely obscured. For this reason, a water-density substance, termed a coupling medium, is used for transmission of the ultrasound waves across the space between the transducer and the body surface, where air pockets frequently occur. This coupling medium is usually a sonographic jelly or lubricant and should be placed between the probe and the rectal surface as well as between the probe and any protective sheaths covering the probe.

Acoustic impedance refers to how resistant a particular structure is to penetration by sound waves.[3,4] As sound waves progress through tissues with varying impedence characteristics, they decrease in amplitude, a process called attenuation. Higher frequencies are attenuated by tissue more than lower frequencies. A key component of successful ultrasound imaging is accurately establishing settings on the ultrasound console to amplify attenuated echoes. This process of amplification is known as time-gain compensation. The goal is increasing amplification of more distant sound waves to generate a uniform image rather than an image that is very bright near the transducer and rapidly becomes too dark to distinguish structures progressively further from the transducer. The appropriate time-gain compensation varies with the location being studied, the organ of interest, the distance from the transducer to the area of interest, and the characteristics of the tissue between the transducer and the area of interest. Most ultrasound consoles with a capacity for transrectal prostate ultrasonography include factory-installed default settings for optimal time-gain compensation in prostate imaging.

Ultrasound Transmission

Ultrasound waves are generated by a transducer. The transducer contains the transmitting element, electrodes, and protective face. The transducer, focusing and steering mechanisms, scanning apparatus, and associated wiring for connection to the ultrasound console are housed in an ultrasound probe which is shaped for the desired application, such as cylindrical for transrectal ultrasonography. Some authors refer to the entire ultrasound probe as the transducer.

The transmitting element, also referred to as the pulser or crystal, is the component that creates the impulses sent to the transducer to generate sound energy. Transmitters were historically composed of crystals, such as quartz. These were replaced by ferro-electric ceramics. Currently, more durable and flexible piezoelectric polymer materials are being used.

The focus of the ultrasound delineates the area where the sound waves are most concentrated. In general, with increasing frequency of the ultrasound waves transmitted by the transducer, the focus becomes closer to the transducer. The location and size of the focus (the focal range) can be further optimized by focusing mechanisms within the ultrasound probe. These focusing mechanisms may be mechanical, annular, linear array, or electronic. Mechanical focusing is performed by placing an acoustic lens on the surface of the transducer or using a transducer with a concave face. With annular focusing, circular or ring-like elements are used to focus the beam. Rather than focusing a single transmitting element, linear array imaging uses a row of elements producing a broad beam. Electronic focusing also utilizes multiple elements; using a process called phased array, the multiple elements are fired sequentially to focus the beam. Most modern transrectal ultrasound probes use electronic, phased array focusing. Unlike mechanical, annular, and linear array probes that can emit ultrasound waves at a fixed frequency and have a fixed focal range, most electronic probes have dynamic, adjustable frequency and focal range.

Phased array transducers have the ability to be steered as well as focused. As with focusing, the beam is directed by sequentially stimulating certain groups of elements. For example, by alternately stimulating elements in two rows perpendicular to each other, some models allow one to display a transverse or longitudinal image of the prostate without moving the transrectal probe. Those probe models with more sophisticated electronics can display both transverse and longitudinal imaging simultaneously (known as bi-plane imaging). Some probe models using mechanical focusing of a single transducer, have a switch that will rotate the transducer at a right angle within the probe to provide both transverse and longitudinal imaging but simultaneous imaging in two planes is not possible. Annular probes are limited to transverse imaging whereas linear array and "side-fire" mechanically focused transducers provide only longitudinal images. The "end-fire" mechanically focused probes (currently more frequently used for transvaginal ultrasound) can produce both transverse and longitudinal images by manually rotating the probe 90° (clockwise, if the patient is in left lateral decubitus position to maintain transverse images in standard right/left orientation).

The scanning apparatus in the probe assures that the sound waves are distributed over adequate area for imaging. Sound waves are emitted from each transducer in a single, very narrow band. To produce a recognizable image in models with a single transducer, the transducer must be mechanically swept across the area of interest producing multiple bands that are combined to form an image. The system for moving the transducer is called a mechanical scanner. As the speed at which the scanner sweeps across the imaged area decreases, the resolution increases. Faster scanner speeds are necessary to detect motion. For example, very rapid scanner rates, at the expense of resolution, are necessary in echocardiography, in which detection of cardiac wall motion and valve characteristics during each heart beat are the goal of imaging. In contrast, the stationary prostate affords the luxury of high-resolution, slow scanner rates. Linear and electronic probes do not require scanners because the multiple transmitting elements generate numerous ultrasound bands that are combined to produce an image.

Electronic scanners allow creation of smaller probes as well as the capacity for bi-plane steering and dynamic focusing described above but are much more expensive than the mechanical and linear array scanners.

Generation of Images

The essential component of diagnostic ultrasound, however, is not the sound wave generated by the transducer, but the sound waves that reflect (or echo) back to the transducer after bouncing off of the tissue of interest.[3,4] In addition to the transmitting element, the transducer also contains a receiving element to detect returning sound waves. In general, transducers transmit sound only 1% of the scanning time and act as a receiver the other 99% of the time. Through a process called acoustic-electric conversion, the transducer transforms the sound energy into electrical energy which is processed by the computer in the ultrasound console to generate an image of minute white dots (pixels) corresponding to the returning signals, displayed on a black background to produce an image of assorted shades of gray on the monitor.

When the sound waves travel easily through uniform substances (water, oil, urine, etc.), no echoes are generated. The ultrasound image seen on the screen is, therefore, black; there are no echoes. When the sound waves encounter a tissue that reflects the sound, a wave is reflected back to the probe. The ultrasound image is white or gray depending on the intensity of the reflection. Unlike plain radiographs or computerized tomography scans, ultrasound does not detect tissue density. Rather, it detects sonotransmission (the passage or reflection of sound). Sonotransmission depends on 1) the angle of incidence of the sound wave to be reflected, and 2) the difference between the acoustic impedance values of adjacent tissues. If the difference is great, a large part of the sound will be reflected back. Tissues with high acoustic impedance such as bone, prostatic calcifications, or brachytherapy implants readily reflect echoes and, therefore, appear bright white on an ultrasound. Air, such as in the bowel, also readily reflects echoes. The edge of the bowel, therefore, appears white on an ultrasound. As a result, substances with widely differing densities (such as air and bone) may both appear bright white on an ultrasound. The range of gray shades generated lends this imaging technique the alternative label "gray-scale imaging" which distinguishes it from color Doppler ultrasonography.

The types of echoes that are converted to sonographic images are divided into two broad categories known as specular echoes and scattered echoes. Specular echoes originate from relatively large, regularly shaped objects with smooth surfaces such as the bladder and the outer capsule of the prostate. These echoes are relatively intense and angle dependent. Scattered echoes that originate from relatively small, weakly reflective, irregularly shaped objects are less angle dependent and less intense. The prostatic parenchyma generally reflects scattered echoes.

Resolution describes how well an imaging technique can distinguish two adjacent objects. In ultrasound imaging, resolution is related to the transducer frequency, the scanner rate, and the focusing mechanism. Two types of resolution are considered: lateral resolution and axial resolution. Lateral resolution is the ability to resolve objects side by side. Lateral resolution is proportionally affected by the frequency; the higher the frequency, the greater the lateral resolution. With higher frequency and higher resolution, however, there is a decrease in the ultrasound depth of penetration. Axial resolution is the ability to resolve objects that lie one above the other. Axial resolution is inversely proportional to the frequency of the transducer, depending on the size of the prostate. The higher the frequency, the lower the axial resolution is in the anterior aspect of large prostates. This state results from the rapid absorption of the ultrasound energy with lower penetration. Lower frequencies can be used to increase depth of penetration and image the anterior aspect of large prostates, but there will be a corresponding decrease in the resolution of the peripheral zone of the gland. The most common frequencies used for prostate imaging are 7–7.5 mHz which have optimal resolution approximately 0.5–4 cm from the surface of the transducer. For imaging larger prostates, lower-frequency transducers can be used; for example, a 4-mHz transducer will produce a focal range of approximately 2–6 mHz.

Normal Appearance

The peripheral zone comprises the posterior and caudal portion (the apex) of the gland, is palpable on digital rectal examination, and is the site of origin of the vast majority of prostate cancers.[5] The central zone is a small, cone-shaped zone at the cephalad aspect of the prostate (the base) surrounding the ejaculatory ducts; cancers arising from this zone are quite rare. The anatomic distinction between central and peripheral zones is not ordinarily visualized by ultrasound, with both zones normally demonstrating a homogeneous light- to medium-gray area occupying the posterior third of the prostate. The echogenicity of structures within the prostate gland is expressed relative to the normal medium-gray echogenicity of the peripheral zone (Figure 10.1). Structures exhibiting the same echogenicity as the normal peripheral zone and central zone are termed isoechoic. Structures brighter than this point of reference are termed hyperechoic whereas darker

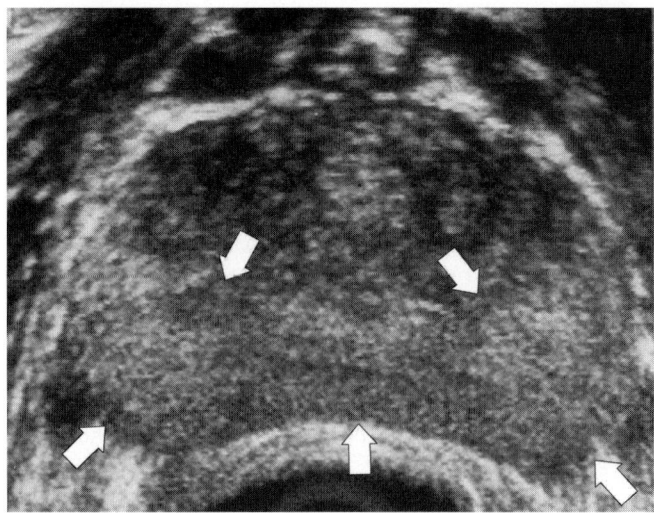

FIGURE 10.1. Transverse ultrasound image of a normal prostate with the medium-gray peripheral zone delineated by arrows.

areas are termed hypoechoic. Areas that sonographically appear completely black are referred to as anechoic.

The transition zone, located anteriorly, on either side of the urethra can exhibit wide variability in size depending on the degree of benign prostatic hyperplasia (BPH), which arises primarily from this zone. Relative to the peripheral zone, the anteriorly located transition zone exhibits moderately heterogeneous hypoechogenicity (Figure 10.2). Hyperplastic nodules in the transition zone can be isoechoic or hyperechoic but are most often hypoechoic. This heterogeneity and hypoechogenicity becomes progressively more prominent with increasing volume of benign hyperplasia and is most likely attributable to variations in the amount of stromal and glandular elements comprising the hyperplasia. With increased size of the transition zone, the peripheral and central zones become progressively more compressed.

The boundary between the transition zone and peripheral is often sharply demarcated on ultrasound images as a hypoechoic convex line. With increasing BPH, this boundary becomes less convex. This margin is often peppered with corpora amylacea, which are markedly hyperechoic; when more calcified and concentrated, these deposits can totally interrupt the ultrasound waves causing posterior shadowing obscuring some or all of the transition zone. The bladder neck and periurethral tissue comprising the preprostatic sphincter are located between the two lobes of the transition zone and demonstrate the dramatic hypoechogenicity typical of muscle because of the concentration of smooth muscle fibers. On transverse images,

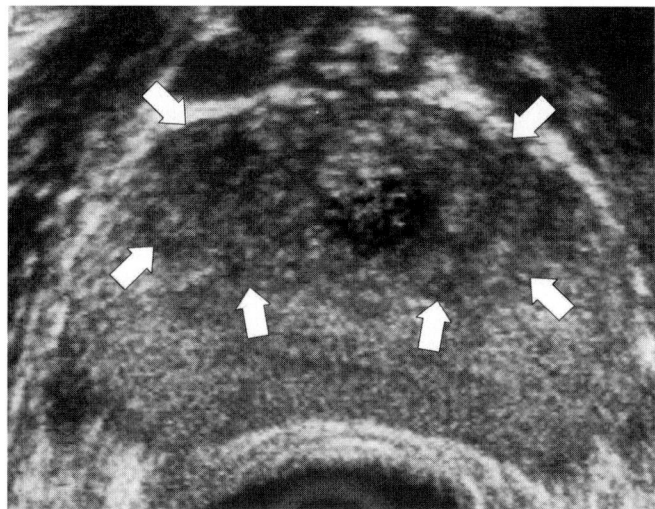

FIGURE 10.2. Transverse ultrasound image of a normal prostate with the hypoechoic transition zone delineated by arrows.

these muscles form an inverted "Y" on either side of the verumontanum, creating an anatomic landmark termed the Eiffel Tower sign (Figure 10.3). The lumen of the prostatic urethra is not visible sonographically unless it has been surgically altered, such as with transurethral resection, or it is distended during sonography. For example, distending the urethra with a urethral catheter is frequently performed during ultrasonography for

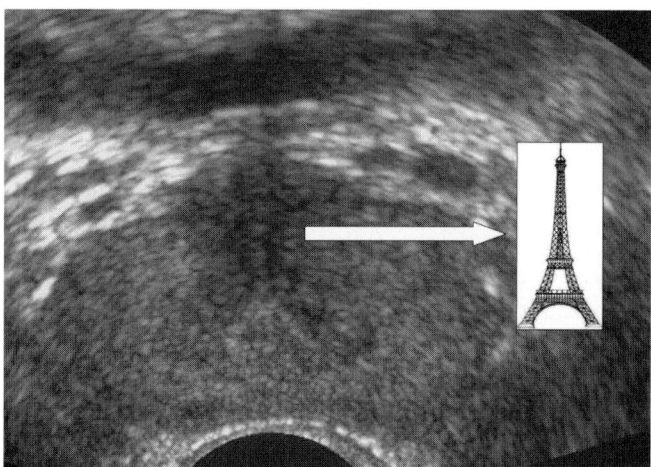

FIGURE 10.3. Transverse ultrasound image of the normal prostate at the level of the verumontanum. The periurethral muscle fibers diverge on either side of the verumontanum in a configuration some authors find reminiscent of the Eiffel Tower.

brachytherapy in order to avoid seed placement near the urethra. Distal to the prostatic apex, the periurethral tissue appears as a hypoechoic inverted horseshoe in the transverse plane. In the sagittal plane, this structure appears tubular and can be followed along its course to the external sphincter and proximal bulbar urethra.

The pubic bone demonstrates a hyperechoic margin with dramatic posterior shadowing. The inner margins of the pubic bone can be recognized and compared with the outer margins of the prostate during evaluation for pubic arch interference during prostate brachytherapy.

The thick muscular wall and fluid-filled lumens of the seminal vesicles, vas deferens, and ejaculatory ducts lend these structures a dark-gray echo pattern. Anterior to the seminal vesicles, the muscular bladder wall is dark gray and of variable thickness. Urine within the bladder is anechoic and can aid in delineating the anterior extent of the prostate and the presence of any median lobe.

Because of their predominantly adipose composition, the periprostatic tissues are generally quite echogenic, appearing almost entirely white on ultrasound images. The posterolateral aspect of the prostate margin where the neurovascular structures enter the gland are generally dark gray with areas that are completely anechoic because of the fluid-filled thin-walled veins. With the patient in left lateral decubitus position, the dependent left neurovascular bundle is often more prominent than the right. The anteromedial venous structure of the dorsal vein complex can also be seen as anechoic, somewhat linear structures within the white periprostatic adipose. Because the scanner rate for prostate sonography is slow, flow in these vascular structures is often not readily apparent. Extending toward the rectum from the dramatic anterior shadowing of the pubic bone, just lateral and distal to the prostate apex, is the levator musculature. This muscle has a distinctive hypoechoic appearance with hyperechoic parallel streaks representing the adipose-containing fascia separating the muscle bundles.

Ultrasonography of Prostatic Malignancy

Peripheral zone prostatic adenocarcinomas are typically considered to demonstrate hypoechogenicity on prostate ultrasound.[5,6] Indeed, an estimated 50%–70% of palpable prostate nodules are hypoechoic. However, few nonpalpable peripheral zone cancers show any abnormal echo patterns. The proportion of newly diagnosed tumors characterized by palpable lesions and/or hypoechogenicity has decreased progressively with the stage migration of prostate cancer. Transition zone malignancies are even more frequently isoechoic than peripheral zone cancers. A small number of transition zone tumors will actually demonstrate hyperechogenicity. The elusive nature of prostatic malignancies on ultrasound imaging has stimulated the development of various extended biopsy schemes.

Appearance after Treatment

External irradiation results in a significant decrease in the calculated volume of the prostate by 6 months after radiotherapy. The rate and degree of reduction correlates significantly with the histologic grade of the tumor (poorly differentiated tumors shrinking most rapidly) and the outcome of treatment but not with stage. The entire prostate is more diffusely hypoechoic and intraprostatic anatomy is poorly defined. There is often associated thickening of the rectal surface which displaces the prostate anteriorly. Larger hypoechoic cancer foci, particularly those that have not responded well to radiation therapy, will show little change in appearance once irradiated but smaller foci and those responding well to therapy tend to become isoechoic. In general, ultrasound findings are poorly correlated with pathologic findings in the irradiated prostate.[5–7]

After brachytherapy, the prostate exhibits many of the same long-term changes in volume and sonographic appearance as with external irradiation. Within the first few weeks after implantation, however, approximately one-third of patients will demonstrate an increase in prostate volume because of postimplant edema. No single parameter, including preimplant prostate volume, preimplant hormonal deprivation, or supplemental external beam radiation therapy, can accurately predict the degree of swelling. The most distinctive characteristic of postbrachytherapy prostate sonography is the appearance of numerous seeds distributed more or less evenly throughout the gland. These seeds are dramatically hyperechoic (Figure 10.4).

Androgen deprivation therapy results in a 30% decrease in prostate volume in patients with and without prostate cancer. The reduction in

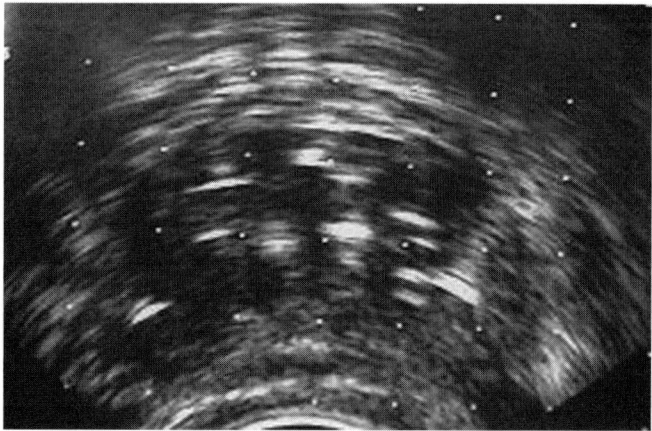

FIGURE 10.4. Transverse ultrasound image of the prostate after brachytherapy. Scattered hyperechoic brachytherapy seeds are readily apparent throughout the prostate.

volume is greatest in the quartile of men with the largest initial gland volume and least in men with smallest glands. The reduction in volume does not correlate with response of the cancer to therapy. After discontinuation of androgen deprivation, the prostate demonstrates gradual regrowth. Any hypoechoic lesions or sonographically apparent extraprostatic extension will progressively diminish in patients with a favorable biochemical response to hormone therapy.

Artifacts

As explained above, sonographic images are generated with the assumption that sound waves propagate through tissue at a constant velocity and reflect back in a narrow straight line. Because the velocity and angle of the ultrasound signal are affected by tissue density and changes in tissue density (abrupt versus gradual), such variations cause deviation of the signal, creating artifacts.[2,7]

Refraction, also called dispersion or scatter, is bending of sound waves in fan-like configuration resulting in a curving and elongation of the structure being imaged. A similar phenomenon can be demonstrated in observed light waves when an object partially submerged in water appears to bend. This is often manifest as an unnaturally curved appearance of the prostate on ultrasound images (Figure 10.5).

Posterior shadowing results from intense reflectors such as calcifications or air. When structures offer sufficiently high impedence that the ultra-

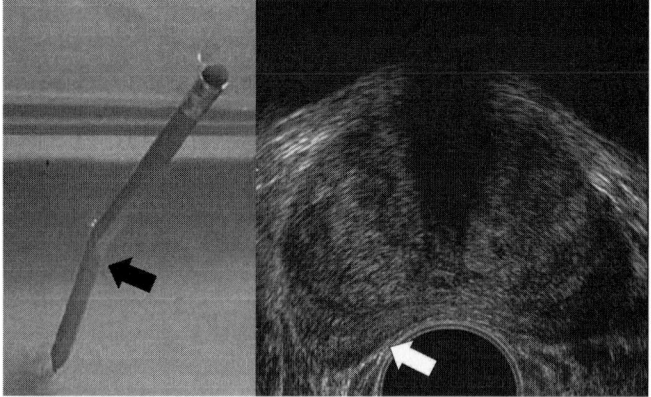

FIGURE 10.5. In the left image, refraction of light waves by the change in density from air to water cause the pencil to appear bent (arrow). In the right image, the posterolateral aspect of the prostate further from the transducer exhibits an artifactual curved appearance (arrow) because of refraction of sound waves.

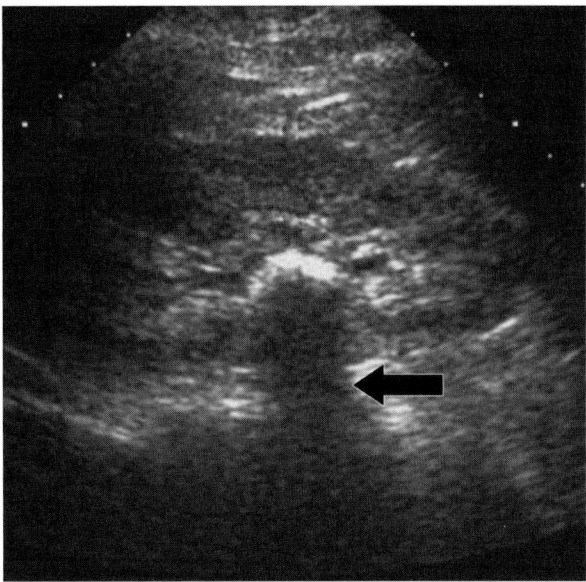

FIGURE 10.6. Although occasionally observed associated with calcifications in the prostate, the best demonstration of posterior shadowing is seen on renal ultrasound (oriented with transducer at the top of the image) imaging in patients with nephrolithiasis. The dense stone results in an intensely hyperechoic border and shadowing of all tissues posterior to the stone (arrow).

sound waves are completely interrupted, no sound waves can be transmitted to the structures on the opposite side of the echogenic structure from the transducer. A dark fan will be displayed on the opposite side of the intense reflector, obscuring any pathology located in that area (Figure 10.6). Note, the term "posterior shadowing" was coined for abdominal imaging and, although still used by convention, is inaccurate for transrectal prostate imaging. The shadowing resulting from echogenic structures encountered while imaging the prostate transrectally will actually be anterior.

Increased through-enhancement is exhibited with fluid-filled, sonolucent structures such as cysts and is manifest as hyperechogenicity posterior to the structure (Figure 10.7). Increased through-enhancement is caused by the ultrasound waves moving rapidly, without reflection, through the low-impedance cyst fluid, then abruptly striking the opposite wall of the cyst; the time-gain compensation and higher concentration of sound waves reaching the opposite wall of the cyst and the tissues beyond it will make these areas appear brighter than the surrounding tissues despite having similar sonotransmission characteristics.

Reverberation is an artifact caused by sound waves striking a very echogenic surface; this signal is ricocheted back and forth between the

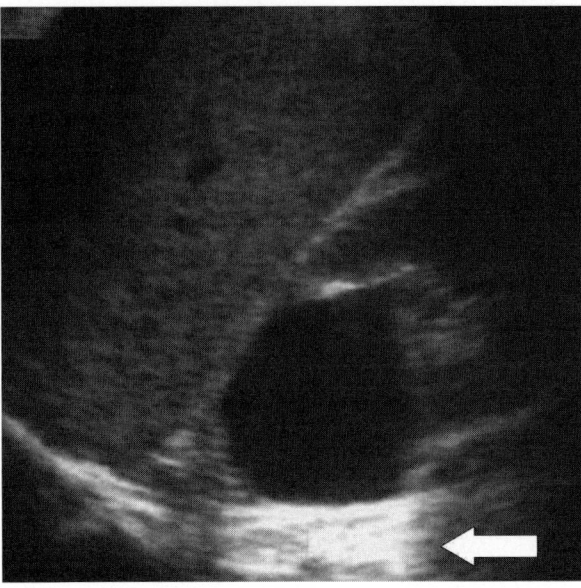

FIGURE 10.7. Cystic structures may occur in the transition zone in conjunction with benign prostatic hyperplasia. As seen in this renal ultrasound with a simple renal cyst, the tissues posterior to the cyst appear hyperechoic because of the unattenuated sound waves that passed through the cyst fluid away from the transducer at the top of the image.

transducer and the reflector. An image is accurately produced representing the echogenic structure but subsequent reflections of the signal, each taking twice as long as the prior signal to reach the transducer, are displayed as equally spaced images of the original reflector of decreasing intensity (Figure 10.8). In transrectal ultrasound imaging, the intense reflector is usually the rectal wall and results in multiple hyperechoic arches evenly spaced between the rectal wall and the anterior aspect of the image. This can be minimized by assuring that there is copious coupling medium and no air between the probe and the rectum.

Phase cancellation can occur when the signal tangentially strikes a curved structure reflecting it laterally rather than back toward the transducer. Also known as "edge" or "side-lobe" effect, this ultrasound phenomenon was capitalized upon in the production of Stealth aircraft which display acute angles rather than flat surfaces, causing phase cancellation of radar waves (Figure 10.9). The lack of signal returning to the transducer is misinterpreted as a lack of tissue and displays a black area on the image. In prostate ultrasonography, this artifact is often encountered during scanning of broad prostates. The sound waves striking the curved posterolateral margin of the prostate are scattered, resulting in a hypoechoic shadow extending from the edge of the prostate (Figure 10.10). Similar shadows may also be

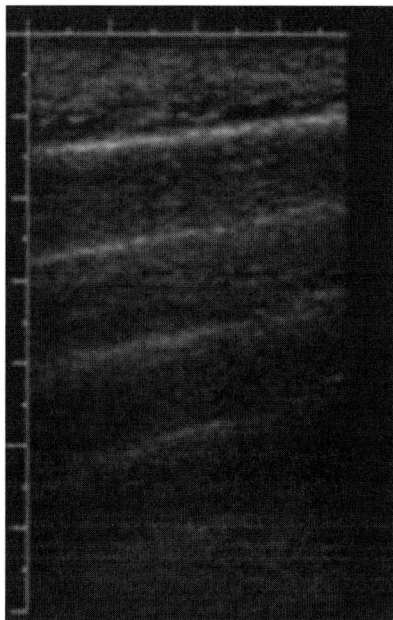

FIGURE 10.8. A hyperechoic line, evenly spaced with progressively decreasing intensity, with increasing distance away from the transducer at the top of the image, is characteristic of reverberation artifact. These lines can be distinguished from hyperechoic structures by their movement in concert with movement of the ultrasound transducer.

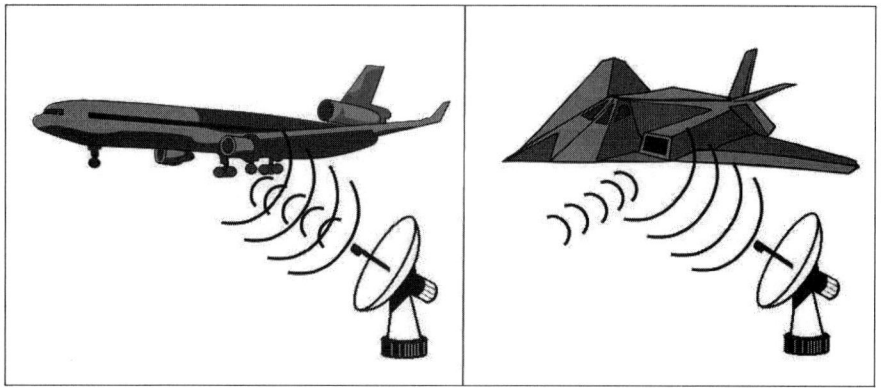

FIGURE 10.9. Sound waves used for radar detection of aircraft are easily reflected by standard construction planes (left). Phase cancellation, caused by the acute angles of stealth aircraft deflecting echoes away from the receiving unit, prevents detection (right).

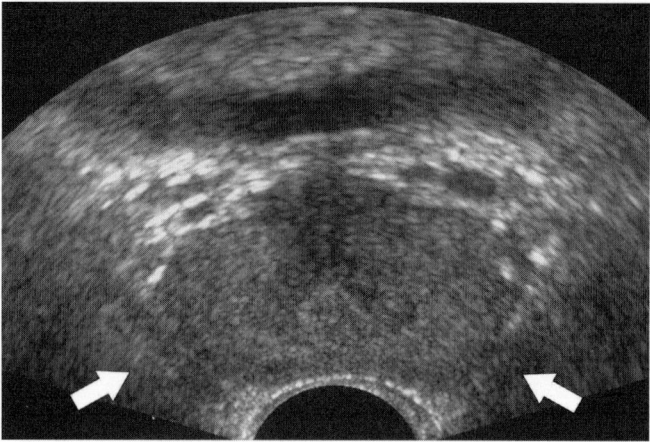

FIGURE 10.10. Transverse ultrasound image of the prostate in which the posterolateral edges of the prostate deflected the echoed ultrasound waves away from the transducer resulting in phase cancellation. On images, this appears as a dark band on either side of the gland (arrows).

generated by the posterolateral margin of the transition zone and even the posterolateral aspect of individual BPH nodules, resulting in multiple bands of shadowing fanning across the prostate producing an appearance that has been likened to a scallop shell (Figure 10.11). These shadows can be minimized by centering the probe under the lateral portions of the gland when inspecting this area.

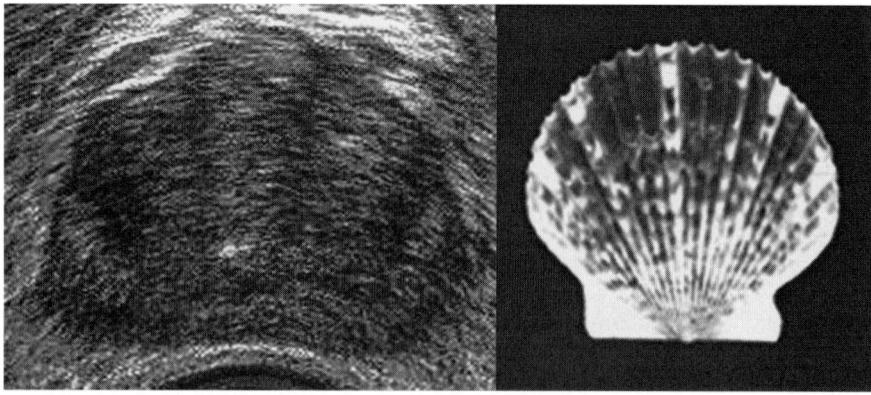

FIGURE 10.11. Transverse ultrasound image of a prostate with benign prostatic hyperplasia (left) causing multiple hypoechoic bands comparable to a scallop shell (right).

References

1. Amiel GE, Slawin KM. Newer modalities of ultrasound imaging and treatment of the prostate. Urol Clin North Am 2006;33(3):329–37.
2. Hulsmans FJ, Castelijns JA, Reeders JW, Tytgat GN. Review of artifacts associated with transrectal ultrasound: understanding, recognition, and prevention of misinterpretation. J Clin Ultrasound 1995;23:483–94.
3. Kossoff G. Basic physics and imaging characteristics of ultrasound. World J Surg 2000;24:134–42.
4. Kremkau FW. Diagnostic Ultrasound: Physical Principles and Exercises. 4th ed. Philadelphia: WB Saunders; 1993.
5. Peterson AC, Terris MK. Urologic imaging without X-rays: ultrasound, MRI, and nuclear medicine. eMedicine.com. 2006. Available at: http://www.eMedicine.com/med/topic.3373.htm.
6. Singer EA, Golijanin DJ, Davis RS, Dogra V. What's new in urologic ultrasound? Urol Clin North Am 2006;33(3):279–86.
7. Terris MK. Prostate ultrasonography. In: Walsh P, Partin, eds. Campbell's Urology. 8th ed. Philadelphia: WB Saunders; 2002:3038–3054.

11
Minimizing Pain and Optimizing Patient Experience During Prostate Biopsy

J. Stephen Jones

Abstract

Pain is not a necessary attribute of prostate biopsy. Respect for the patient's comfort, modesty, and well-being greatly improves his experience. Periprostatic lidocaine injection should be standard for the reduction of pain and discomfort. Lidocaine injection at the basilar "Mount Everest" notch is advocated because of the ease of administration as well as the short learning curve for the procedure. More-experienced surgeons may find injection at the apex more effective. Local anesthesia of the prostate and anus allows for better probe positioning crucial to obtaining diagnostic needle cores especially of the anterior horn region. New residents should be trained to respect the patient's concerns and administer periprostatic block to minimize the discomfort of transrectal ultrasound biopsy.

Keywords: periprostatic block, visual analog pain scores, rectal sensation test, Mount Everest sign

Until recently, almost all efforts at improving prostate biopsy revolved around increasing detection rates. It was assumed that the potential indignity and pain were worthwhile to achieve the goal of cancer detection, especially after transrectal biopsy became the norm.

Local anesthetic injection into the perineum was standard during the era of transperineal biopsy, but was abandoned when transrectal biopsy became possible under ultrasound guidance. Because the rectal mucosa was neither easily accessible to direct injection nor sensate above the dentate line, urologists readily accepted the idea that anesthesia was unnecessary.

It was not until 1996 that the first paper emphasized that transrectal biopsy is painful for most men. Investigators at the University of California

From: *Current Clinical Urology: Prostate Biopsy: Indications, Techniques, and Complications*
Edited by J.S. Jones © Humana Press, Totowa, NJ

San Francisco (UCSF), under the direction of senior author Dr. Katsuto Shinohara, injected lidocaine into the periprostatic nerves on one side and found that pain control was significantly better in the side injected with lidocaine compared with the side injected with saline.[1] Disappointingly, their landmark study had little impact on practice patterns as urologists chose to ignore this pain and to continue to do business as usual for the next few years.

Drs. Mark Soloway and Cän Obek confirmed the findings of the UCSF group in 2000, and encouraged urologists to heed the reality that pain was not a necessary evil accompaniment of biopsy.[2] Dr. Michael O. Koch, Chairman of Urology at Indiana University Medical Center, brought the concept to this author's attention. One case was all it took to become convinced that the previously ignored pain could rapidly, easily, and reproducibly be essentially eliminated by periprostatic block. We explored the concept through a randomized, prospective investigation that was such a success that it was closed before completing accrual. The results were overwhelming and statistically unequivocal, so the coinvestigators refused to further randomize patients to the control arm. The era of nonanesthetized prostate biopsy at the Cleveland Clinic had ended convincingly.[3]

Eliminating pain and other measures to improve patient experience are the topics of this chapter.

Improving Patient Experience Through Room Setup

A pleasant atmosphere can improve any patient experience, including transrectal ultrasound and prostate biopsy. This begins with the room setup. The procedure room layout should minimize the possibility that someone opening the door will be able to see the patient in a compromising position. Respect for modesty is medicolegally advisable and simply the right thing to do. Entrances ideally open in a manner that puts the door between someone entering and the patient until completely opened. Curtains in front of the door provide additional privacy, and undoubtedly make the patient feel less vulnerable. When possible, the examining table should be placed such that the patient in an exposed position is not left in a manner that private body areas are visible from the entry. Sheets to cover the legs allow the patient to feel some control over an embarrassing situation.

Finally, the traditional Spartan patient room is conducive to neither a relaxed patient nor a satisfied client. Patients go to the physician for medical expertise, but they should be able to assume high-level skills in the modern era. Thus, they have the right to expect to be treated as if the healthcare provider wants their patronage as well. Room temperature should accommodate the comfort of the partially clothed patient. Simple touches such as uncompromising cleanliness, comfortable chairs, and hooks for clothing enhance the atmosphere. We have found that décor as simple as freshly coated (paint or wallpaper) surfaces, unscuffed floors, and prints on the walls reduce anxiety and improve patient satisfaction scores. Although not strictly medical in nature, we believe these measures create a sense of value for the patient, and improve the doctor–patient relationship.[4]

Patient Positioning

Patient positioning on the examination table is influenced by the type of ultrasound probe to be used. There are two types of prostate ultrasound probes—side-fire and end-fire. Side-fire probes project laterally from the probe axis (Figure 11.1). For this reason, twisting the probe while keeping its axis neutral with respect to the sagittal plane enables lateral visualization (Figure 11.2). In contrast, end-fire probes project an imaging plane either directly or at a slight angle from the end of the probe (Figure 11.3) This requires that the probe handle be directed away from the side of interest in order to visualize the lateral areas, using the anus as a fulcrum to gain accurate placement (i.e., the handle is moved downward, toward the patient's dependent left side, in order to visualize the right side of the

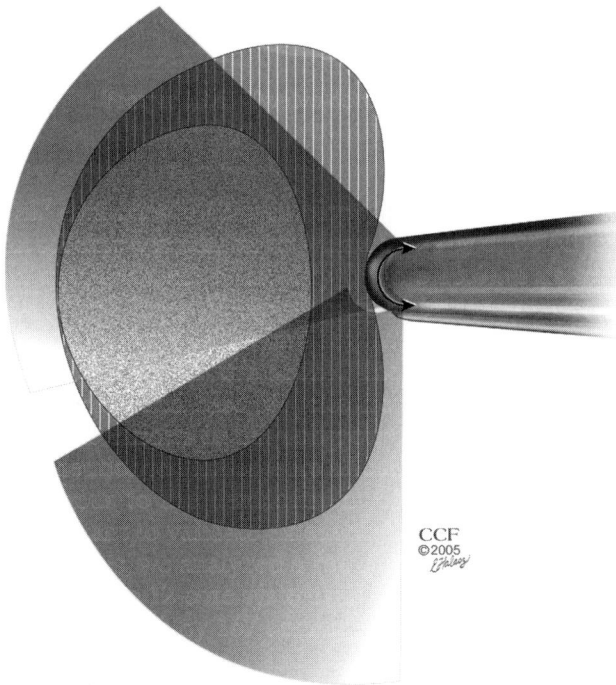

FIGURE 11.1. The side-fire probe projects its image at or nearly at a right angle to the probe in the transverse plane.

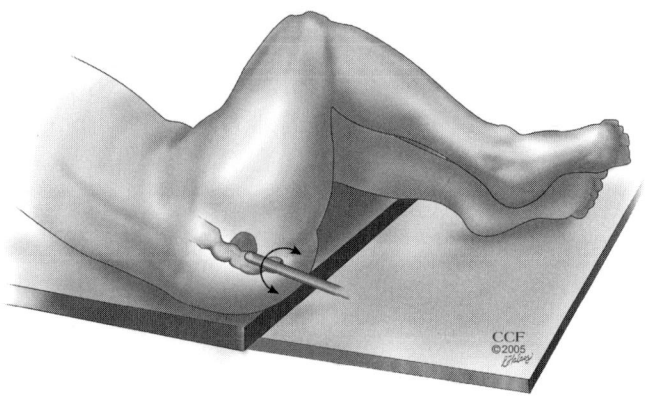

FIGURE 11.2. Because of its geometry, twisting the side-fire probe allows lateral visualization. Thus, the patient does have to be at the edge of the bed, although this position may still be more convenient for the urologist. Because twisting allows lateral visualization, the probe remains essentially in the same axis throughout the procedure.

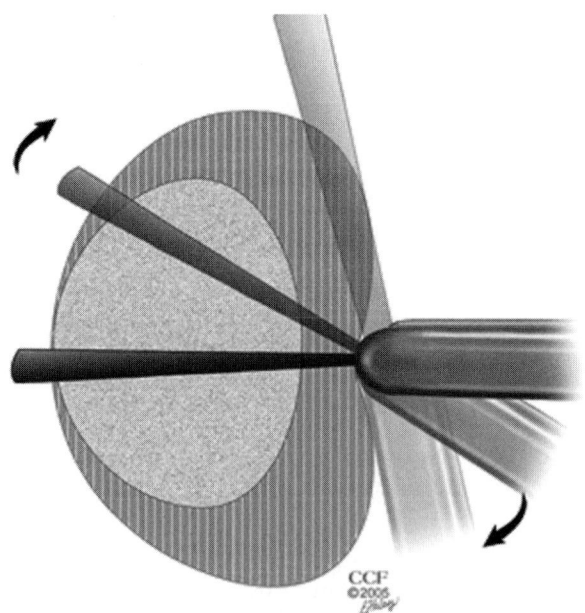

FIGURE 11.3. The end-fire probe projects almost directly off the tip of the probe. Thus, visualization of the lateral aspects of the prostate necessary for anesthetic injection and to biopsy the areas where cancer occurs most frequently are identified by moving the probe handle laterally away from the side of interest (handle toward floor for the right side, toward ceiling for left side).

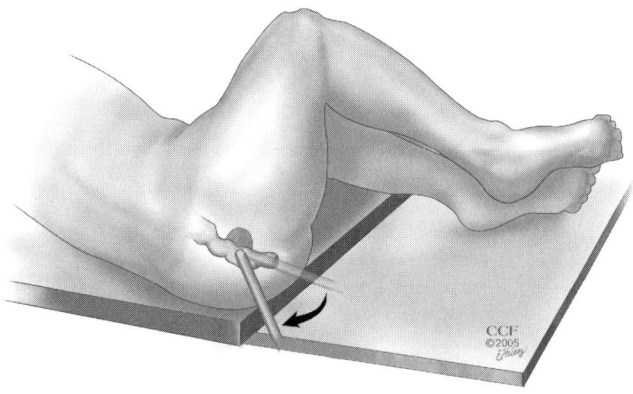

FIGURE 11.4. Moving the probe handle up and down to point toward the left or right side of the prostate maintains orientation with the end-fire probe and allows visualization of the lateral aspects of the prostate. This makes patient positioning on the examination table important, because if the patient is not all the way back to the edge of the table and with his buttocks at the corner at the location where the leg extension protrudes, the probe handle will hit the examination table when visualizing the right side of the prostate and preclude both anesthetic injection and adequate lateral biopsy.

prostate, and vice versa), as shown in Figure 11.4. Failure to recognize the impact of this geometry will create disorientation if one uses one type of probe in the manner that is appropriate for the other type.

Thus, a man undergoing prostatic ultrasound using a side-fire probe should have the probe remain essentially in the midline, twisting to reach the lateral aspects. This makes patient positioning relatively unimportant, as long as the anus is accessible. However, the man undergoing ultrasound using an end-fire probe must be positioned with his buttocks on the edge of the examination table to allow the ultrasound probe handle to be lowered far enough to reach beneath the plane of the examination table when visualizing the right lateral border of the prostate. This is most readily accomplished if his buttocks are directly over the corner of a table that has a leg extension (Figure 11.4). Pillows under the legs are usually helpful.

Limited visualization of the lateral aspects of the prostate using either style probe can result in two problems. First, periprostatic block as described below is performed laterally where the periprostatic nerves approach the prostate. As importantly, the lateral aspects of the peripheral zone are the areas most likely to harbor cancer, so limiting such access risks inadequate biopsy.

We find that lateral visualization is most readily achieved using an end-fire probe, although we routinely perform biopsies successfully using either style. Another advantage of the end-fire probe is that the needle exits its

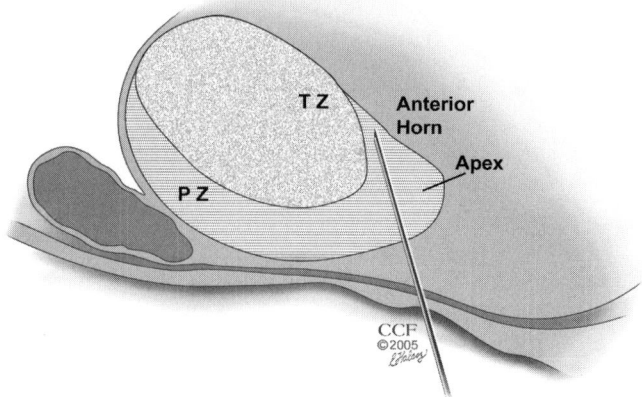

FIGURE 11.5. The apex is entirely composed of peripheral zone (PZ) tissue, where cancer is most likely to occur. Studies also demonstrate that this is the most likely area where cancer is overlooked by initial biopsy. TZ = transition zone.

guide in a trajectory more directly toward the prostate instead of tangentially. This allows easier biopsy of the apex and anterior horn of the peripheral zone (Figures 11.5 and 11.6), further minimizing the possibility of false-negative biopsy. This is likely to explain the potentially higher cancer detection rate when the end-fire probe is used.[5]

The final issue on positioning involves body orientation, which is more important when using the end-fire probe. Some patients wish to see the

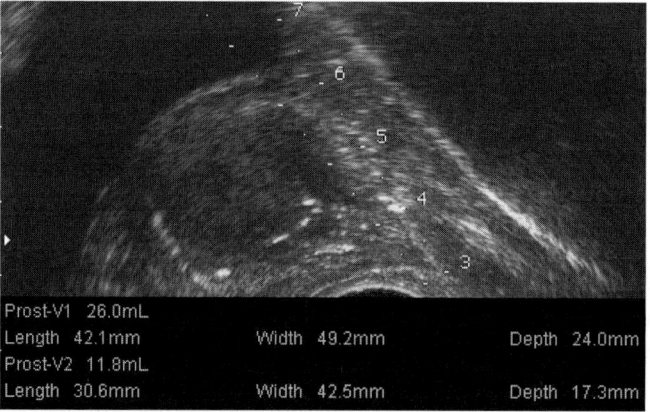

FIGURE 11.6. Ultrasound image demonstrates the same area as shown on Figure 11.5. Assuring the needle is placed in the isoechogenic peripheral zone tissue of the apex maximizes cancer detection. Transition zone can be readily identified as the darker, heterogeneous sphere cranial to the anterior horn (i.e., to the left of the biopsy needle).

examiner, so lean backward slightly. This makes it difficult to lower the probe far enough to visualize the right side. Similarly, leaning forward makes it difficult to raise the probe far enough to visualize the left side. Simply noting this axis allows the examiner to orient the patient in the right direction.

Optimizing Probe Placement

The pain of intrarectal probe placement has traditionally been an overlooked aspect of transrectal ultrasound. Most modern ultrasound probes are reasonably sized—some no larger than an examining finger—so size alone should not cause undue pain. However, biopsy guides and irregularly shaped ends create pain for many men, which is approximately one-third higher than the pain of biopsy—visual analog scale (VAS) 29 versus 20 in a recent review from our clinic.[6]

Lubrication for urologic instruments is vital. The value of anesthetic-based lubricants has not been demonstrated, but the role of lubrication to minimize the shearing forces of friction against rectal mucosa is undeniable. Respectful recognition of the embarrassing nature of the procedure can help relax the patient. Gentle finger dilation (followed by a change of examination glove) sometimes facilitates sphincter relaxation. Placement can be facilitated by asking the patient to breathe in and out slowly, or by asking him to bear down in a manner similar to having a bowel movement.

Probe placement should be controlled, applying light but slowly increasing pressure against the probe as its tapered end dilates the sphincter during entry. Holding the end of the probe between the thumb and forefinger allows greater range of motion than does a tight-fisted ("tennis racquet") grip and makes biopsy easier on the surgeon. The anus is usually oriented slightly off the axis of the spine, so the probe handle moves ventrally as it initially enters. Once through the sphincter, the probe is pulled toward the examiner in order to point the tip toward the prostate's position immediately behind the pubis. The anal canal may be oriented slightly in varying anatomic configurations. The probe can find the route of least resistance by altering its orientation slightly in each direction until it enters easily.

The physician should remain mindful of the topical anatomy throughout the procedure. Just as the laparoscopic surgeon observes the body during instrument entry and exit, the urologist or ultrasonographer should be observant that the probe should point in the direction of the rectal course during probe placement, and firmly against the prostate during imaging and biopsy.

Analgesia for the sphincter has been elusive because of the circuitous route of the inferior rectal nerve. It exits through Alcock's canal and divides into branches that pass beneath the levator ani, so injection of adequate amounts of local anesthetic would cause more pain than probe insertion. Topical analgesics and intrarectal diclofenac have been described, but their role remains undefined.

Evidence that Prostate Biopsy Is Painful

Although urologists for years thought little about the need for analgesia, patients had a different assessment. Initially, biopsies were only performed by taking a limited number of cores from a palpable nodule. The sextant biopsy technique became standard for most urologists in the 1990s.[7] Although wanting to believe that transrectal ultrasound was painless, most urologists stuck to the limit of six cores regardless of how large the gland was, based on a clear appreciation that few patients were willing to tolerate more sticks.

With the acceptance that at least 8 and up to 14 cores were optimal to minimize the chance of overlooking cancer, many patients voiced dissatis-faction. Whereas many urologists continued to state that prostate biopsy was painless, up to 96% of patients disagreed.[8] This author has long inter-preted the difference in patient and physician observation to mean that the perception of pain during prostate biopsy is largely dependent on which end of the needle one is on.

Most urologists have observed that it is much easier to convince a patient to have an initial biopsy than it is to convince him to undergo a repeat biopsy, and published reports suggest that up to one third of patients will refuse the recommendation for repeat biopsy because of this pain, despite concern that cancer is present.[9]

Prostatic Anesthesia Options

Before the description of periprostatic block, the only reliable way to elimi-nate the pain of prostate biopsy was to place the patient under general or regional anesthesia. Some centers, particularly in Europe, continue to do so, or to use systemic Entonox.[10] However, the cost, time, operating room resources, and paperwork required when doing so are rarely worthwhile. Moreover, employed patients must take off work, and must have a driver to do so as well. The only study to compare inhalational agents to peripros-tatic block found no advantage to the more complex systemic option.[11]

Issa et al.[12] reported pain control using intrarectal lidocaine, but subse-quent investigators[13,14] have found little benefit. In a prospective, random-ized, double-blind trial, Chang and associates[15] at Vanderbilt found no benefit to its use compared with placebo. The theory behind using intrar-ectal lidocaine seems flawed. Many medications are administered via the intrarectal route, but the mechanism of action involves absorption of the medication into the hemorrhoidal circulation. Thus, it is unlikely that the medication will cross through the rectal wall and into the periprostatic nerves. A 2005 review published in both *BJU International* and the *Journal of Urology* determined that, in seven of the eight comparative studies, intrarectal lidocaine was ineffective, or at least inferior to periprostatic block.[16,17]

As noted, intrarectal diclofenac has also been described, but results are indeterminate on its effectiveness. It offers little benefit as a single agent, but may help with postbiopsy pain if used in addition to periprostatic block. Further study will be needed to determine whether it has any role.[18] Intrarectal administration of 40% dimethyl sulfoxide for 10 minutes before biopsy has been advocated to control pain of probe insertion and biopsy, but has not been confirmed by other studies.[19]

These agents will potentially decrease pain sensation from *anal* sensory fibers, but these nerves do not exist in the *rectum* (above the dentate line in most patients), so are not involved in pain sensation at most of the biopsy sites (see below). We have found that an occasional patient can sense *rectal* mucosal pain apparently as a result of atypical sensation above the dentate line. Anecdotally, intrarectal lidocaine has allowed a more comfortable biopsy in these patients, which have been well less than 0.5% of cases. As a means to address the pain of both biopsy and probe insertion, Adsan et al.[20] injected the pudendal nerves, but the injection required a rectally placed finger for guidance, so its use seems limited.

Periprostatic injection of local anesthetic as described in the next section has found the most acceptance, and is supported by more than 50 peer-reviewed publications. The short-acting agent, lidocaine, is the subject of most, but we have also demonstrated that bupivacaine (Marcaine®) or a combination of bupivacaine and lidocaine is as effective as lidocaine alone, and onset of action is as rapid as in the lidocaine group.[21] Whether the longer duration of action of bupivacaine offers a benefit has not yet been demonstrated, although the combination has been reported to decrease the pain 1 hour after biopsy.[22] This agent may have a role in local anesthesia for more-involved prostatic procedures.

Periprostatic Block: Mount Everest Technique

All current periprostatic block techniques are based on that originally reported by Nash et al.[1] Our minimally modified preferred technique is described as follows:

1. The probe is adjusted to the sagittal plane with the onscreen biopsy guide operational before placement.

2. A 22-gauge, 7-inch spinal needle is placed through the biopsy guide channel under ultrasound guidance into the area where the prostatic inner-

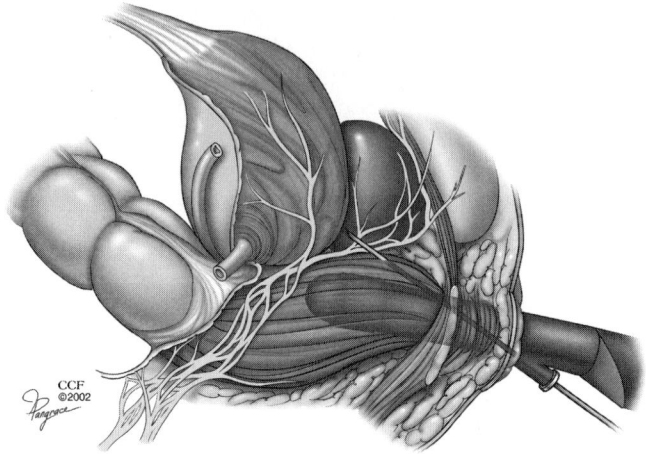

FIGURE 11.7. Injection at the base of the prostate or anywhere along the course of the periprostatic nerves will anesthetize the sensory input to the prostate. Their distribution is demonstrated.

vation enters the gland (Figure 11.7). Although this can be identified in a number of locations, we find the Mount Everest sign as described below to identify the easiest location to inject.

3. Our preferred technique based on simplicity and reproducibility involves injection of the nerve as it enters the prostate at its base. This is identified by angling laterally until the notch between prostate and seminal vesicle is visualized. The fat in this notch is present in 100% of patients, and creates what we describe as the "Mount Everest sign" based on its white, pyramidal appearance (Figure 11.8).[3] Plain lidocaine, 5 cc, is injected on each side.

4. Successful placement is confirmed by observing the injectate cause separation of the seminal vesicles and prostate from the rectal wall (the "ultrasonic wheal") as shown in Figure 11.9.

5. Getting the anesthetic into the proper plane is facilitated by injecting as the needle enters the space in order to expand its boundaries, and then pulling back slightly in order to open up the potential space until anesthetic is seen dissecting caudally (Figures 11.10–11.12). Note in the figures that the space between the rectal wall and prostate widens when this fluid dissects into this plane. This can be accomplished by injection at the base, midgland, or apex as described below.

6. Ultrasound examination and volume calculation are then performed per routine. There is no reason to delay biopsy because lidocaine has an onset of action that is essentially immediate.

Difficulty finding this "Mount Everest" notch immediately upon probe placement is usually either attributable to inadequate depth of probe

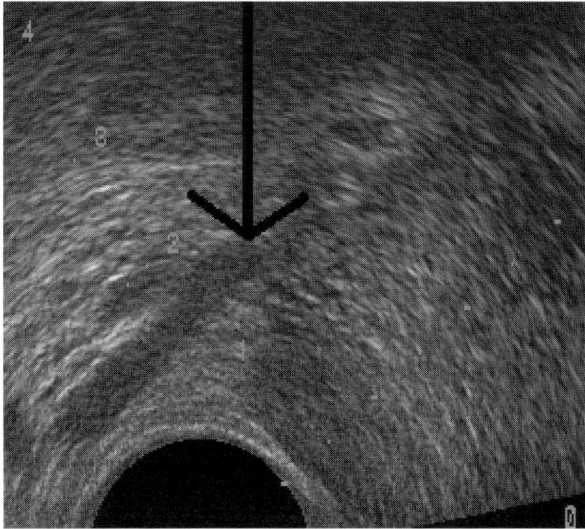

FIGURE 11.8. The Mount Everest sign is a hyperechoic area symbolizing the junction of the seminal vesicle and prostate as demonstrated by the arrow. This hyperechoic pyramid is identified on all patients in varying triangular formations.

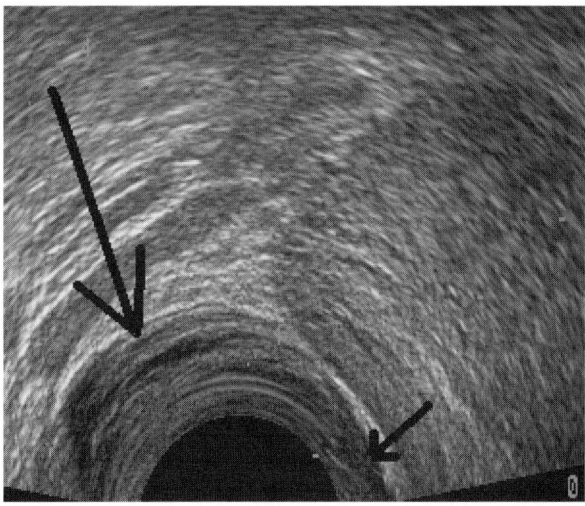

FIGURE 11.9. Injection of the lidocaine at the Mount Everest area of the same patient as shown in Figure 11.8 demonstrates the ultrasonic wheal. This is the hypoechoic fluid collection that is elevating the seminal vesicle away from prostate (large arrow). Lidocaine is seen dissecting along the periprostatic nerves toward the apex on the right side (small arrow).

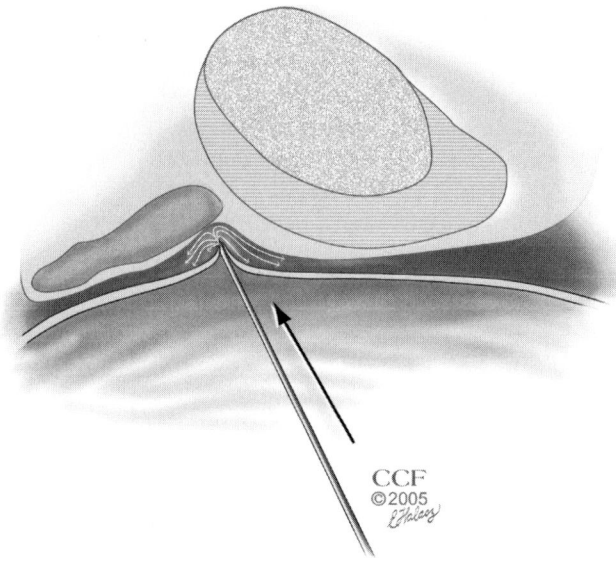

FIGURE 11.10. As the needle enters the Mount Everest space, it closes the space temporarily by dragging rectal wall ventrally; injection during placement helps avert this and expands the potential space.

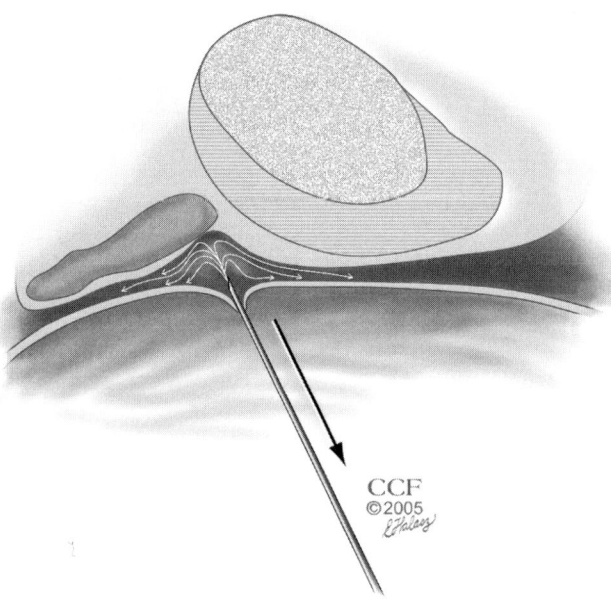

FIGURE 11.11. Continuing to inject as the needle pulls back into the proper plane, the space opens up as the needle drags rectal mucosa toward the probe.

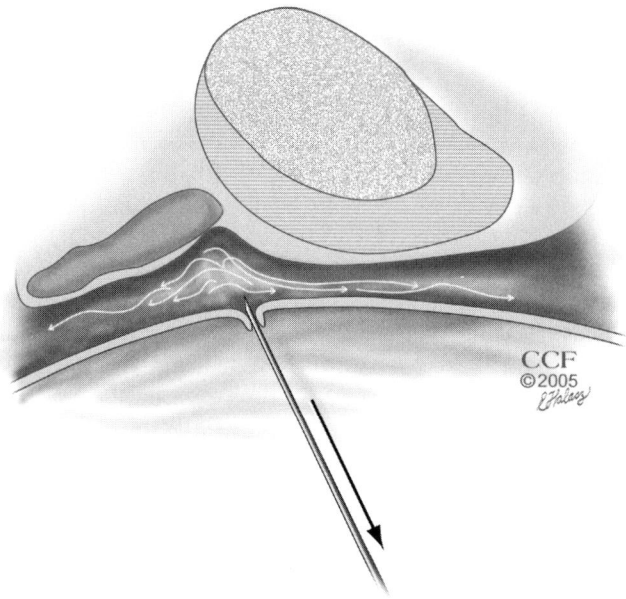

FIGURE 11.12. The proper plane is identified during pulling back on the needle when the anesthetic is seen dissecting along the length of the prostate. This ensures the entire periprostatic nerve is bathed in lidocaine and assures prostatic anesthesia; once this plane is reached, the needle remains in position until 5 cc of injectate is placed on each side.

placement (easily remediable) or inadequate visualization laterally, often because the novice is twisting the end-fire probe or angling the side-fire probe, which leads to loss of bearings and perspective for either as described above. We find that newcomers to the technique often do not place the probe deeply enough to easily position the biopsy guide into the large target area the Mount Everest sign affords. Additionally, failure to maintain direct contact of the probe against the rectal wall limits visualization, and also sacrifices the benefits of improved hemostasis through probe tamponade. Whenever disorientation or difficulty occurs, simply noting the topical anatomy and placing the probe firmly against the prostate usually clarifies the situation.

Results with Periprostatic Block

After the landmark report by Nash et al.[1], more than 50 published reports have demonstrated the effectiveness of periprostatic block. The single study failing to report an advantage involved injection at the tip of the seminal vesicle instead of periprostatic injection, explaining why this was the only study unable to find success.[23,24]

A prospective, randomized, controlled trial at our institution demonstrated a threefold difference in VAS pain scores using periprostatic block. VAS scores (10 denoting the worst pain ever experienced and 0 denoting no pain) for men who received a block were 1.4, compared with 4.5 in men who had biopsy without the benefit of local anesthetic ($p < 0.0001$). A majority of patients reported VAS scores in the moderate (28.6%) or severe (28.6%) ranges unless local anesthesia was administered. However, only 1 of 27 patients (3.7%) receiving local anesthetic reported moderate pain (VAS 4, which was less than the mean of the control group), and none reported severe pain. These findings are consistent with the consensus of the literature, where biopsy pain is typically between 4 and 5, and is notably consistent among studies.

A review published in two major journals assessed representative peer-reviewed publications reporting the impact of periprostatic block. Every periprostatic injection method described, regardless of injection site, was found to be effective at elimination of biopsy pain.[16,17] This accumulation of evidence leads to the inescapable conclusion that periprostatic block is the standard of care for prostate biopsy. The learning curve is short, and this author is unaware of a single urologist who has tried the technique and decided to discontinue its use. The step-by-step instructions above should preclude the need for formal training. The American Urological Association supports a course at its annual meeting each year for anyone desiring instruction as well.

Complications

No major complications have been attributed to periprostatic block. There is the potential that injection into the area of the periprostatic nerves could make nerve sparing more difficult during radical retropubic prostatectomy. This has not been observed in the only two published series to address the question,[3,25] or in more than 1000 patients operated on at our institution after periprostatic block. The lack of reports including this theoretic complication signifies it is not a significant concern.

There is a possibility that these additional injections through the rectal wall could add to infection or bleeding risk. This has not been our observation, nor has it been demonstrated in multiple reports. A single report showed an increase in bacteriuria when periprostatic block was placed (including two patients who developed clinical infections), but also showed less rectal bleeding in the periprostatic block group.[26] The authors attributed the increased bacteriuria to the additional two punctures through the rectal mucosa, and decreased rectal bleeding to the decreased discomfort of biopsy. It is feasible that additional injections are more likely to introduce bacteria than two additional biopsies because of the nature of injection versus noninjecting needle passes of a biopsy. Multiple other reports have shown no impact on either bleeding or pain, which is consistent with our findings in more than 3000 biopsies.

Alternative Injection Techniques

The optimal site of injection is a matter of debate. Alavi et al.[27] described the ultrasonic wheal as the visualization of anesthetic into the area of the periprostatic nerve bundle, and suggested that three separate injections on each side assured adequate anesthesia. However, we have determined that injection anywhere along the course of the periprostatic nerves is successful as discussed below; the ultrasonic wheal indicates complete nerve blockade regardless of where injection is performed as long as the injectate dissects along the course of the nerve.

The vast majority of reports describing successful periprostatic block have involved injection at the base of the prostate as described above. Occasionally, authors have described variations, such as injection near the apex on either side,[28,29] direct injection into the prostate,[30,31] pericapsular,[32] or a single injection of anesthetic into the midline at the level of the apex.[33] Our observation from performing all of these variations is that pain relief is reliable regardless of the location or number of injections if the agent dissects along the course of both periprostatic nerves. As long as this dissection is visualized, the nerves have received lidocaine and will be without pain sensory input. This is more difficult with a single injection in the apical midline, but the agent will still dissect to the necessary location bilaterally in the majority of cases. Similarly, injection on one side in either the Mount Everest basilar location or at the level of the lateral apex will exhibit dissection of agent all the way to the contralateral nerve bundle in many cases. We have anecdotally noted this dissection crossing the midline to the other nerve bundle to be more likely to occur with apical injection, but this remains under study at this point.

It is usually easy to identify a pyramidal space lateral to the apex and above the levator ani that is similar to the Mount Everest sign (Figure 11.13). In a randomized trial of 143 patients at our institution, patients with traditional basilar injection had VAS scores averaging 28.7, compared with apical injection (identified by the above apical pyramid) patients whose VAS scores averaged 17.6 ($p = 0.0004$). Pain during injection was comparable in each group (22.0 vs. 21.1, respectively). Placement of the ultrasound probe (by definition before periprostatic block) was more painful than either biopsy or injection in each group: 28.5 and 30.2, respectively.[6] Although the apical injection yielded slightly better pain control, it is subjectively more difficult to teach to residents. We have also observed that

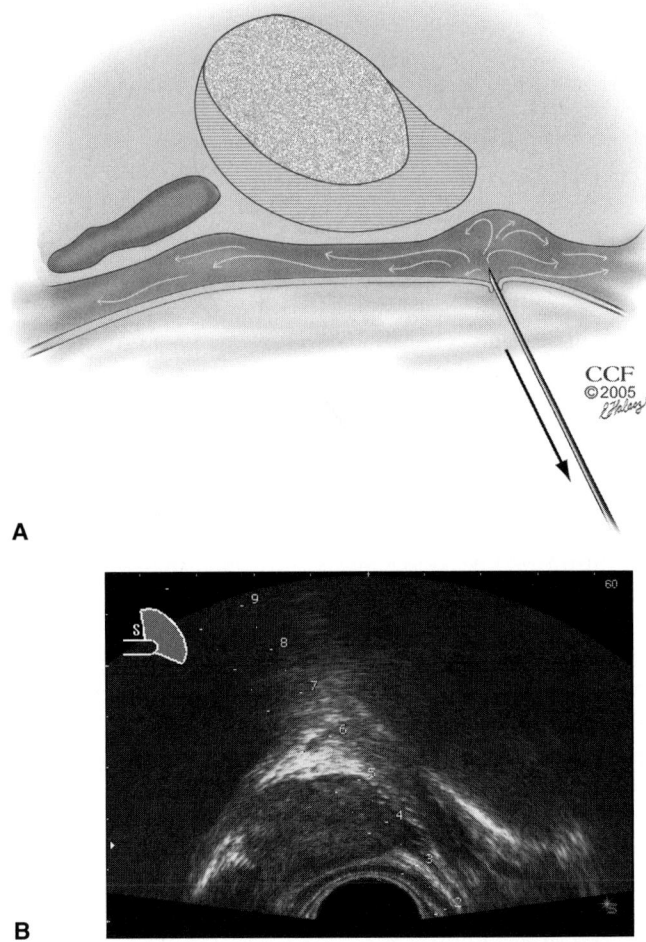

A

B

FIGURE 11.13. **A**: Ultrasound reveals a hyperechoic pyramidal area lateral to the apex as well. This is between the apex and the levator ani (dark line between the 2- and 3-cm measurement on the onscreen needle guide). **B**: Schematic of the pyramidal area for injection in order to achieve cranial dissection of an ultrasonic wheal during apical periprostatic block.

antegrade dissection of the ultrasonic wheal after injection at the Mount Everest site is easier to achieve than is retrograde injection at the apex (Figure 11.14). We continue to study these concepts to determine the optimal periprostatic block, and to determine the impact of residents performing prostate biopsy.

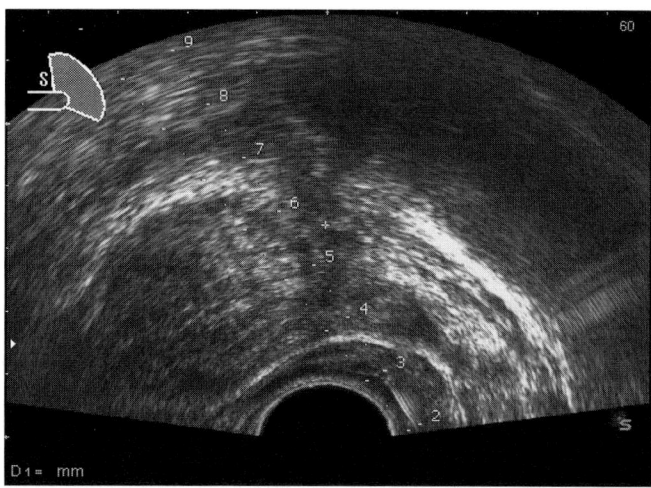

FIGURE 11.14. Dissection in the hyperechoic area demonstrated in Figure 11.13 (different patient) allows lidocaine to dissect cranially along the course of the periprostatic nerves. This accomplishes the same distribution as injecting at the Mount Everest site. We find this somewhat more difficult to inject, but there is no greater pain with injection and we have found that analgesia may be slightly better.

Based on these observations, we believe that the location or number of injections is of limited consequence as long as the anesthetic agent is visualized dissecting to the proper location bilaterally. The basilar Mount Everest offers the largest and easiest to define location, so remains our slightly preferred technique despite the findings above of improved pain control with apical injection. As our residents become more familiar with basilar injection, it will potentially become the standard.

Apical Biopsy Pain

Attempts to inject the level of the apex or directly into the apex as described above have been based on the observation that apical biopsy is more painful than biopsy of the remainder of the gland even if periprostatic block is applied. When we query attendees at Continuing Medical Education (CME) or American Urological Association (AUA) courses, this observation is confirmed by essentially all urologists. However, the reason for this increased pain in the apex was not understood until 2003, when we reported that this pain seemed to be related to stimulation of anal pain fibers, not the apex itself. By performing the rectal sensation test as described below, the apical pain fibers may be bypassed to achieve a painless apical biopsy.

Apical biopsy is crucial because of the predominance of cancers in this location, especially in the anterior portion of the apex (Figures 11.5 and

11.6). This area is named the anterior horn because of its beaked appearance as it wraps around the transition zone. This is the most likely site of cancer that has been missed during a false-negative previous biopsy.[34] We believe this is attributable to two factors. The first is that it is difficult to reach, especially using side-fire probes because of their tangential needle tract. The second is the above-noted perception by urologists that apical biopsy is more painful than biopsy of other areas of the prostate, so they may be tempted to avoid the area in exchange for improved patient tolerance.

Based on anatomic study in collaboration with our colorectal surgery colleagues, we determined that pain of apical biopsy is not attributable to prostatic pain; rather, it is attributable to anal pain fibers below the dentate line of the rectum, which approximately corresponds to the superior limit of such sensory pain fibers. Because this is often near the level of the prostatic apex, a needle often traverses such areas, resulting in significant anal—not prostatic—pain.

The dentate line, identified by the "rectal sensation test" is shown with arrows in Figure 11.15. During this test, the needle is lightly applied against mucosa. It is immediately and strikingly obvious upon even light touch whether anal pain fibers are present at this level. If the patient answers affirmatively that he feels sharpness, the needle is repositioned 1–2 mm higher until reaching an asensate area. He usually does not have to state such perception, because its noxious stimulation is enough to elicit his noticeable movement with even light touch of the needle.

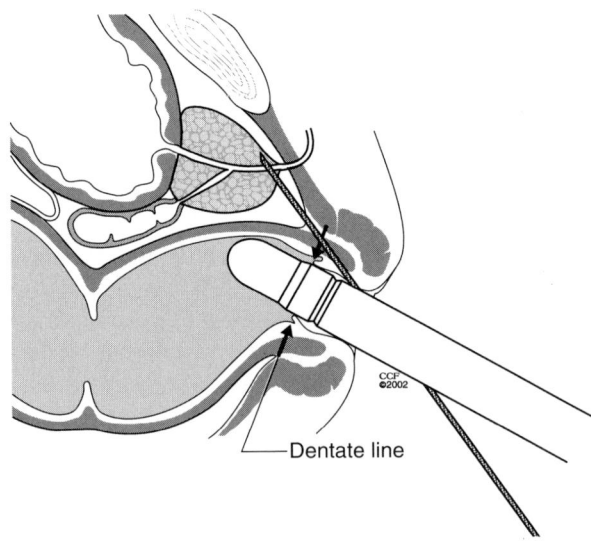

FIGURE 11.15. Increased pain during apical biopsy is attributed to piercing anal pain fibers below the dentate line.

When the needle is advanced cranially above the dentate line, the trajectory is often toward the midgland, precluding adequate apical biopsy (Figure 11.16). This is especially problematic because of the need to biopsy the "anterior horn" or peripheral zone tissue as described above.

Angling the probe handle craniodorsally as indicated by curved arrows in Figure 11.17 allows the needle to pull rectal mucosa caudally. Painless apical biopsy may then be obtained, bypassing the sensory fibers below the dentate line. This must be performed carefully to avoid dragging the needle against hemorrhoidal vessels in the rectum, which could lead to excessive bleeding. Using the needle tip as the pivot point instead of dragging allows this to occur safely.

VAS scores for apical biopsy in patients who have already undergone periprostatic block show improvement from 2.28 to 1.25 using this approach.[35]

The implications of these anatomic observations are obvious for injection of periprostatic block at the level of the apex instead of our preferred location at the base. However, as noted above, injection at this site does not seem to cause increased pain compared with injection at the base.[28] We continue to study these issues in order to more fully understand the neuroanatomy of the prostatic sensory innervation.

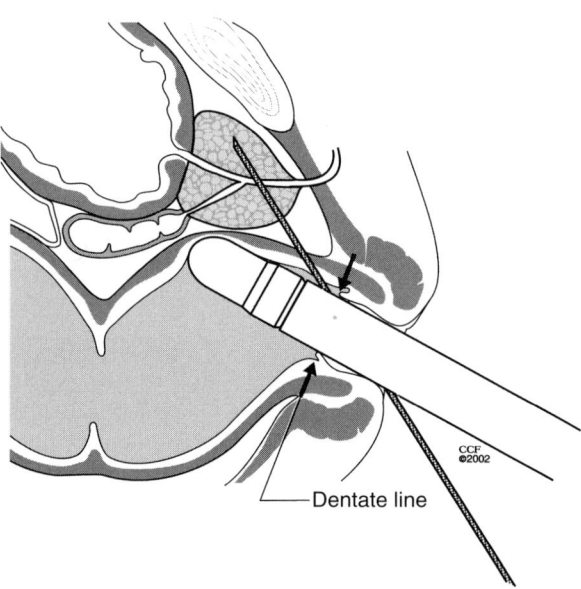

FIGURE 11.16. The patient will feel the sharp tip of the needle when it touches the intensely sensitive anal pain fibers. Marching 1–2 mm cranially allows the needle to reach an insensate area above the dentate line. However, this often results in the needle being directed at the midgland instead of apex as shown.

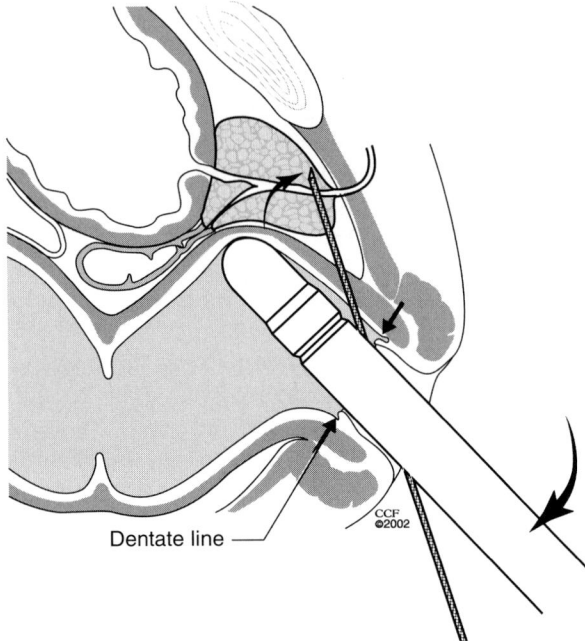

Dentate line

FIGURE 11.17. Once above the sensation limit of the dentate line, the needle may be advanced through rectal wall painlessly. The probe can be rotated as shown taking care not to drag the needle against the mucosa, in order to obtain a painless apical biopsy.

Conclusions

We believe that the demonstration of its efficacy in more than 50 publications to date clearly has placed periprostatic block for prostate biopsy into the status of standard of care. Patients should expect this level of concern for their comfort and well-being. We have found that the technique is of minimal consequence, although injection at the apex seems to be more effective than injection at the base. Injection into the Mount Everest sign at the base is easier to learn initially. Further efforts into improving the pain of probe placement are particularly pertinent, because nothing has been demonstrated to date to optimize this specific maneuver.

References

1. Nash P, Bruce J, Indudhara R, et al. Transrectal ultrasound guided prostatic nerve blockade eases systemic needle biopsy of the prostate. J Urol 1996; 155:607.
2. Soloway MS, Obek C. Periprostatic local anesthesia before ultrasound guided prostate biopsy. J Urol 2000;163(1):172–3.

3. Jones JS, Ulchaker JC, Nelson D, et al. Periprostatic local anesthesia eliminates pain of office-based transrectal prostate biopsy. Prostate Cancer Prostatic Dis 2003;6(1):53–5.

4. Jones JS. Office procedures. In: Novick AC, Jones JS, eds. Operative Urology at the Cleveland Clinic. Totowa, NJ: Humana Press; 2006, pp. 236–7.

5. Paul R, Korzinek C, Necknig U, et al. Influence of transrectal ultrasound probe on prostate cancer detection in transrectal ultrasound-guided sextant biopsy of prostate. Urology 2004;64(3):532–6.

6. Jones JS, Nguyen C. Apical injection of periprostatic block gives better pain control than traditional basilar injection. Société Internationale d'Urologie Annual Meeting, Capetown, South Africa. November 2006.

7. Hodge KK, McNeal JE, Terris MK, Stamey TA. Random systematic versus directed ultrasound-guided core biopsies of the prostate. J Urol 1989;142: 71–5.

8. Zisman A, Leibovich D, Kleinmann J, Siegel YI, Lindner A. The impact of prostate biopsy on patient well-being: a prospective study of pain, anxiety, and erectile dysfunction. J Urol 2001;165:445–54.

9. Roehl KA, Atenor JAV, Catalona WJ. Serial biopsy results in prostate cancer screening study. J Urol 2002;67(6):2435–9.

10. Masood J, Shah N, Lane T, Andrews H, Simpson P, Barua JM. Nitrous oxide (Entonox) inhalation and tolerance of transrectal ultrasound guided prostate biopsy: a double blind randomized controlled study. J Urol 2002;168:116–20.

11. Manikandan R, Srirangam SJ, Brown SC, O'Reilly PH, Collins GN. Nitrous oxide vs periprostatic nerve block with 1% lidocaine during transrectal ultrasound guided biopsy of the prostate: a prospective, randomized, controlled trial. J Urol 2003;170(5):1881–3.

12. Issa MM, Bux S, Chun T, et al. A randomized prospective trial of intrarectal lidocaine for pain control during transrectal prostate biopsy: the Emory University experience. J Urol 2000;164:397–9.

13. Desgrandchamps F, Meria P, Irani J, Desgrippes A, Teillac P, Le Duc A. The rectal administration of lidocaine gel and tolerance of transrectal ultrasonography-guided biopsy of the prostate: a prospective randomized placebo-controlled study. BJU Int 1999;83:1007–9.

14. Cevik I, Ozveri H, Dillioglugil O, Akdas A. Lack of effect of intrarectal lidocaine for pain control during transrectal prostate biopsy: a randomized prospective study. Eur Urol 2002;42(3):217–20.

15. Chang SS, Alberts G, Wells N, Smith JA Jr, Cookson MS. Intrarectal lidocaine during transrectal prostate biopsy: results of a prospective double-blind randomized trial. J Urol 2001;166(6):2178–80.

16. Autorino R, De Sio M, Di Lorenzo G, et al. How to decrease pain during transrectal ultrasound guided prostate biopsy: a look at the literature. J Urol 2005;174(6):2091–7.

17. De Sio M, D'Armiento M, Di Lorenzo G, et al. The need to reduce patient discomfort during transrectal ultrasonography-guided prostate biopsy: what do we know? BJU Int 2005;96(7):977–83.

18. Ragavan N, Philip J, Balasubramanian SP, Desouza J, Marr C, Javle P. A randomized, controlled trial comparing lidocaine periprostatic nerve block, diclofenac suppository and both for transrectal ultrasound guided biopsy of prostate. J Urol 2005;174(2):510–3.

19. Kravchick S, Peled R, Ben-Dor D, Dorfman D, Kesari D, Cytron S. Comparison of different local anesthesia techniques during TRUS-guided biopsies: a prospective pilot study. Urology 2005;65(1):109–13.
20. Adsan O, Inal G, Ozdogan L, Kaygisiz O, Ugurlu O, Cetinkaya M. Unilateral pudendal nerve blockade for relief of all pain during transrectal ultrasound-guided biopsy of the prostate: a randomized, double-blind, placebo-controlled study. Urology 2004;64(3):528–31.
21. Rabets JC, Jones JS, Patel AR, Zippe CD. Bupivacaine provides rapid, effective periprostatic anaesthesia for transrectal prostate biopsy. BJU Int 2004;93(9): 1216–7.
22. Lee-Elliott CE, Dundas D, Patel U. Randomized trial of lidocaine vs. lidocaine/bupivacaine periprostatic injection on longitudinal pain scores after prostate biopsy. J Urol 2004;171(1):247–50.
23. Wu CL, Carter HB, Naqibuddin M, et al. Effect of local anesthetics on patient recovery after transrectal biopsy. Urology 2001;57:925–9.
24. Jones JS. Technique determines efficacy of local anesthetic for outpatient prostate biopsy. Urology 2001;58:635–6.
25. Vaidya A, Soloway MS. Periprostatic local anesthesia before ultrasound-guided prostate biopsy: an update of the Miami experience. Eur Urol 2001;40:135–8.
26. Obek C, Onal B, Onder AU, et al. Is periprostatic local anesthesia for transrectal ultrasound guided prostate biopsy associated with increased infectious or hemorrhagic complications? A prospective randomized controlled trial. J Urol 2002;168:558–61.
27. Alavi AS, Soloway MS, Lynne CM, Gheiler El. Local anesthesia for ultrasound guided prostate biopsy: a prospective randomized trial comparing two methods. J Urol 2001;166:1343–5.
28. Kaver I, Mabjeesh NJ, Matzkin H. Randomized prospective study of periprostatic local anesthesia during transrectal ultrasound-guided prostate biopsy. Urology 2002;59(3):405–8.
29. Rodriguez A, Kyriakou G, Leray E, Lobel B, Guille F. Prospective study comparing two methods of anaesthesia for prostate biopsies: apex periprostatic nerve block versus intrarectal lidocaine gel: review of the literature. Eur Urol 2003;44(2):195–200.
30. Emiliozzi P, Longhi S, Scarpone P, Pasadoro A, et al. The value of a single biopsy with 12 transperineal cores for detecting prostate cancer in patients with elevated prostate specific antigen. J Urol 2001;166:845–50.
31. Mutaguchi K, Shinohara K, Matsubara A, Yasumoto H, Mita K, Usui T. Local anesthesia during 10 core biopsy of the prostate: comparison of 2 methods. J Urol 2005;173(3):742–5.
32. Walker AE, Schelvan C, Rockall AG, Rickards D, Kellett MJ. Does pericapsular lignocaine reduce pain during transrectal ultrasonography-guided biopsy of the prostate? BJU Int 2002;90(9):883–6.
33. Schostak M, Christoph F, Muller M, et al. Optimizing local anesthesia during 10-core biopsy of the prostate. Urology 2002;60:253–7.
34. Hong YM, Lai FC, Chon CH, McNeal JE, Presti JC Jr. Impact of prior biopsy scheme on pathologic features of cancers detected on repeat biopsies. Urol Oncol 2004;22(1):7–10.
35. Jones JS, Zippe CD. Rectal sensation test helps avoid pain of apical prostate biopsies. J Urol 2003;170(6 Pt 1):2316–8.

12
Prostate Biopsy Techniques

Katsuto Shinohara

Abstract

Prostate biopsy has evolved to the current transrectal ultrasound–guided, multiple systematic biopsy scheme. In this chapter, the basics of prostate biopsy, and various current biopsy procedures including transrectal, transperineal, and transurethral are discussed. Biopsy techniques in special patient groups, such as biopsy after radical prostatectomy and abdominoperineal resection of the rectum, are also discussed.

Keywords: prostate, biopsy, transrectal ultrasonography, transrectal biopsy, transperineal biopsy, local recurrence, anesthesia, abdominoperineal resection

Prostate cancer continues to be the most frequently diagnosed cancer in men. The American Cancer Society estimated that there would be 230,000 newly diagnosed cases and 29,900 deaths from prostate cancer in 2006.[1] Significant decreases in prostate cancer mortality have been achieved, likely with screening efforts involving blood testing and with detection efforts in the form of ultrasound-guided biopsy of the prostate.[2] Transrectal ultrasound (TRUS)-guided needle biopsy of the prostate is the current gold standard for the detection of prostate cancer. In this chapter, the current optimal strategies for TRUS-guided needle biopsy of the prostate, highlighting special scenarios, and newer, adjunctive techniques for prostate needle biopsy are described.

From: *Current Clinical Urology: Prostate Biopsy: Indications, Techniques, and Complications*
Edited by J.S. Jones © Humana Press, Totowa, NJ

History of Prostate Biopsy

Prostate biopsy was first described in 1930 when Ferguson[3] successfully obtained cancer cells by aspirating prostate tissue through a transperineally introduced 18-gauge needle. In 1937, Astraldi[4] described the first transrectally performed core needle biopsy of the prostate. In the late 1980s, TRUS-guided prostate biopsy using an 18-gauge needle loaded in a spring-action device was first introduced.[5] Since then, prostate biopsy under ultrasound guidance using an automated device has become standard procedure. In 1989, Hodge et al.[6] proposed the modern model of performing biopsy of defined areas of the prostate, namely, the "sextant" method of prostate biopsy. Technologic developments that have improved prostate biopsy and its role in prostate cancer detection include an automated spring-loaded prostate biopsy device, multiaxial planar imaging, and a better understanding of prostate zonal anatomy.[7]

Equipment

Transrectal Ultrasound Device

Transrectal ultrasonography is currently the gold standard for prostate biopsy guidance. This imaging modality not only guides the needle in the designated area of the prostate, but also gives information regarding prostate size and shape, localized lesion, tumor extension, seminal vesicle pathology, etc. Currently, either a biplane probe or an end-fire probe with a variable frequency of 5–10 MHz is used for transrectal prostate biopsy (*see* Figure 12.3A,B). Depending on the type of probe, the images obtained are slightly different, and sonographers must be familiar with the differences.

Biopsy Device

For prostate biopsy, an 18-gauge needle loaded in a spring-action, automated biopsy device is frequently used. When the trigger button of this device is pushed, the inner needle advances 23 mm, followed by the outer needle advancement in the same distance. The prostate tissue is caught between the inner and outer needle. It is designed to obtain about a 15- to 17-mm length of tissue from the tip of the needle before the activation (Figure 12.1). Therefore, the needle tip must be right at the target before the activation of the device. On transrectal ultrasonography, a needle tract may appear longer than the biopsy specimen that is actually taken. Cancer is frequently located along the capsule of the gland. When the anterior biopsy is performed, the needle tip must be advanced into prostate tissue about 15 mm from the anterior capsule in order to sample the tissue where cancer is located (*see* Figure 12.5).

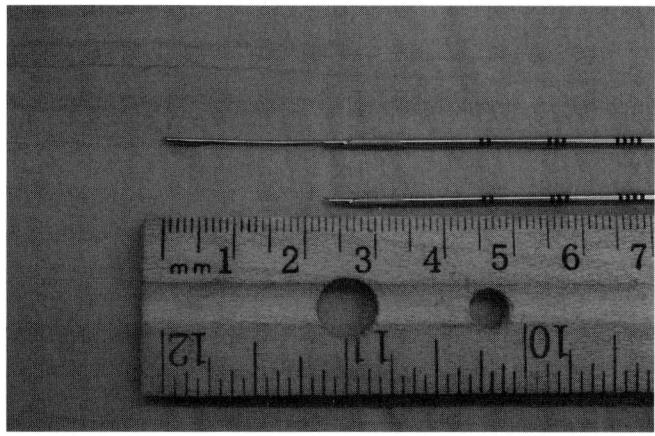

FIGURE 12.1. The bottom needle is before activation, and the top needle is after the inner needle is advanced. The automated biopsy needle is designed to obtain a 15-mm-long tissue sample from the tip of the needle. Note that total needle advancement is 23 mm.

Preparation for Biopsy

Bowel Preparation

Generally, no diet restriction is necessary before biopsy. A Fleet enema is given 1 hour before the procedure. This will evacuate rectal contents including gas and fecal matter, which causes interference on ultrasound imaging. An enema also reduces the incidence of infectious complications.[8]

Antibiotics

Antibiotics, usually fluoroquinolones, are given starting 12 hours before biopsy and continue for a total of 72 hours. Recent study by Lindstedt et al.,[9] however, showed that a single dose of ciprofloxacin 750 mg at the time of prostate biopsy equally achieved low septicemia events of about 1%. Use of antibiotics significantly reduces the risk of septicemia.[10] This subject will be further discussed in the complication section. If a patient is known to have heart valve disease or is susceptible to endocarditis, appropriate antibiotics, usually ampicillin and gentamicin, should be given according to the American Heart Association's recommendation.[11] Patients with artificial joints or prosthesis need to be appropriately covered with parenteral antibiotics as well.

Special Precaution for Patients with Anticoagulation

Any anticoagulation medications or antiplatelet function medication, such as aspirin, nonsteroidal antiinflammatory drugs, or clopidogrel (Plavix), are generally stopped for an appropriate length before biopsy. However, aspirin use at the time of biopsy has shown no statistical difference in incidence of bleeding in some reports.[12,13]

Anesthesia

Local Anesthesia

The administration of anesthetic agents during the performance of TRUS biopsy is now well known to reduce patient discomfort. This may be important because a study from the Netherlands examining the reasons why men refuse to attend a prostate cancer screening showed that 18% of men believed that the prostate biopsy would be painful.[14] Nash et al.,[15] at University of California at San Francisco (UCSF), first conducted a randomized, double-blinded study of local infiltration of 1% lidocaine around the prostate vascular pedicle of 64 patients. Mean pain scores were significantly lower on the side injected with lidocaine compared with the saline control. Previously reported nerve block technique to the vascular pedicle was occasionally associated with systemic circulation of lidocaine caused by injecting the agent in the vascular-rich area. This results in such sensations as strange taste, ear tingling, or vertigo. At the same time, the local anesthetic effect is not achieved because the majority of the anesthetic circulates in the body rather than stays locally. Also, nerve block does not completely anesthetize the anterior part of the gland. Currently, a 1% lidocaine 10 cc and 7.5% sodium bicarbonate 1 cc solution mixture is used to reduce the burning sensation. The solution is injected directly into the prostate at three locations in each lobe by inserting a 22-gauge needle all the way to the anterior capsule at the base, midgland, and the apex, and as the needle is pulled back, 1–2 cc of anesthetic is infiltrated in the prostate parenchyma at each location. By doing this, systemic circulation of anesthetic can be avoided, and the entire gland is anesthetized including the anterior part. A recent study compared this technique with conventional nerve block and concluded that the anesthetic effect in the intraprostatic injection group was superior.[16]

Intrarectal Application of Anesthetics

Issa et al.[17] reported the benefit of 2% Xylocaine jelly injected in the rectum before biopsy. Pain associated with biopsy is generally from the prostate capsule and parenchyma, and not from the rectal wall. The sensation of the ultrasound device being in the anus is another component of discomfort during the biopsy. Anesthetic jelly generally anesthetizes the anal ring and proctocanal, achieving a more comfortable biopsy procedure. However, the intrarectal injection of anesthetic jelly alone does not completely block the pain because of needle penetration into the prostate. The same anesthetic effect of Xylocaine jelly can be achieved by 20% benzocaine cream (Hurricaine; Beutlich Pharmaceuticals, Waukegan, IL) applied at the time of the digital rectal examination before biopsy. Benzocaine is a faster-acting mucosa anesthetic that achieves effective anesthesia in 30 seconds. Combining intrarectal anesthesia with a prostate block seems to provide maximum comfort during prostate biopsy.

Biopsy Procedure

Transrectal Prostate Biopsy

Patient Positioning

The left lateral decubitus position is usually preferred for transrectal prostate biopsy. The patient's buttocks should be placed on the closest edge of the table to the operator. The hip and knee joints are flexed to right angle, and the legs are placed along the far edge of the table from the operator in order to create a wide area below the buttocks for the TRUS probe and biopsy device maneuver. The pelvis should be slightly tilted front. This will also allow more freedom of probe movement during biopsy.

Location of Biopsy

In 1989, Hodge et al.[6] proposed the modern model of performing biopsy of defined areas of the prostate, namely, the "sextant" method of prostate biopsy. After the initial introduction of the sextant, systematic prostate biopsy, little refinement of the technique was made until, in an editorial, Stamey suggested moving the biopsies more laterally to better sample the anterior horns of the peripheral zone and avoid sampling error.[18–20] Such recommendations were supported by the meticulous whole-mount analyses of radical prostatectomy specimens, which helped to further delineate the zonal anatomy of the prostate and the spatial origin of prostate cancers as well.[21] Extended sextant biopsy obtaining two specimens from each sextant totaling 12 samples is now common practice. Within each sextant, one biopsy is obtained from the medial part close to the median furrow of the gland, and the other from the lateral part close to the lateral edge of the gland. Each biopsy entry site has to be separated well in order to cover the gland widely. However, frequently the apex and base biopsies are obtained close to the mid portion of the gland. This results in all three biopsies, apex, mid portion, and base, coming from almost the same area

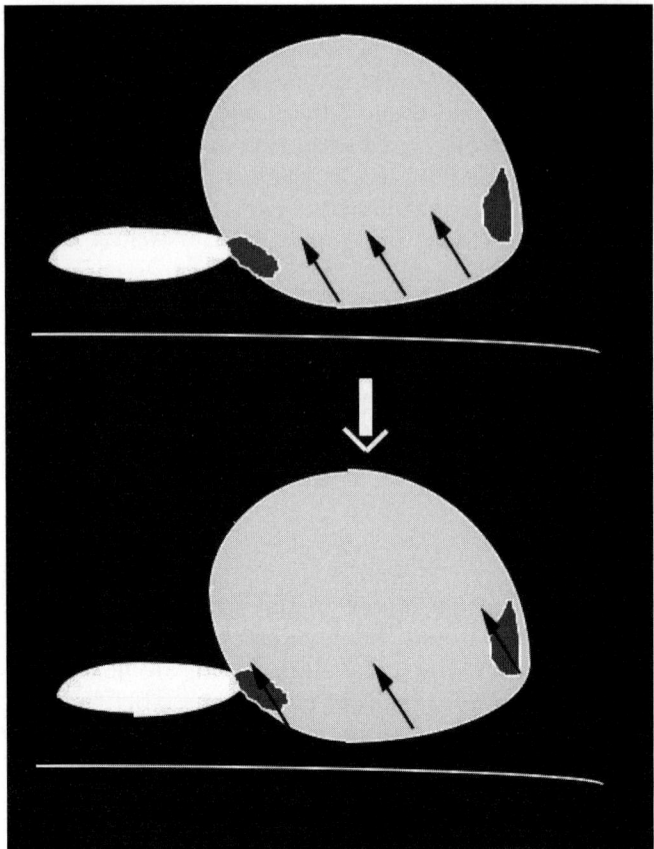

FIGURE 12.2. **Top:** Diagram showing a common mistake of the apex and base biopsy being too close to the midgland, sparing the tissue at apex and base. **Bottom:** The entry site of the biopsy needle should be widely separated to cover the prostate homogeneously.

(Figure 12.2). When the needle is advanced through the biopsy guide, the first resistance noticed is from the rectal wall. With further advancement of the needle, the second resistance from the prostate capsule is recognized. At this point, the TRUS image should show the needle tip to be slightly indenting the prostate capsule. If the needle tip is still not reaching the capsule or the tip is already in the prostate parenchyma, satisfactory biopsy sampling cannot be achieved.

When the very apex of the prostate is biopsied, a needle may enter in the proctocanal distal to the dentate line. In such case, a patient may experience significant pain even with local anesthesia, because the mucosa distal to the dentate line is very sensitive to pain. A needle tip must be advanced above the dentate line, and then the needle tip should be redirected to the apex within the rectum in order to avoid such pain. Some ultrasound probes have a biopsy guide traversing through the probe itself (Figure 12.3A,B). Such probes have less flexibility in maneuvering the biopsy direction, because the angle of the biopsy guide to the prostate is almost fixed. Apical biopsy with this probe can be challenging, because the needle may go through the proctocanal distal to the dentate line more often than an end-fire probe with a needle guide attached on the side of the probe (Figure 12.4A,B). It is also important to note that biopsy of the base or anterior part of the gland frequently resulted in the needle penetrating the bladder wall, because the needle advances a total of 23 mm. If the bladder wall is penetrated, ultrasonography can show the severity of the bleeding from the bladder wall. If continuous pumping blood is noticed at the end of the

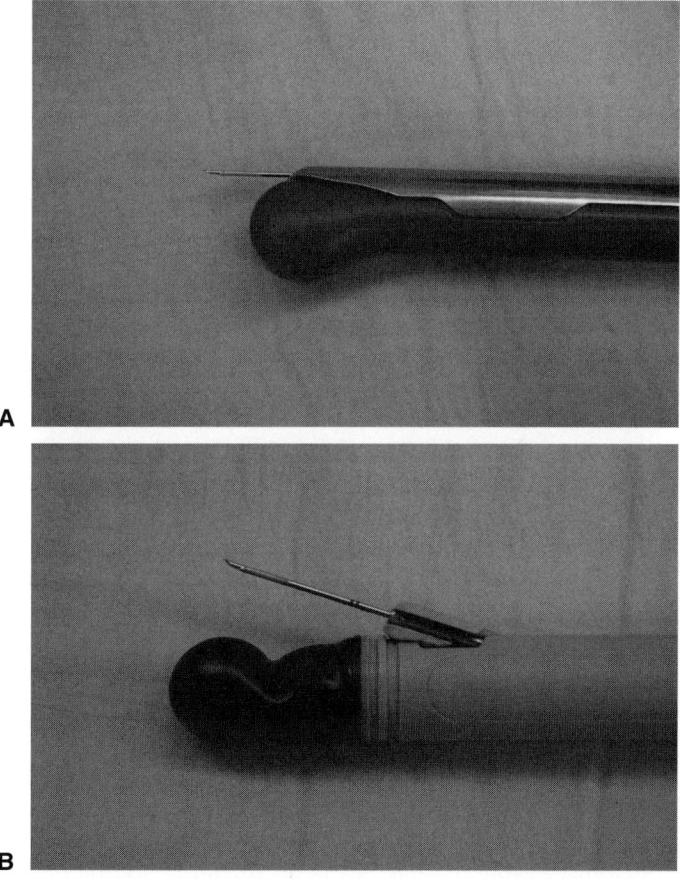

A

B

FIGURE 12.3. **A**: End-fire probe with the biopsy guide attached on the side of the probe. A biopsy needle is advanced parallel to the probe. **B**: A biplane transrectal probe with needle guide built in the probe.

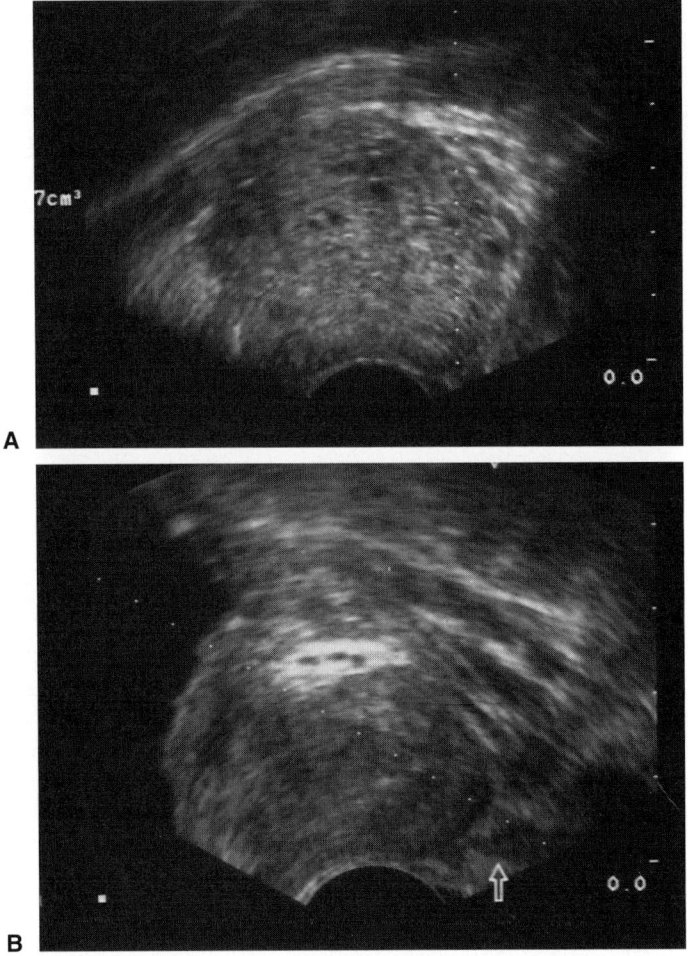

FIGURE 12.4. **A**: With an end-fire probe, an apex biopsy is easily done without compromising the proctocanal. **B**: Using a biplane probe with built-in guide, a very-apex biopsy is challenging with the needle going through the area distal to the dentate line. The dotted line on both pictures indicates the needle path.

procedure, Foley catheterization should be considered in order to monitor and stop further bleeding.

Number of Biopsies

Extensive or "saturation" biopsy has been recommended by some investigators to maximize cancer detection rates in patients with clinical criteria that put them at high risk for prostate cancer despite a previous benign biopsy [e.g., increasing prostate-specific antigen (PSA) in a patient with a first-degree family history of prostate adenocarcinoma]. This type of biopsy scheme has been performed in the office using periprostatic block, with intravenous sedation, or in the outpatient surgery center with general or spinal anesthetic.[22–25] Although most of the saturation biopsy protocols are done transrectally, there are also reports of transperineal saturation biopsy.[26] Generally, irrespective of anesthetic used, these saturation biopsy protocols obtain 22–24 cores per patient. Borboroglu et al.[24] found 17 of 57 men (30%) of their cohort had adenocarcinoma identified using a six-region biopsy pattern. Interestingly, 41% of these men had only one positive biopsy core. Complications included urinary retention in 11%, but it is unclear how much the anesthetic contributed to this complication. Stewart et al.[25] used a radial biopsy pattern separated by 20–30 degrees and found a similar detection rate of 34% in 224 patients. The overall complication rate was 12%, which included 5% of men requiring hospitalization for hematuria. Finally, Rabets et al.[27] recently published a 29% overall positive biopsy rate in 116 consecutive patients who underwent a 24-core saturation biopsy regimen in the office after previous negative biopsies. This 29%–34% rate of cancer detection is similar to repeat extended (10- or 12-core) prostate biopsy, which is generally accomplished with less morbidity. In summary, these data suggest a threshold over which cancer yield is not increased. Furthermore, the use of intravenous or greater anesthesia may be necessary and complications might be increased. Recently, Eichler et al.[28] conducted a meta-analysis of various extended biopsy procedures and concluded that a 12-core biopsy scheme strikes the balance between cancer detection and adverse events. Finally, it seems likely, as extended biopsy schemes become more frequently performed for initial diagnosis, rather than initial sextant biopsy, there will be less need for such saturation biopsy protocols.

Transition Zone Biopsy

According to McNeal's study,[29] prostate cancer frequently originates from the peripheral zone, but approximately 24% of cancers arise from the transition zone. Chang et al.[30] evaluated the role of a routine transition zone biopsy in patients with a large prostate gland more than 50 cc and concluded that there is little benefit to adding a transition zone biopsy in such patients. Takashima et al.[31] carefully examined radical prostatectomy specimens in 62 T1c cancer patients and reported that T1c cancer is densely located at the apex to mid portion in the anterior half of the gland. At UCSF, in addition to an extended sextant biopsy, a pair of samples along the anterior capsule of the apex/midgland is routinely taken (Figure 12.5). With this biopsy scheme, two anterior biopsies are obtained not from the transition zone but from the peripheral zone located anterior to the urethra at the apex and extending anteriorly along the lateral edge of the midgland. Meng et al.[32] reported that adding anterior apical biopsy to the extended

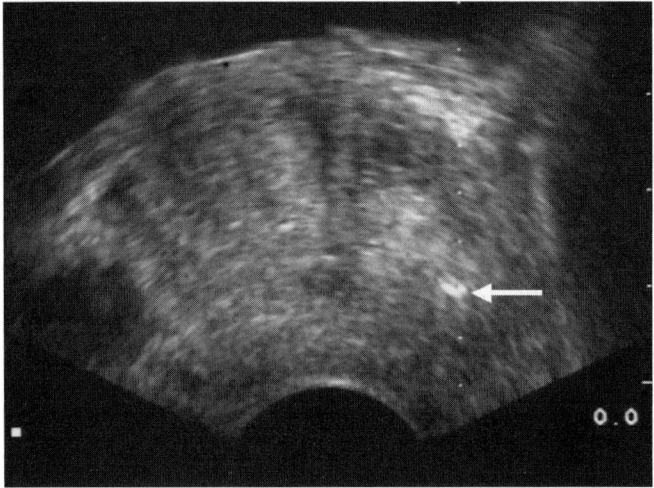

FIGURE 12.5. Anterior apical biopsy is obtained by a needle advanced into the gland from the apex along the anterior capsule from the apex. The needle tip before sampling is about 15 mm from the anterior capsule (arrow).

sextant biopsy scheme increased cancer detection, especially in patients with normal digital rectal examination. Biopsy in the middle of the transition zone is less likely to yield positive results. The biopsy must be taken from the tissue along the anterior capsule. When the anterior part of the gland is biopsied, the needle tip must be located 1.5 cm from the anterior capsule in order to sample the tissue along the anterior capsule where cancer is frequently located.

Repeat Biopsy

With conventional TRUS technology, sampling errors are inevitable and a negative biopsy does not rule out malignancy with certainty. The management of the patient with repeatedly negative prostate biopsies and clinical characteristics suggestive of cancer, such as an elevated PSA or abnormal digital rectal examination remains a challenging problem for physicians and patients. Repeat prostate biopsies will detect cancer in 16%–41% of cases in which an initial biopsy is negative, but the majority of patients will have a repeat negative biopsy. At UCSF, 325 men with a history of two or more negative biopsies were studied. The mean age of this patient population was 61 years with a mean serum PSA of 13.8. Overall percent positive biopsy for patients with two or more prior negative biopsies was 38%. The percentage of patients with a positive biopsy decreased as the number of previous negative biopsies increased: 40% in patients with 2–3 prior negative biopsies, 36% in patients with 4–5 prior negative biopsies, and 17% in

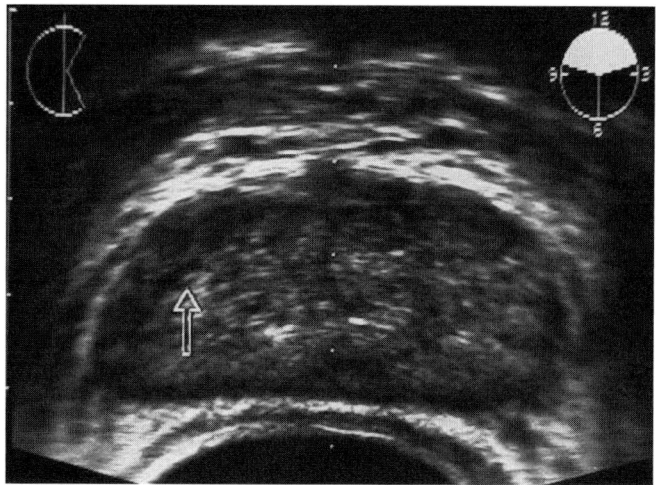

FIGURE 12.6. This patient had a steady PSA increase of 4 to 9 in 3 years. Three sessions of prostate biopsies were done showing all benign tissue. Abnormal hypoechoic tissue was noted at the right anterior part of the midgland on referral (arrow). Biopsy revealed a Gleason grade 3+4 cancer in this location.

patients with 6 prior negative biopsies. Using a Cox proportional hazards model, we identified predictors of positive biopsy, which were higher PSA, gradually increasing PSA rather than stable PSA, increased age, hypoechoic lesions on ultrasound, and smaller prostate. Abnormal pathology [prostatic intraepithelial neoplasia (PIN), atypical small acinar proliferation (ASAP)] on previous biopsy, abnormal digital rectal examination, and transition zone volume were not significant predictors of a positive biopsy (unpublished data).

The most common areas to be missed on initial biopsy are at the apices as well as in the anterior prostate. It is common that the biopsy entry site tends to be sparing of the very apex of the gland (Figure 12.2). In fact, positive biopsy cores in cases with previously multiple, negative biopsies are frequently found at apex biopsy and anteriorly directed biopsy (Figure 12.6). On repeat biopsy, taking samples from the same location is unlikely to detect cancer. The biopsy should be directed to a previously unsampled area, such as the very apex, very base, very lateral edges, midline, and along the anterior capsule.

Strategy for High-Grade Prostatic Intraepithelial Neoplasia and Atypical Small Acinar Proliferation

Although current biopsy strategies provide an extensive sample of the prostate, the histology of biopsy samples may not be conclusive for either the presence or the absence of adenocarcinoma. High-grade PIN (HGPIN) is found on a varying, but significant fraction of prostate biopsies (1%–25%), with most modern series having an average of 5%.[33] PIN is characterized by architecturally benign prostate acini which are lined by cytologically atypical cells. The significance of discovering HGPIN on prostate biopsy has received much attention. Varying results from repeat biopsy have been reported with prostate cancer detection ranging from 0% to 100%. Historically, the probability of detecting prostate cancer on repeat biopsy after HGPIN diagnosis is reported to be 30%–50%.[34,35] However, Lefkowitz et al.[36] reported that with an extended biopsy scheme showing HGPIN, repeat biopsy showed cancer in only 2.3% of the cases. Recent recommendation is that immediate repeat biopsy is not necessary after a 12-core biopsy showing HGPIN.[37]

ASAP, which has also previously been termed atypical adenomatous hyperplasia or atypia, is characterized by the crowding and proliferation of small glands; however, cytologic atypia is minimal.[38] This lesion has been less well characterized as compared with HGPIN, but ASAP alone is identified in 5% of patients undergoing needle biopsy. This lesion could be a part of a cancer focus sampled by the needle, but is not sufficient enough to call cancer because the amount is so small. Another possibility is that the lesion could represent a group of atrophic prostatic acini. Importantly, the association of ASAP with prostate cancer is higher than that of HGPIN. A contemporary biopsy series looking at the influence of ASAP has shown a 40%–50% probability of detecting adenocarcinoma. Having both HGPIN and atypia together on the first biopsy may increase the rate of cancer detection on the second biopsy to as high as 75%.[39] In a study by Park et al.,[40] between 1991–1998, 45 men with atypia underwent rebiopsy and 23 of 45 (51%) men were found to have cancer. Ninety-one percent of these patients had a positive biopsy for cancer on their repeat biopsy, whereas 9% required two or more biopsy sessions. Cancer is more likely to be detected in the sextant where HGPIN or ASAP is found. Moreover, Allen et al.[41] reported that subsequent cancer was found 88% of the time in the sextant or its adjacent area. This implies that each biopsy specimen should be labeled separately and submitted for pathology in case the results show HGPIN or ASAP. In addition to the routine random biopsy, one or two samples should be obtained from the sextant with abnormality and its adjacent sextants during the repeat biopsy.

Seminal Vesicle Biopsy

Routine seminal vesicle biopsy is usually not necessary. However, patients with significant disease found at the base of the prostate or an abnormal seminal vesicle appearance should undergo seminal vesicle biopsy. Seminal vesicle abnormality is not apparent in patients treated in the past with radiation therapy. Seminal vesicle biopsy should be performed regardless of findings in this population. To obtain a meaningful pathology specimen,

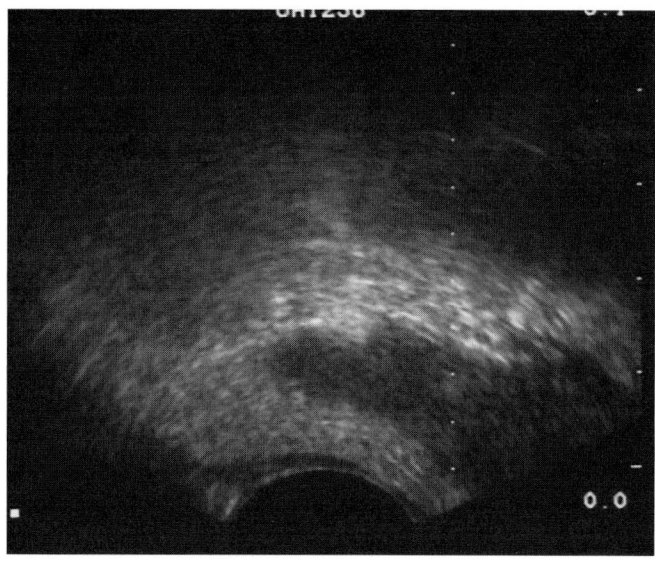

FIGURE 12.7. Seminal vesicle biopsy should be obtained from the base of the organ near the junction of the prostate.

the base of the seminal vesicle near the junction of prostate should be biopsied, because tumor invasion always occurs from the base (Figure 12.7). To avoid confusion of cancer in the prostate next to the seminal vesicle, rather than seminal vesicle invasion, the needle tip must be pushed up against the seminal vesicle base before taking the biopsy.

Transperineal Prostate Biopsy

Patients with multiple negative biopsies are almost always undersampled at the anterior part, and the multiple biopsies should be obtained from the tissue along the anterior capsule, as stated before. Recently, a series of TRUS-guided transperineal template prostate biopsies showed significant apicoanterior cancer detection in patients with normal digital rectal examination.[42] The procedure is generally performed under general or spinal anesthesia. The patient is placed in the lithotomy position. A biplane TRUS probe is frequently used. The probe is fixed on a brachytherapy stand and a brachytherapy template is used to guide a needle in the appropriate location.[26] Depending on the report, the number of the cores obtained varies but is generally approximately 20 cores.[43] Satoh et al.[44] reported their procedure in detail. In their report, four samples are taken from each quadrant in the coronal plane at midgland, then at the apex, three cores are obtained at each of anterior and posterior halves, totaling 22 cores. At UCSF, transperineal biopsy is performed only in cases with multiple negative biopsies.

In these patients, the prostate gland is divided into eight regions defined by following characteristic combinations, right or left, posterior or anterior, and apex or base. In each region, four cores are obtained along the prostate capsule, totaling 32 core samples. Using a brachytherapy stand and template, an apical coronal image is obtained. In this plane, four biopsy locations in each quadrant are chosen and a needle is advanced through the preselected hole in the template. The needle is then identified in the longitudinal view and advanced until the tip reaches the prostatic capsule. Biopsy is taken from this point in each location. After completing the 16 biopsies in this plane, the TRUS probe is advanced to the mid portion of the gland. New biopsy locations on the template are chosen, and the needle is advanced to the midgland in the longitudinal view. A biopsy is taken from the midgland to the base by advancing the needle to the midgland in the longitudinal view. In any method, transperineal biopsy will completely change the direction and location of needle puncture from the transrectal approach. Therefore, it may be reasonable to consider this procedure for patients with previously multiple negative biopsies with continuous PSA elevation. At present, this method is considered to be better in mapping a tumor, and has been proposed for focal treatment of prostate cancer using ablative therapy.[45]

Transurethral Biopsy

There has been no transurethral needle biopsy procedure described in the past. In this chapter, transurethral biopsy of the prostate refers to transurethral resection of prostate (TUR-P). Patients with multiple negative biopsies are often offered TUR-P to obtain anterior prostate tissue regardless of urinary symptoms. Puppo et al.[46] reported that 14 men with three negative prostate biopsies and increasing PSA were offered both TUR-P and transrectal biopsy. Eight cancers (57%) were detected in this population, and of those, six cancers were detected only by TUR-P. The authors stressed the importance of a combined procedure to achieve a maximum detection rate of cancer in this population. Whether those cancers are detectable by anterior-directed transrectal biopsy or transperineal template biopsy could not be answered by this report.

Digitally Guided Prostate Biopsy

In the era of TRUS-guided extended systematic random biopsy, digitally guided prostate biopsy is rarely performed.[47] A palpable nodule is usually identifiable by careful TRUS imaging, and if so, TRUS-guided biopsy will more accurately sample the area of interest than digitally guided biopsy. However, occasionally a clearly palpable nodule may not be seen on TRUS imaging. In this scenario, one can decide to perform a digitally guided biopsy. A biopsy needle's protective sheath can be cut short and placed on the index finger covered with another glove. This sheath provides good needle access to the tip of the finger for digitally guided biopsy. This biopsy should be performed before the TRUS-guided random biopsy, because the palpable nodule could be obscured by a hematoma that developed after the random biopsy.

Biopsy in Special Populations

Patients after Radical Prostatectomy

Biochemical failure with detectable PSA after radical prostatectomy can be seen in 30%–40% of cases in follow-up. Patients with slow PSA increase and evidence of a positive surgical margin at the time of radical prostatectomy are more likely to have local recurrence. Biopsy in this setting is generally not considered to be mandatory before radiation therapy. However, pathologic confirmation and fiduciary marker placement could help to improve the outcome.

Anatomy of Anastomotic Site after Radical Prostatectomy

To accurately perform a biopsy, recognition of TRUS-based anatomy of the anastomotic site is important. In a sagittal view in the midline, the anastomotic site is clearly identifiable as the area where the membranous urethra's low echogenicity suddenly changes to more echogenic tissue[48] (Figure 12.8). Local recurrence is frequently located proximal to this area and often on the side or posterior aspect of the tubularized segment of bladder neck.[49] Identifying the membranous urethra, as described in the normal transrectal prostate biopsy section, also helps in orienting the true midline of the patient.

Biopsy Technique

On TRUS image, the bladder neck tissue can be seen as a tubularized segment. A local recurrence is frequently seen on the side or posterior aspect of this tubularized segment of the bladder neck as hypoechoic tissue. When the probe is slightly tilted to obtain an off-midline image, hypoechoic tissue can be seen isolated from the bladder neck. This finding is very suspicious for local recurrence. The same lesion can be seen as an asymmetrical thickening of tissue around the anastomotic site or behind the bladder on coronal image (Figure 12.9). Local anesthesia is usually not necessary, because only a few samples are taken. However, similar to the apex biopsy, a needle can stimulate the proctocanal when this area is biopsied. The needle tip can easily penetrate through the bladder wall in these patients. Observation of the bladder wall by TRUS and confirming the degree of hematuria after biopsy are always necessary for this procedure, because bladder wall bleeding is quite common.

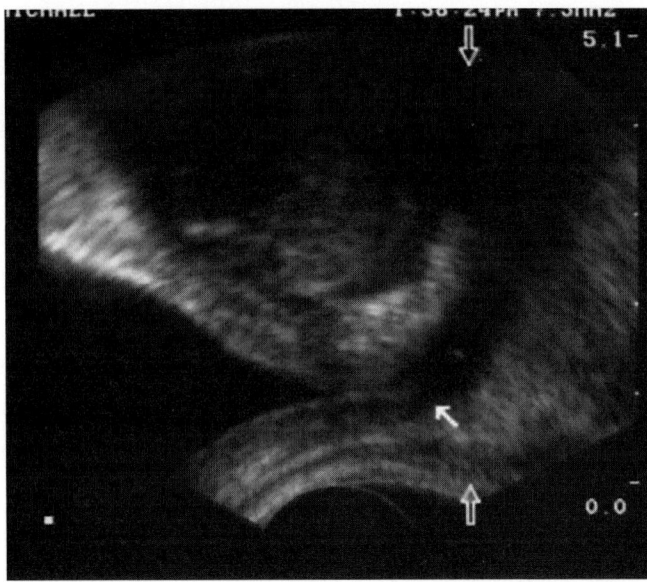

FIGURE 12.8. Midline sagittal view of the anastomotic site after radical prostatectomy. Note that echogenicity of the urethra suddenly changes at the anastomotic site (arrow). Membranous urethra is low echogenic, but the tubularized segment of the bladder neck is always more echogenic. Local recurrence should be located proximal to the anastomotic site.

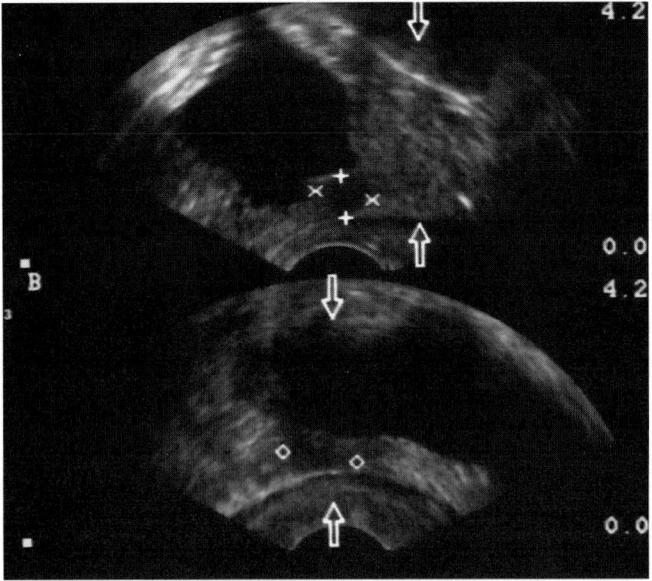

FIGURE 12.9. Local recurrence is seen as a hypoechoic mass (marked by cursors) off the midline at the bladder neck on the right side (top, sagittal view; bottom, coronal view).

Patients after Abdominoperineal Resection of the Rectum

After abdominoperineal resection of the rectum, there is no access to the rectum. Digital rectal examination or transrectal ultrasonography cannot be performed, and often prostate cancer diagnosis can be delayed. PSA elevation is the only sign for screening prostate cancer in this population. Trans-

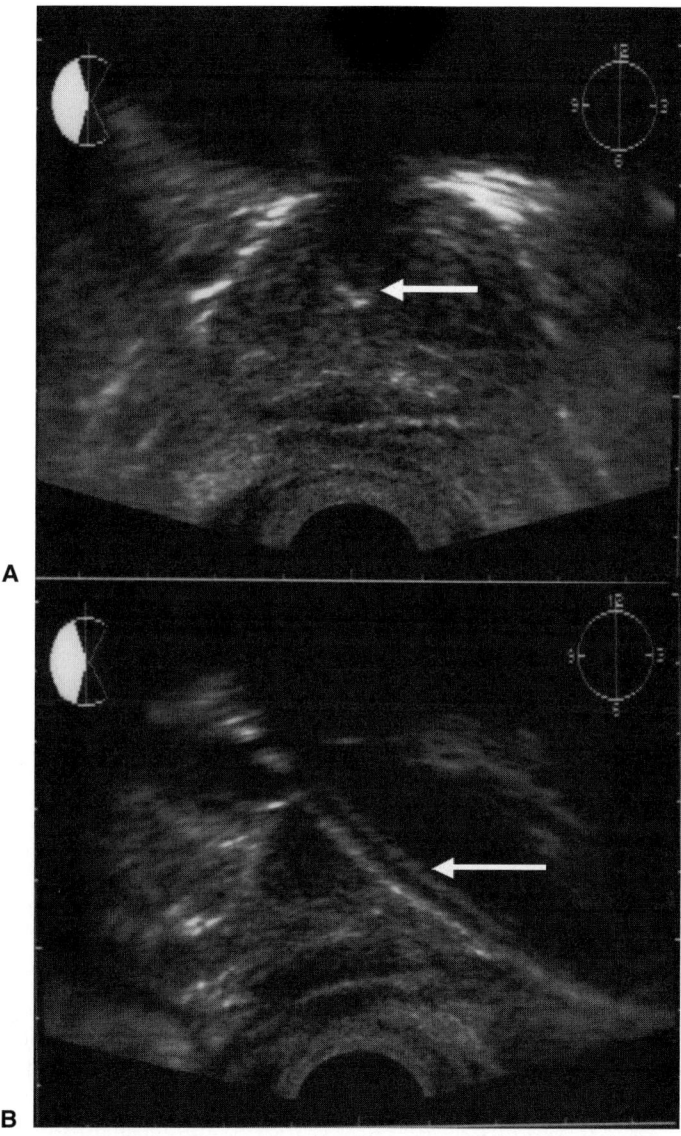

FIGURE 12.10. Transperineal scanning shows an oblique frontal view of the prostate gland **(A)** and sagittal view **(B)** in patient after abdominoperineal resection of rectum. A Foley catheter (arrow) guides the location of the prostate and urethra.

perineal ultrasound-guided prostate biopsy can be performed.[50] Generally, the procedure is performed with the patient in lithotomy position. To clearly visualize the urethra and bladder, placement of a Foley catheter is recommended. Intraprostatic information is very difficult to obtain by transperineal ultrasound, and the more important task of TRUS in this procedure is localization and delineation of the prostate boundary. For this purpose, a lower-frequency, 5- to 6-MHz, end-fire probe is ideal for scanning, because better penetration and visualization of deeper tissue are required. After preparation of the skin with an antiseptic solution, a probe is applied on the previous anus location, which is frequently identifiable by a small skin dimple. When the Foley catheter is identified, following the catheter will identify the balloon. At this point, the prostate is seen next to the balloon. The prostate can be visualized as either a longitudinal or cross-sectional image (Figure 12.10A,B). Local anesthesia is given in the perineal skin, pelvic floor, and all the way to the prostate gland by ultrasound guidance. Prostate biopsy can be done in either a sagittal or coronal view. A needle is advanced until it reaches the prostate capsule, confirmed by ultrasound and a tactile sensation. After the needle tip reaches the pro-static capsule, a biopsy specimen is taken. An extended sextant biopsy of 12 samples can be obtained. Seminal vesicles are frequently biopsied as a staging purpose whenever they are visible, because local staging cannot be performed by either digital rectal examination or transrectal ultrasonography.

Future Directions

Current biopsy techniques allow us to make a diagnosis of prostate cancer much more sensitive than before. Febrile complication and postbiopsy bleeding seem to be rare, and the procedure can be safely done in the clinic setting.

Even though high-tech imaging, such as magnetic resonance imaging/magnetic resonance spectroscopic imaging or power Doppler imaging, are available, prostate cancer diagnosis still heavily relies on the random biopsy. Prostate cancer is hence a unique malignancy that is detected by multiple, blind punctures of the organ, in the hope that some of the biopsy will find the cancer area. Despite taking more needle cores, biopsy is much less painful than ever before by using local anesthesia. However, patient discomfort associated with the biopsy is still tremendous. Obviously, a future direction of prostate cancer diagnosis will be to find a more noninvasive method. It could be a super-accurate tumor marker, ultrasensitive imaging modality, or a newer, tissue-diagnostic tool to detect a minor field effect specific to prostate cancer. Until such a method is established, prostate biopsy must continue to be performed.

References

1. Estimated new cancer cases and deaths by sex for all sites, US, 2006. Available at: http://www.cancer.org/downloads/stt/caff06escsmc.pdf. 2006.
2. SEER cancer statistics review 1975–2001. Available at: http://seer.cancer.gov/csr/a975_2001/results_merged/sect_22_prostate.pdf. 2006.
3. Ferguson RS. Prostatic neoplasms: their diagnosis by needle puncture and aspiration. Am J Surg 1930;9:507–11.
4. Astraldi A. Diagnosis of cancer of the prostate: biopsy by rectal route. Urol Cutan Rev 1937;41:421.
5. Torp-Pedersen S, Lee F, Littrup PJ, et al. Transrectal biopsy of the prostate guided with transrectal US: longitudinal and multiplanar scanning. Radiology 1989;170(1 Pt 1):23–7.
6. Hodge KK, McNeal JE, Terris MK, Stamey TA. Random systematic versus directed ultrasound guided transrectal core biopsies of the prostate. J Urol 1989;142(1):71–4; discussion 74–5.
7. Lee F, Torp-Pedersen ST, Siders DB, Littrup PJ, McLeary RD. Transrectal ultrasound in the diagnosis and staging of prostatic carcinoma. Radiology 1989;170(3 Pt 1):609–15.
8. Lindert KA, Kabalin JN, Terris MK. Bacteremia and bacteriuria after transrectal ultrasound guided prostate biopsy. J Urol 2000;164(1):76–80.
9. Lindstedt S, Lindstrom U, Ljunggren E, Wullt B, Grabe M. Single-dose antibiotic prophylaxis in core prostate biopsy: impact of timing and identification of risk factors. Eur Urol 2006;50(4):832–7.
10. Crawford ED, Haynes AL Jr, Story MW, Borden TA. Prevention of urinary tract infection and sepsis following transrectal prostatic biopsy. J Urol 1982;127(3):449–51.
11. Dajani AS, Taubert KA, Wilson W, et al. Prevention of bacterial endocarditis. Recommendations by the American Heart Association. JAMA 1997;277(22): 1794–801.
12. Herget EJ, Saliken JC, Donnelly BJ, Gray RR, Wiseman D, Brunet G. Transrectal ultrasound-guided biopsy of the prostate: relation between ASA use and bleeding complications. Can Assoc Radiol J 1999;50(3):173–6.
13. Maan Z, Cutting CW, Patel U, et al. Morbidity of transrectal ultrasonography-guided prostate biopsies in patients after the continued use of low-dose aspirin. BJU Int 2003;91(9):798–800.
14. Nijs HG, Essink-Bot ML, DeKoning HJ, Kirkels WJ, Schroder FH. Why do men refuse or attend population-based screening for prostate cancer? J Public Health Med 2000;22(3):312–16.
15. Nash PA, Bruce JE, Indudhara R, Shinohara K. Transrectal ultrasound guided prostatic nerve blockade eases systematic needle biopsy of the prostate. J Urol 1996;155(2):607–9.
16. Mutaguchi K, Shinohara K, Matsubara A, Yasumoto H, Mita K, Usui T. Local anesthesia during 10 core biopsy of the prostate: comparison of 2 methods. J Urol 2005;173(3):742–5.
17. Issa MM, Bux S, Chun T, et al. A randomized prospective trial of intrarectal lidocaine for pain control during transrectal prostate biopsy: the Emory University experience. J Urol 2000;164(2):397–9.

18. Stamey TA. Making the most out of six systematic sextant biopsies. Urology 1995;45(1):2–12.
19. Freedland SJ, Amling CL, Terris MK, et al. Is there a difference in outcome after radical prostatectomy between patients with biopsy Gleason sums 4, 5, and 6? Results from the SEARCH database. Prostate Cancer Prostatic Dis 2003;6(3):261–5.
20. Chang JJ, Shinohara K, Bhargava V, Presti JC Jr. Prospective evaluation of lateral biopsies of the peripheral zone for prostate cancer detection. J Urol 1998;160(6 Pt 1):2111–14.
21. Freiha FS, McNeal JE, Stamey TA. Selection criteria for radical prostatectomy based on morphometric studies in prostate carcinoma. NCI Monogr 1988(7): 107–8.
22. Eskew LA, Woodruff RD, Bare RL, McCullough DL. Prostate cancer diagnosed by the 5 region biopsy method is significant disease. J Urol 1998; 160(3 Pt 1):794–6.
23. Jones JS, Oder M, Zippe CD. Saturation prostate biopsy with periprostatic block can be performed in office. J Urol 2002;168(5):2108–10.
24. Borboroglu PG, Comer SW, Riffenburgh RH, Amling CL. Extensive repeat transrectal ultrasound guided prostate biopsy in patients with previous benign sextant biopsies. J Urol 2000;163(1):158–62.
25. Stewart CS, Leibovich BC, Weaver AL, Lieber MM. Prostate cancer diagnosis using a saturation needle biopsy technique after previous negative sextant biopsies. J Urol 2001;166(1):86–91; discussion 91–2.
26. Bott SR, Henderson A, McLarty E, Langley SE. A brachytherapy template approach to standardize saturation prostatic biopsy. BJU Int 2004;93(4): 629–30.
27. Rabets JC, Jones JS, Patel A, Zippe CD. Prostate cancer detection with office based saturation biopsy in a repeat biopsy population. J Urol 2004;172(1): 94–7.
28. Eichler K, Hempel S, Wilby J, Myers L, Bachmann LM, Kleijnen J. Diagnostic value of systematic biopsy methods in the investigation of prostate cancer: a systematic review. J Urol 2006;175(5):1605–12.
29. McNeal JE, Redwine EA, Freiha FS, et al. Zonal distribution of prostatic adenocarciinoma. Correlation with histologic pattern and direction of spread. Am J Surg Pathol 1988;12(12):897–906.
30. Chang JJ, Shinohara K, Hovey RM, Montgomery C, Presti JC Jr. Prospective evaluation of systematic sextant transition zone biopsies in large prostates for cancer detection. Urology 1998;52(1):89–93.
31. Takashima R, Egawa S, Kuwao S, Baba S. Anterior distribution of Stage T1c nonpalpable tumors in radical prostatectomy specimens. Urology 2002;59(5): 692–7.
32. Meng MV, Franks JH, Presti JC Jr, Shinohara K. The utility of apical anterior horn biopsies in prostate cancer detection. Urol Oncol 2003;21(5):361–5.
33. Meng MV, Shinohara K, Grossfeld GD. Significance of high-grade prostatic intraepithelial neoplasia on prostate biopsy. Urol Oncol 2003;21(2): 145–51.
34. Oyasu R, Bahnson RR, Nowels K, Garnett JE. Cytological atypia in the prostate gland: frequency, distribution and possible relevance to carcinoma. J Urol 1986;135(5):959–62.

35. Prange W, Erbersdobler A, Hammerer P, et al. Significance of high-grade prostatic intraepithelial neoplasia in needle biopsy specimens. Urology 2001; 57(3):486–90.
36. Lefkowitz GK, Sidhu GS, Torre P, Lepor H, Taneja SS. Is repeat prostate biopsy for high-grade prostatic intraepithelial neoplasia necessary after routine 12-core sampling? Urology 2001;58(6):999–1003.
37. Epstein JI, Herawi M. Prostate needle biopsies containing prostatic intraepithelial neoplasia or atypical foci suspicious for carcinoma: implications for patient care. J Urol 2006;175(3 Pt 1):820–34.
38. Helpap BG, Bostwick DG, Montironi R. The significance of atypical adenomatous hyperplasia and prostatic intraepithelial neoplasia for the development of prostate carcinoma. An update. Virchows Arch 1995;426(5):425–34.
39. Alsikafi NF, Brendler CB, Gerber GS, Yang XJ. High-grade prostatic intraepithelial neoplasia with adjacent atypia is associated with a higher incidence of cancer on subsequent needle biopsy than high-grade prostatic intraepithelial neoplasia alone. Urology 2001;57(2):296–300.
40. Park S, Shinohara K, Grossfeld GD, Carroll PR. Prostate cancer detection in men with prior high grade prostatic intraepithelial neoplasia or atypical prostate biopsy. J Urol 2001;165(5):1409–14.
41. Allen EA, Kahane H, Epstein JI. Repeat biopsy strategies for men with atypical diagnoses on initial prostate needle biopsy. Urology 1998;52(5):803–7.
42. Kawakami S, Kihara K, Fujii Y, Masuda H, Kobayashi T, Kageyama Y. Transrectal ultrasound-guided transperineal 14-core systematic biopsy detects apico-anterior cancer foci of T1c prostate cancer. Int J Urol 2004;11(8):613–18.
43. Pinkstaff DM, Igel TC, Petrou SP, Broderick GA, Wehle MJ, Young PR. Systematic transperineal ultrasound-guided template biopsy of the prostate: three-year experience. Urology 2005;65(4):735–9.
44. Satoh T, Matsumoto K, Fujita T, et al. Cancer core distribution in patients diagnosed by extended transperineal prostate biopsy. Urology 2005;66(1): 114–18.
45. Crawford ED, Wilson SS, Torkko KC, et al. Clinical staging of prostate cancer: a computer-simulated study of transperineal prostate biopsy. BJU Int 2005;96(7):999–1004.
46. Puppo P, Introini C, Calvi P, Naselli A. Role of transurethral resection of the prostate and biopsy of the peripheral zone in the same session after repeated negative biopsies in the diagnosis of prostate cancer. Eur Urol 2006;49(5): 873–8.
47. Turkeri L, Tarcan T, Biren T, Kullu S, Akdas A. Transrectal ultrasonography versus digitally guided prostate biopsies in patients with palpable lesions on digital rectal examination. Br J Urol 1995;76(2):184–6.
48. Foster LS, Jajodia P, Fournier G Jr, Shinohara K, Carroll P, Narayan P. The value of prostate specific antigen and transrectal ultrasound guided biopsy in detecting prostatic fossa recurrences following radical prostatectomy. J Urol 1993;149(5):1024–8.
49. Connolly JA, Shinohara K, Presti JC Jr, Carroll PR. Local recurrence after radical prostatectomy: characteristics in size, location, and relationship to prostate-specific antigen and surgical margins. Urology 1996;47(2):225–31.
50. Shinohara K, Gulati M, Koppie TM, Terris MK. Transperineal prostate biopsy after abdominoperineal resection. J Urol 2003;169(1):141–4.

13
Biopsy Strategies—How Many and Where?

Joseph C. Presti, Jr.

Abstract

Definitive prostate cancer diagnosis can only be made through histologic evaluation of prostate tissue. Transrectal ultrasound–guided, 10- to 12-core biopsy is the gold standard for practicing urologists and should be routinely used in initial evaluation because this examination contributes significantly to risk stratification models for men with localized cancer. Anterior biopsies may be less significant than other samples in extended biopsy schemes. A greater number of lateral and transition zone–directed needle biopsies may be recommended in men with critical risk factors such as advanced age, substantially elevated prostate-specific antigen (PSA) level, or prostate volume >50 cc. PSA density and PSA transition zone density are also useful in distinguishing prostate cancer from benign prostatic hyperplasia.

The diagnostic value of needle cores is greatly increased if the cores are divided into separate sample bottles, thus pathologic results would be more informative and useful in determining the prognosis of prostate cancer. Simply separating cores into two bottles by laterality has important clinical significance, serving as a guide for repeat biopsy and/or focal therapy if its role becomes established. However, many clinicians do not practice these measures because they increase the cost of biopsy screening.

Keywords: prostate biopsy, biopsy strategy, repeat biopsy, extended core biopsy, PSA density

Brief History of Prostate Biopsy

The diagnosis of prostate cancer can only be established after histologic evaluation of prostate tissue. Before the use of prostate-specific antigen (PSA), "early" diagnosis of prostate cancer resulted from the detection of

From: *Current Clinical Urology: Prostate Biopsy: Indications, Techniques, and Complications*
Edited by J.S. Jones © Humana Press, Totowa, NJ

prostatic induration on digital rectal examination and subsequent biopsy. Transperineal biopsies performed under digital guidance were the predominant method of prostate cancer detection used until the 1980s. The introduction of serum PSA testing for prostate cancer screening resulted in the indication for a prostate biopsy in the absence of any abnormality on digital rectal examination. Thus, the need for "random sampling of the prostate" arose and systematic biopsy was born. When introduced in 1989, systematic sextant biopsies under transrectal ultrasound guidance revolutionized our ability to detect prostate cancer.[1] Traditional systematic sextant biopsies were usually performed in the parasagittal plane halfway between the lateral border and midline of the prostate on both right and left sides from the base, midgland, and apex (Figure 13.1). From the meticulous

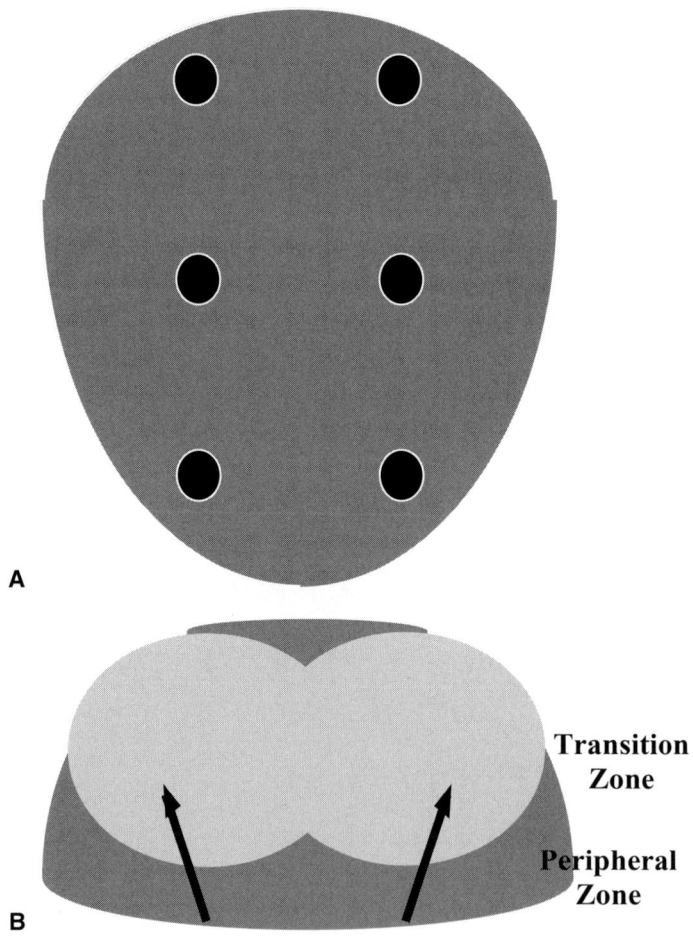

FIGURE 13.1. **A**: Standard sextant biopsy in coronal plane showing apex, mid, and base biopsies. **B**: Standard sextant biopsy in cross-sectional plane at level of midgland showing needle placement halfway between the midline and the lateral edge of prostate.

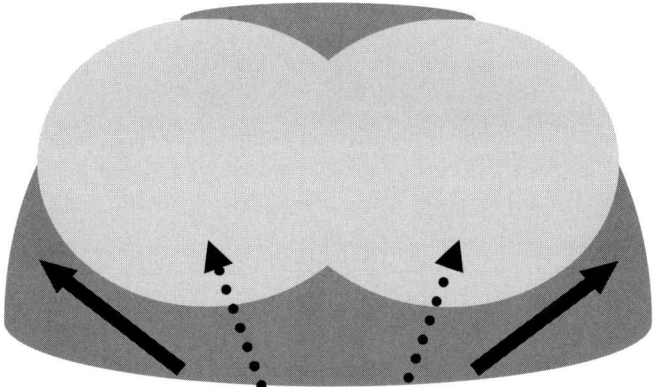

FIGURE 13.2. Needle cores are directed more laterally to better sample the anterior horn of the peripheral zone (solid arrows) compared with standard sextant needle cores (dashed arrows).

analyses of radical prostatectomy specimens, it was clear that the majority of prostate cancers (approximately 80%) originated in the peripheral zone.[2] With a better understanding of the zonal anatomy of the prostate, Stamey[3] suggested a modification of the standard sextant biopsy scheme by directing the biopsy needle more laterally to better sample the anterior horns of the peripheral zone (Figure 13.2). However, the sextant biopsy scheme remained the "gold standard" for prostate cancer detection for several more years.

Evolution of the Extended Biopsy Schemes

One of the first studies to assess the utility of extended peripheral zone biopsy schemes came from Eskew et al.[4] who reported on their five-region biopsy scheme (Figure 13.3). The five regions included the standard sextant biopsy regimen obtained halfway between the lateral border and midline of the prostate on both right and left sides (regions 2 and 4) but in addition obtained two biopsies from each lateral aspect of the prostate (regions 1 and 5) and three biopsies from the midline at the apex, midgland, and base (region 3). Of the 119 patients, 48 (40%) had cancer detected by biopsy, of which 17 (35% of cancers detected) were only detected in regions 1, 3, and 5. Of note, only two cancers were detected solely by the three centrally placed biopsies of region 3. With respect to complications, these investigators reported an 80% incidence of gross hematuria, which they attributed to the region 3 biopsies, which probably penetrated the urethra.

The work of Eskew et al. prompted us to investigate the utility of adding four lateral biopsies of the peripheral zone to the routine sextant biopsy

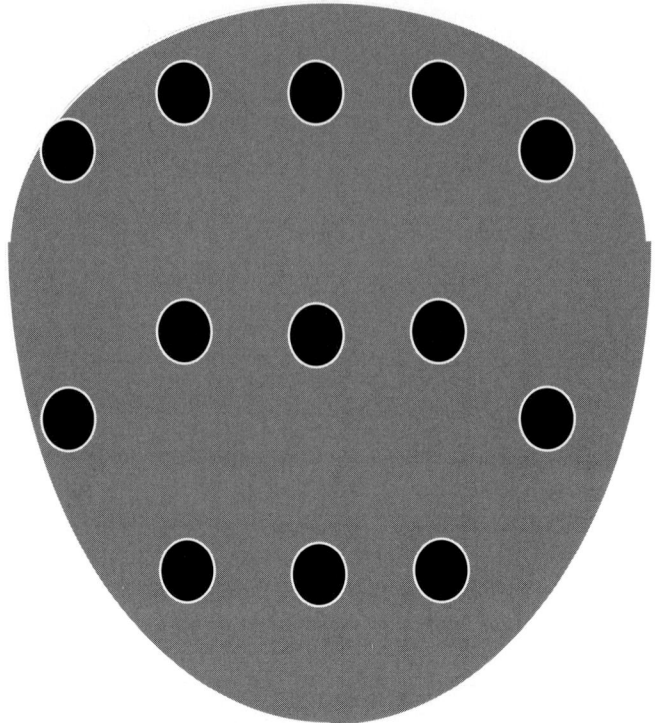

FIGURE 13.3. Five-region biopsy scheme, including a total of 13 cores form the standard sextant (regions 2 and 4), the lateral aspect of the gland (regions 1 and 5), and the midline (region 3).

regimen (10-core biopsy scheme).[5] Because the midline biopsies, as described above, had a very low unique cancer detection rate and resulted in a high complication rate, they were deleted from our biopsy template (Figure 13.4). This prospective study evaluated 483 consecutive patients who had not been previously biopsied and were referred because of an abnormal digital rectal examination or an elevated PSA. All identified hypoechoic lesions were first biopsied before obtaining systematic biopsies. Sextant biopsies were obtained in the midlobar parasagittal plane, halfway between the lateral edge and midline of the prostate gland, at the base, midgland, and apex. The lateral biopsies were performed by positioning the probe just medial to the lateral edge of the prostate at the mid and base portions of the gland. In patients with prostate sizes exceeding 50 cc, in addition to this 10-core biopsy scheme, six additional anteriorly directed biopsies were performed in the midlobar parasagittal plane at the apex, mid, and base (16-core systematic biopsy). For these additional cores, the needle was advanced to within 1.5 cm of the anterior prostate capsule before firing the biopsy gun. Forty-two percent of the patients had cancer on biopsy (202 of 483). Routine sextant biopsies detected 161 cancers (80% of all cancers detected) whereas the combination of sextant and lateral biopsies, for a total of 10 peripheral zone biopsies, detected 194 cancers (96% of all cancers detected). The eight missed cancers were detected by the lesion-directed (n = 5) or the anteriorly directed biopsies in glands >50 cc (n = 3). We noted several important results from this study: 1) traditional sextant biopsies may miss more than 20% of cancers; 2) a lateral sextant regimen (apex, lateral mid, lateral base) outperforms the traditional midlobar sextant regimen (89% vs. 80%, respectively; p = 0.027); 3) regardless of the number of systematic biopsies performed (6 vs. 8 vs. 10), variations in cancer detection rates were most pronounced in patients with PSA levels <10 ng/mL or in patients with prostate sizes ≥50 cc, reflecting the importance of sampling because patients with lower PSA levels or larger prostates more often may have smaller cancer volumes per unit of prostate tissue; 4) anteriorly directed biopsies rarely uniquely identify cancers in men undergoing initial biopsies with an extended peripheral zone scheme; 5) when performed in conjunction with extended peripheral zone biopsy

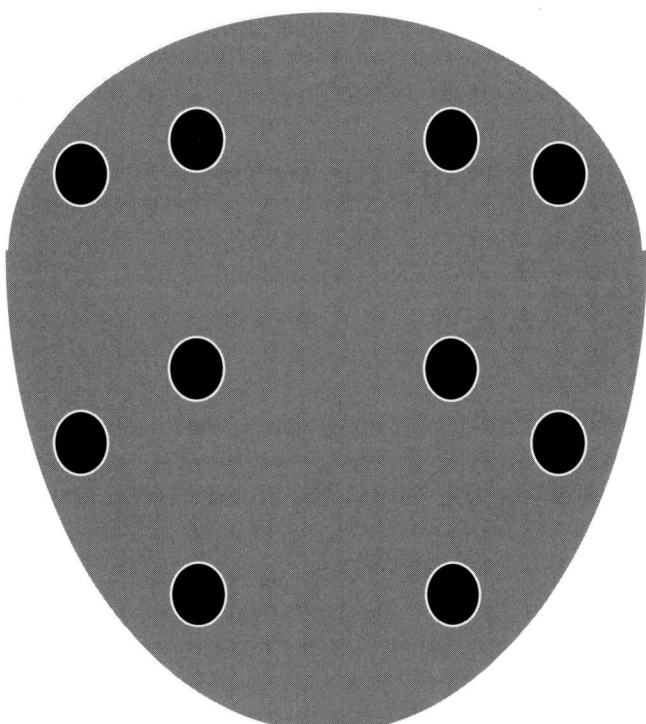

FIGURE 13.4. Ten-core biopsy scheme consisting of standard sextant laterally directed cores at mid and base.

schemes, lesion-directed biopsies provide little unique cancer identification; 6) when comparing the detection rates of the five systematic peripheral zone regions in the 10-biopsy scheme, the midlobar base region demonstrated the lowest detection rate as well as the lowest unique cancer detection rate. From the latter observation, we believed that the midlobar base biopsy could be omitted from the systematic biopsy scheme. The low yield from this site might be because this biopsy site may, in part, be sampling the central zone, where the incidence of cancer is low (<5%).

Several other investigators have reported on various extended biopsy schemes. Babaian et al.[6] evaluated an 11-core biopsy strategy in 362 patients. Of note, only 85 of these patients (23%) were first-time biopsy patients. The biopsy scheme included the standard sextant along with bilateral anterior horn biopsies, bilateral transition zone biopsies, and a midline biopsy (Figure 13.5). The detection rate for patients undergoing initial biopsy was 34% (29 of 85) and nine cancers were uniquely identified by nonsextant sites (31% increase in cancer detection rate). Of the nonsextant, uniquely identified cancers, seven were identified by the anterior horn biopsies and two by the transition zone biopsy.

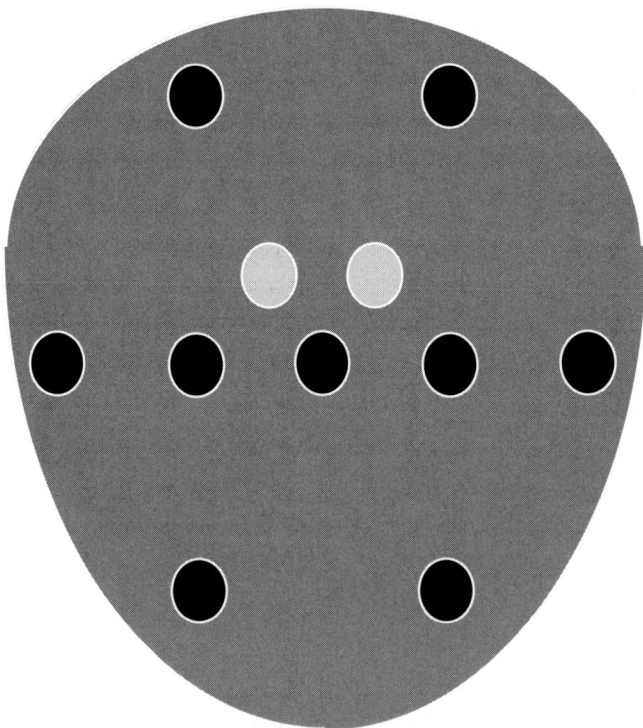

FIGURE 13.5. Eleven-core biopsy scheme. The two lighter sites are transition zone biopsies.

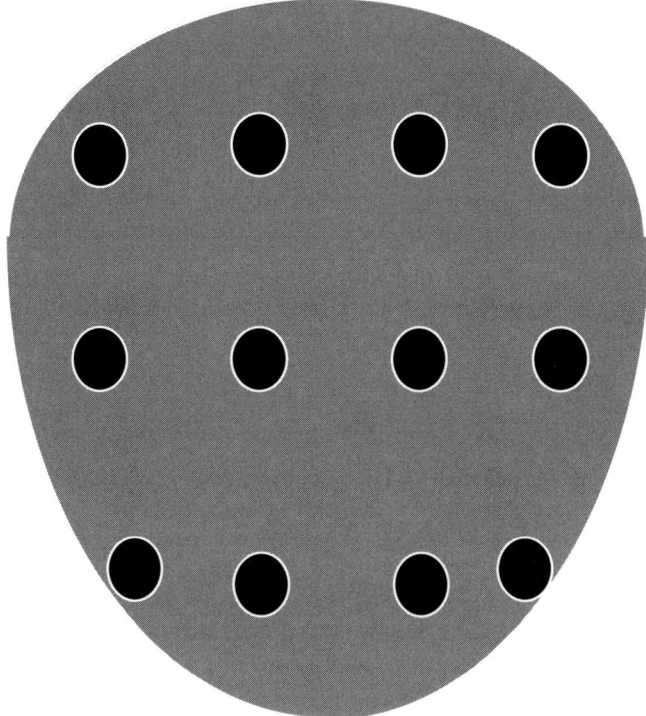

FIGURE 13.6. Twelve-core biopsy scheme.

Gore et al.[7] evaluated a 12-core biopsy scheme in 396 patients. A standard sextant scheme was combined with a laterally directed sextant scheme at the apex, mid, and base bilaterally (Figure 13.6). This series was comprised of 264 (67%) first-time biopsy patients and the cancer detection rate in this subgroup was 42%. Standard sextant biopsies would have detected only 71% of the cancers in this group. The lateral sextant biopsy scheme along with the apical and base biopsies from the standard sextant scheme detected all of the cancers in this subgroup.

The above-mentioned studies were all single-site, academic center, experiences. Analogous to the development of therapeutic clinical trials, we thought it important to validate extended biopsy schemes in a multicenter situation. To do this, we analyzed a retrospective data set of 2299 patients who had undergone a 12-core systematic biopsy scheme (similar to what is depicted in Figure 13.6) by 167 community-based urologists.[8] All patients were first-time biopsy patients and the overall cancer detection rate was 44%. This large series demonstrated the reproducibility of extended biopsy schemes in the hands of practicing urologists and it is interesting to note that the overall detection rates were essentially identical to those

TABLE 13.1. Age-stratified detection rates.

Age	No. of patients	No. of cancers	Detection rates (%)	% with grade 4 or 5
≤59	516	171	33	46
60–64	338	133	39	56
65–69	465	211	45	62
70–74	441	214	49	63
75–79	332	177	53	68
≥80	207	114	55	81

demonstrated by several of the above-mentioned studies. It is obvious that detection rates in referral-based populations (patients referred because of an abnormal digital rectal examination or an elevated PSA level) will vary as a function of the patient population, and this large series enabled analyses that could be stratified for age and PSA. Table 13.1 demonstrates the detection rates as a function of age. Note that the detection rate increases with increasing age; however, also note that the percentage of patients with high-grade cancer on the biopsy (presence of grade 4 or 5) also increases with increasing age. Similar observations are seen when the data are stratified for PSA (Table 13.2). Increasing PSA levels are associated with higher detection rates as well as a higher percentage of patients harboring high-grade cancer. Table 13.3 shows the overall and unique cancer detection rates for each of the specific biopsy sites in the 12-core biopsy scheme. In general, the lowest yield comes from the midlobar-mid and midlobar-base biopsy from the standard sextant scheme. When various biopsy schemes were retrospectively simulated and then compared with the "gold-

TABLE 13.2. Prostate-specific antigen (PSA)-stratified detection rates.

PSA (ng/mL)	No. of patients	No. of cancers	Detection rates (%)	% with grade 4 or 5
<2	86	16	19	36
2–4	145	50	35	36
4.1–7	800	350	44	59
7.1–10	313	157	50	64
10.1–20	227	110	49	72
>20	112	76	68	80

TABLE 13.3. Site-specific overall and unique cancer detection rates in multipractice initial biopsy study (n = 2299).

Site	Overall detection rate (%)	Unique detection rate (%)
Apex	50	5.8
Mid	48	3.1
Base	42	4.2
Lateral apex	52	7.0
Lateral mid	54	5.6
Lateral base	49	3.7

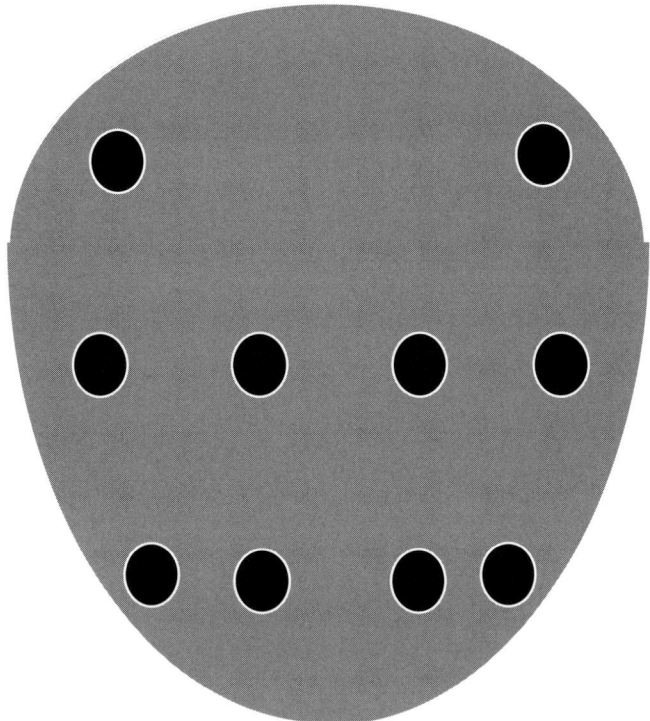

FIGURE 13.7. Optimal 10-core scheme. Similar to 12-core scheme, deleting the biopsies at the base from the standard sextant scheme.

standard" 12-biopsy scheme (assume it detects 100% of the cancers in the population), the following rates were observed: standard sextant had 78%; lateral apex, lateral mid, lateral base (lateral sextant) had 83%; apex, lateral apex, lateral mid, lateral base (optimal 8-core scheme) had 92%; apex, mid, lateral apex, lateral mid, lateral base (optimal 10-core scheme, Figure 13.7) had 96%.

The above studies have resulted in an acceptance of extended biopsy schemes by most urologists as the standard. Despite this advancement, more work needs to be done in better tailoring the biopsy scheme to prostate size and shape. It is possible that the number of cores should be adjusted for the cephalocaudad length of the prostate. It is well established that in a referral-based biopsy population, cancer detection rates are inversely proportional to prostate size. As with any situation that involves sampling, the possibility of sampling error exists. This notion was supported in prostate biopsy series by a study demonstrating an inverse relationship between prostate gland size and cancer detection rates as determined by sextant biopsies (Figure 13.8).[9] It is now recognized that sextant biopsies

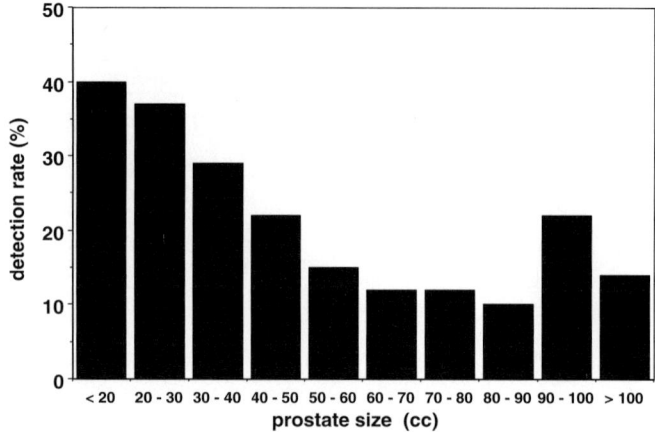

FIGURE 13.8. Relationship between prostate gland size and cancer detection rates as determined by sextant biopsies.

could miss up to 30% of cancers.[10,11] The notion of sampling error has been further supported by the novel study by Levine et al.[12] In this study, two consecutive sets of sextant biopsies of the prostate in a single office visit in 137 consecutive patients were performed. A total of 43 cancers were detected in the entire study population (31% cancer detection rate). Using the first sextant biopsy set as the reference set, 30 cancers were detected (70% of all cancers) so the second biopsy set increased the detection rate by 30%. However, if the second biopsy set had been used as the reference, 40 cancers were detected (93% of all cancers), whereas the first biopsy set would have only increased the detection rate by 7%.

Number and Location for Repeat Biopsy

One of the most challenging dilemmas facing urologists is the management of patients who have had a prior negative biopsy, yet have persistently increasing PSA levels or other indicators heightening one's suspicion for the presence of prostate cancer. It is important in this evaluation to first address the adequacy of the initial biopsy. Factors to consider include the location and number of cores taken as well as the size of the prostate. We have previously reported that in a repeat biopsy population, detection rates vary as a function of how many cores were obtained.[13] In the Stanford series, cancer detection rates were higher in patients who had undergone a prior sextant biopsy compared with a prior extended biopsy scheme. Of the 153 patients who had undergone a prior sextant biopsy, 59 patients (39%) had cancer on repeat biopsy. Of the 65 patients who had undergone a prior extended biopsy, 18 patients (28%) had cancer on repeat biopsy. In this

TABLE 13.4. Overall and unique site-specific cancer detection rates by type of prior negative biopsy (n = 218).

Site	Overall detection rate (%)		Unique detection rate (%)	
	Prior sextant	Prior extended	Prior sextant	Prior extended
Apex	49	56	6.8	27.8
Mid	41	17	0	5.6
Base	32	22	1.7	5.6
Lateral mid	51	0	6.8	0
Lateral base	56	28	13.6	11.1
Six anterior biopsies	32	33	3.4	5.6

Note: Anterior biopsies include anterior apex, anterior mid, and anterior base sites.

study, we also further analyzed the utility of each of the individual core sites. Site-specific detection rates are shown in Table 13.4 stratified by the type of prior negative biopsy. In general, apical and laterally directed biopsies resulted in the highest overall and unique cancer detection rates. The yield from laterally directed biopsies decreased in patients who had undergone prior extended biopsy schemes because these regions had been previously sampled by this negative biopsy. A subset of 139 patients underwent six additional anteriorly directed, transition zone biopsies. Note that unique cancer yields in the anterior biopsies (cumulative for a total of six cores per patient) were low regardless of type of prior biopsy scheme (3.4% for prior sextant biopsy and 5.6% for prior extended biopsy). This further confirmed the lack of utility of transition biopsies in these patients.

Unfortunately, despite the use of extended biopsy schemes, some patients in whom we have a high index of suspicion for cancer, fail to show cancer on repeat biopsy. Such patients might warrant saturation biopsies. This approach is discussed elsewhere in this book.

Utility of Individual Core Labeling and Risk Stratification

As we have increased the number of needle cores obtained, the question of whether these cores need to be individually labeled (site-specific labeling) has been raised. Certainly, from a research perspective, individual core labeling was critical in the evolution of the extended core biopsy scheme. Only then could we uniquely identify the individual contribution for each site to the extended biopsy scheme. However, for the practicing urologist, is it necessary to individually identify each core? This is not only a matter of convenience for the urologist, it often also impacts the charges generated by the pathologist. In most pathology departments, a charge is generated for each separate sample bottle. Thus, if 12 cores are placed into one bottle, a charge is generated, yet if those same 12 cores are now placed into 12 separate bottles, the charge is 12-fold increased. At a minimum, the cores should be divided into right and left sides of the prostate. We should recognize that the utility of the needle cores goes well beyond the presence or absence of cancer. In addition, these needle cores contribute to risk assessment in patients found to have cancer. Several investigators have demonstrated that either the percentage of positive cores or the cumulative measured cancer length contributes to the risk of pathologic end points, such as extracapsular extension, and also to the risk of serologic relapse after radical prostatectomy.[14–17] Knowing the laterality of the pathologic needle data contributes to plans for ipsilateral nerve preservation or wide excision at radical prostatectomy. Extended biopsy schemes also result in more accurate prediction of tumor grade within the prostate. In one series, we showed that clinically significant upgrading occurred in 38% of patients if a standard sextant scheme was used compared with 23% of patients if data from an extended biopsy scheme were available (p = 0.039).[18] One disadvantage of separating the cores into just right and left sides is that if a biopsy shows atypical small acinar proliferation, then the site of the abnormality is lost for the direction of additional needle cores at repeat biopsy. Certainly, irrespective of the number of cores obtained, the number of bottles submitted can at least be half the number of cores, by applying a dye to the tissue before placement in the fixative. In this scenario, one color corresponds to the right side and the second color corresponds to the left side and thus the individual needle core site is preserved.

Utility of Prostate-Specific Antigen and Its Indices for the Indications for Biopsy

PSA density (PSAD) has been popularized by Benson and associates[19,20] in its ability to distinguish between PSA elevations resulting from prostate cancer versus benign prostatic hyperplasia. PSAD is calculated by dividing the total serum PSA level by the entire volume of the prostate as determined by transrectal ultrasound. Typically, the prostate volume is estimated using a prolate ellipse formula, the volume equals $\pi/6 \times$ length $\times$ width $\times$ height where length is obtained in the longitudinal plane and height and width are obtained in the axial plane. A further refinement of this index has been the realization that as a prostate enlarges with age, most of the enlargement occurs in the transition zone. Thus, one can calculate a transition zone density (PSAD-TZ). These indices have been studied by numerous investigators; however, in most cases, these have relied on sextant biopsy sampling as the gold standard for the determination of the presence or absence of prostate cancer. One of the larger studies analyzed 974 consecutive patients with total PSA levels between 4 and 10 ng/mL and applied both age and prostate-volume stratifications.[21] These authors concluded that for total prostate volumes ≤30 cc, a cut point of 0.18 and 0.44 should be used for PSAD and PSAD-TZ, respectively. For prostates >30 cc, corresponding cut points of 0.11 and 0.26 should be used for PSAD and PSAD-TZ, respectively. Although intriguing, these cut points need to be further validated in a large series of patients undergoing extended biopsy schemes. In addition, the disadvantage of such indices is that they require either total or transition zone volume measurement by transrectal ultrasound. Thus, biopsy decisions would have to be made only after insertion of the ultrasound probe. I currently use these indices as part of a decision algorithm in determining the need of a *repeat* biopsy rather than in patients being evaluated for an *initial* biopsy.

Conclusions

Extended biopsy schemes have increased our ability to detect prostate cancer and significantly contribute to risk stratification models for men with localized prostate cancer. In addition, they provide more reliable results with respect to predicting the grade of cancer and facilitate treatment planning. A 10- or 12-core extended biopsy scheme should routinely be used in the initial evaluation of patients for prostate cancer.

References

1. Hodge KK, McNeal JE, Terris MK, Stamey TA. Random systematic versus directed ultrasound guided transrectal core biopsies of the prostate. J Urol 1989;142:71–5.
2. McNeal JE, Redwine EA, Freiha FS, Stamey TA. Zonal distribution of prostatic adenocarcinoma: correlation with histologic pattern and direction of spread. Am J Surg Pathol 1988;12:897–906.
3. Stamey TA. Making the most out of six systematic sextant biopsies. Urology 1995;45:2–12.
4. Eskew LA, Bare RL, McCullough DL. Systematic 5 region prostate biopsy is superior to sextant method for diagnosing carcinoma of the prostate. J Urol 1997;157:199–203.
5. Presti JC Jr, Chang JJ, Bhargava V, Shinohara K. The optimal systematic prostate biopsy scheme should include 8 rather than 6 biopsies: results of a prospective clinical trial. J Urol 2000;163:163–6.
6. Babaian RJ, Toi A, Kamoi K, et al. A comparative analysis of sextant and an extended 11-core multisite directed biopsy strategy. J Urol 2000;163:152–7.
7. Gore JL, Shariat SF, Miles BJ, et al. Optimal combinations of systematic sextant and laterally directed biopsies for the detection of prostate cancer. J Urol 2001;165:1554–9.
8. Presti JC Jr, O'Dowd G, Miller MC, Mattu R, Veltri RW. Extended peripheral zone biopsy schemes increase cancer detection rates and minimize variance in prostate specific antigen and age related cancer rates: results of a community multi-practice study. J Urol 2003;169:125–9.

9. Karakiewicz PI, Bazinet M, Aprikian AG, et al. Outcome of sextant biopsy according to gland volume. Urology 1997;49:55–9.
10. Rabbani F, Stroumbakis N, Kava BR, Cookson MS, Fair WR. Incidence and clinical significance of false-negative sextant prostate biopsies. J Urol 1998;159:1247–50.
11. Norberg M, Egevad L, Holmberg L, Sparén P, Norlén BJ, Busch C. The sextant protocol for ultrasound-guided core biopsies of the prostate underestimates the presence of cancer. Urology 1997;50:562–6.
12. Levine MA, Ittman M, Melamed J, Lepor H. Two consecutive sets of transrectal ultrasound guided sextant biopsies of the prostate for the detection of prostate cancer. J Urol 1998;159:471–6.
13. Hong YM, Lai FC, Chon CH, McNeal JE, Presti JC Jr. Impact of prior biopsy scheme on pathologic features of cancers detected on repeat biopsies. Urol Oncol 2004;22:7–10.
14. D'Amico AV, Whittington R, Malkowicz SB, et al. Clinical utility of the percentage of positive prostate biopsies in defining biochemical outcome after radical prostatectomy for patients with clinically localized prostate cancer. J Clin Oncol 2000;18:1164.
15. Freedland SJ, Aronson WJ, Csathy GS, et al. Comparison of percent of total prostate needle biopsy tissue with cancer to percent of cores with cancer for predicting PSA recurrence following radical prostatectomy: results from the SEARCH database. Urology 2003;61:742–7.
16. Freedland SJ, Presti JC Jr, Terris MK, et al. Improved clinical staging system combining biopsy laterality and TNM stage for men with T1c and T2 prostate cancer: results from the SEARCH database. J Urol 2003;169:2129–36.
17. Freedland SJ, Aronson WJ, Terris MK, et al. Percent of prostate needle biopsy cores with cancer is a significant independent predictor of PSA recurrence following radical prostatectomy: results from the SEARCH database. J Urol 2003;169:2136–41.
18. King CR, McNeal JE, Gill HR, Presti JC Jr. Extended prostate biopsy scheme improves reliability of Gleason grading: implications for radiotherapy patients. Int J Radiat Oncol 2004;59:386–91.
19. Benson MC, Whang IS, Olsson CA, et al. The use of prostate-specific antigen density to enhance the predictive value of intermediate levels of serum prostate-specific antigen. J Urol 1992;147:817–21.
20. Benson MC, Whang IS, Pantuck A, et al. Prostate-specific antigen density: a means of distinguishing benign prostatic hypertrophy and prostate cancer. J Urol 1992;147:815–6.
21. Djavan B, Zlotta AR, Remzi M, et al. Total and transition zone prostate volume and age: how do they affect the utility of PSA-based diagnostic parameters for early prostate cancer detection? Urology 1999;54:846–52.

14
Transperineal Prostate Biopsy

Paolo Emiliozzi and Vito Pansadoro

Abstract

Transperineal prostate biopsy is receiving renewed scientific interest. Although neglected for several decades in favor of transrectal ultrasound biopsy, the transperineal procedure continues to have a minor, but defined and specific role in prostate cancer diagnosis. It is an effective procedure for detection and has a low incidence of infective complications. This chapter illustrates the technique and surgical approach for transperineal biopsy. Comparison of the two procedures is offered.

Keywords: transperineal, prostate biopsy, transrectal, saturation biopsy

With the increasing and extensive use of prostate-specific antigen (PSA) screening, prostate cancer detection has gained a major role in urologic oncology. Prostate biopsy is the mainstay of prostate cancer diagnosis.

The transperineal route for prostate biopsy is not new. In 1972, Peck[1] found prostate cancer in 55 of 190 patients with transperineal biopsy under digital rectal guidance. In 1993, Webb et al.[2] studied 171 patients undergoing transperineal biopsy and found very low incidence of infective complications (0.5%). They proposed to reserve the transperineal approach to high-risk or elderly patients.

With the increasing use of transrectal ultrasound (TRUS), transrectal prostate biopsy with the needle passing through the probe, under the direct control of the needle marker, has rapidly gained popularity, because of the ease of the procedure. After the 1989 report of Hodge and coworkers,[3] showing that a six-core random biopsy was more effective than lesion-directed biopsy for prostate cancer detection, transrectal sextant biopsy

From: *Current Clinical Urology: Prostate Biopsy: Indications, Techniques, and Complications*
Edited by J.S. Jones © Humana Press, Totowa, NJ

became the standard procedure for prostate biopsy for nearly a decade. However, because of a high incidence of false negatives with sextant prostate biopsy, further protocols including an increased number of cores to improve cancer detection rate have been introduced in recent years.[4]

The transrectal prostate biopsy is the favorite approach in the United States, where only 2% of urologists[5] perform transperineal biopsy regularly. The transperineal approach was long neglected in the urologic literature in the 1990s. However, in some European countries (especially Italy) and in some Asian countries (mainly Japan), the procedure was and is still performed.[4,6] An increase of papers dealing with prostate biopsy in 2005 created a new scientific interest in the transperineal procedure. Transperineal biopsy has a minor, but defined and specific place in urology for prostate cancer diagnosis.

Technique

Anticoagulant therapy should be stopped 7 days before the procedure. If needed, low-molecular-weight heparin can be administered to the patient. A cleansing enema is not strictly required. Antibiotic cover is not routinely provided, unless there is a history of recent genitourinary infection, or an indwelling catheter.

The patient is in the lithotomy position. The scrotum is held above the perineum by the patient's hand. In case of general anesthesia, which is very rarely required, the scrotum is fixed upward with adhesive tape. It is important to instruct the patient to maintain the same position of the scrotum for all the procedure. If the scrotum is stirred upward and downward by the patient, the perineal planes can move and the anesthesia can be less effective. Digital rectal examination (DRE) is performed. A transrectal longitudinal probe is inserted. The perineum is disinfected. The local anesthesia is accomplished with a solution of 20 cc of 2% mepivacaine plus 1 cc of sodium bicarbonate, to decrease the burning sensation during the injection. Two points above the anus, at 45° on each side, and at 15 mm from the anus, are selected (Figure 14.1).

Under ultrasound control, a 22-gauge spinal needle is inserted. The local anesthetic is slowly released under the skin. The needle is advanced through the perineum, and directed toward the space between the prostatic apex and the rectum, under constant ultrasound guidance. It is easy to move the needle in the direction desired, as long as the probe and the needle are maintained exactly parallel. The probe must follow the needle through rotating and tilting movements. They are both parallel when the whole needle can be seen on the screen, for all its length. If only a part of the needle is shown, the position of the probe must be corrected until the full length of the needle is visible. When the needle and the probe are perfectly parallel, an artifact double image of the needle can be seen (Figure 14.2).

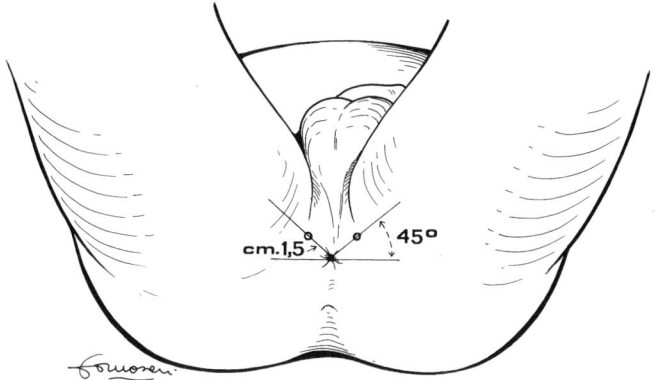

FIGURE 14.1. The position of the patient, and the points of anesthetic injection.

Although the description may seem complicated, the procedure is easily performed with a short learning curve. Once the space between the rectum and the prostate is reached, near the prostatic apex, the anesthetic is gently injected and the needle is pushed toward the base of the prostate (Figure 14.3A–C), at the insertion of the seminal vesicle. With this maneuver, the

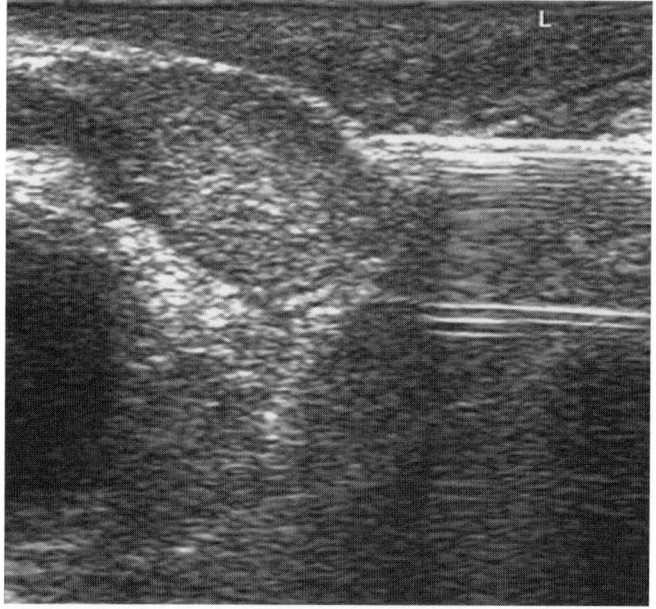

FIGURE 14.2. When the transrectal probe and the needle are exactly parallel, a double needle image can be seen. The lower image is an artifact.

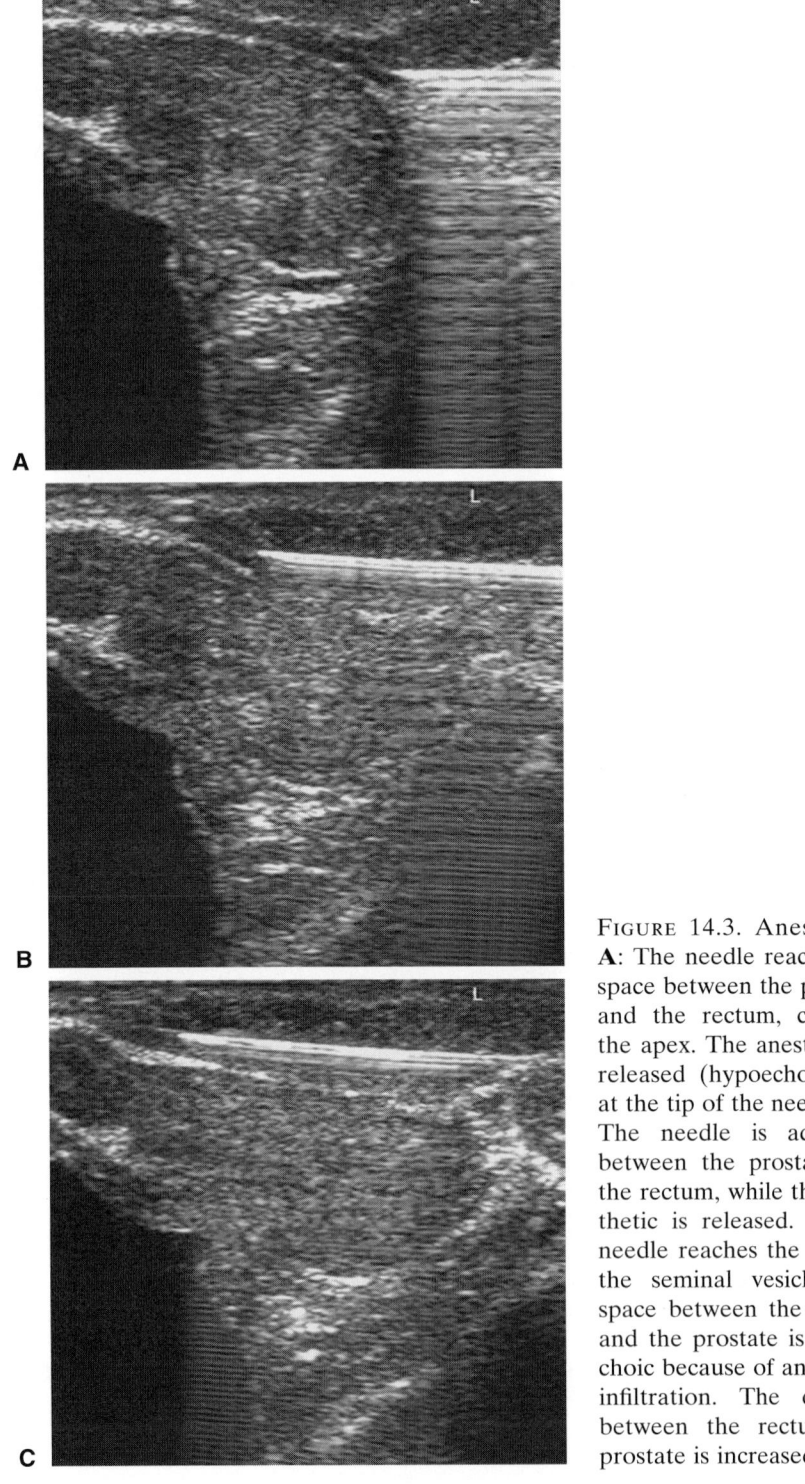

FIGURE 14.3. Anesthesia.
A: The needle reaches the
space between the prostate
and the rectum, close to
the apex. The anesthetic is
released (hypoechoic area
at the tip of the needle). **B**:
The needle is advanced
between the prostate and
the rectum, while the anesthetic is released. **C**: The
needle reaches the base of
the seminal vesicle. The
space between the rectum
and the prostate is hypoechoic because of anesthetic
infiltration. The distance
between the rectum and
prostate is increased.

space between the rectum and the prostate is infiltrated and the prostate is raised above the rectum (Figure 14.3C).

The anesthetic is constantly released while the needle is slowly retracted backward. A sudden and instantaneous discomfort may be felt by the patient when the anesthetic is released in the levator ani muscle. The anesthesia is repeated on the contralateral side with the same technique.

After 60–120 seconds, the biopsy procedure is started. Each lobe of the prostate is ideally divided into six sections in a fan shape (far lateral, lateral, lateral midlobe, medial midlobe, paramedian, close to midline). The needle is advanced toward the peripheral area of the prostate. The ultrasound probe is maintained exactly parallel to the needle, and every "sextant" of each lobe is targeted and reached (Figures 14.4 and 14.5), with a fan

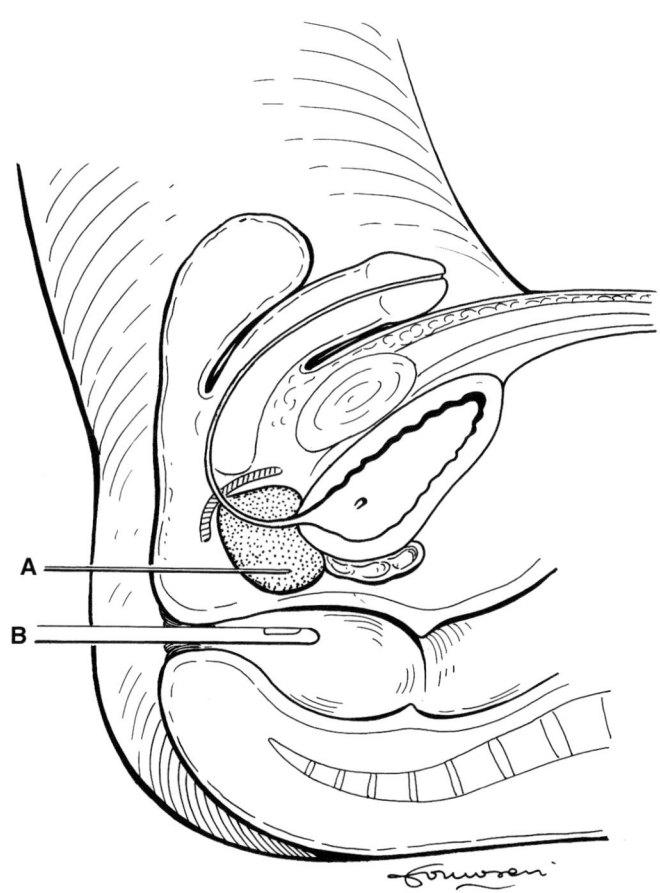

FIGURE 14.4. The **(A)** biopsy needle is inserted and maintained exactly parallel to the transrectal probe **(B)**.

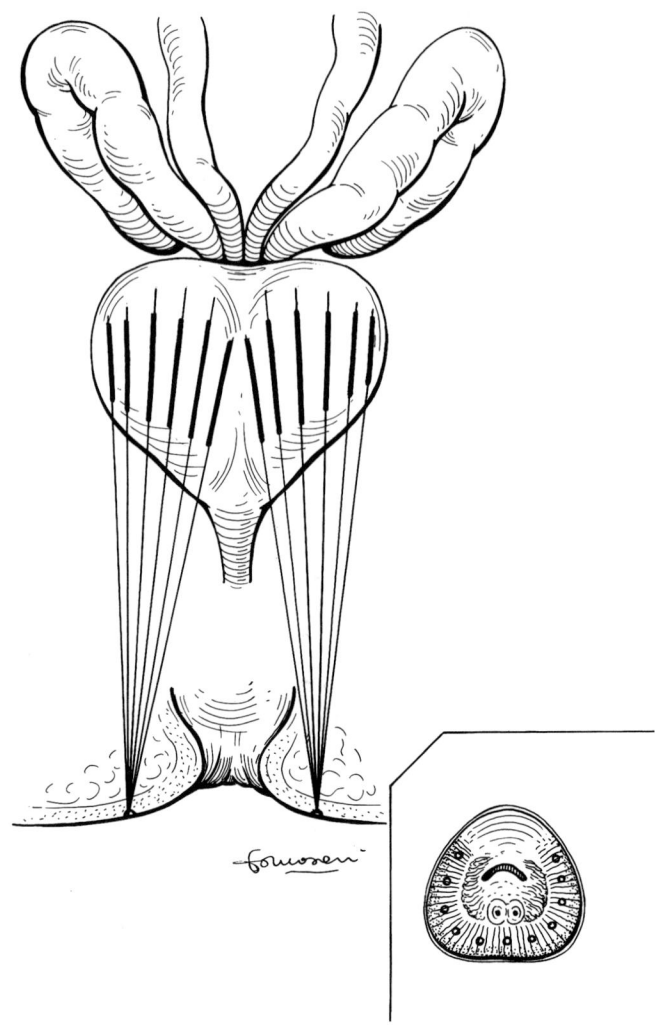

FIGURE 14.5. Six cores with a fan technique are obtained from each lobe of the prostate.

technique. The skin point of insertion of the needle is the same as the anesthetic injection for all the cores on each side (Figures 14.1 and 14.5). Although this technique may seem complex, after the first few procedures, each step is accomplished in a few seconds.

The Steps of the Technique

1. The needle is inserted in the perineum, at the point described.
2. The transrectal ultrasound probe is placed exactly parallel to the needle. The probe must be rotated and tilted to obtain the exact position.
3. The likely direction of the needle is then visualized.
4. The probe is rotated to detect if the chosen target area is medial or lateral, compared with the present direction.
5. The needle is angulated if a correction of direction is required.
6. The new direction is checked with the probe parallel to the needle and the core is obtained (Figure 14.6A and B).

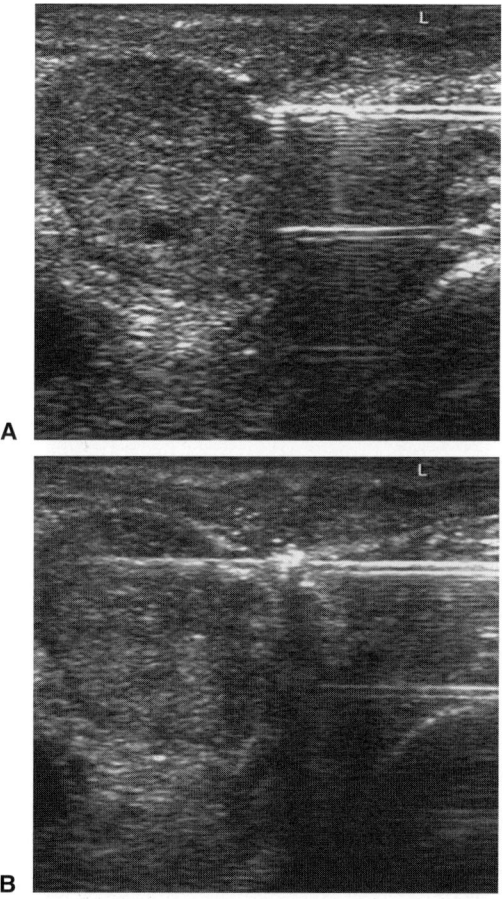

FIGURE 14.6. **A**: The desired area is targeted. **B**: The core is obtained.

The axis of the perineal route is the same as the peripheral area, so each whole core will be obtained exclusively from the peripheral area, where most cancers occur. Care must be taken to avoid the spongiosum of the bulbar urethra, to avoid the risk of perineal hematoma. However, even when the needle is passed through the spongiosum, significant bleeding will rarely occur. With the fan technique, it is difficult to pass through the urethra, but some care must be taken when obtaining a core from the midline in patients with very large adenomas, where the peripheral area is compressed and thin.

At the end of the procedure, a few drops of blood may leak from the skin injection point(s). Moderate perineal compression for 1–2 minutes is usually effective to stop the bleeding. The patient should avoid standing immediately after the biopsy. Because of the stress of the procedure, the lithotomy position, and the local anesthesia, the patient could experience a sudden decrease of blood pressure and/or heart rate. We advise keeping the patient sitting for 1 minute; after that, if he feels good and does not feel any "fainting" sensation, he can walk away. We dismiss the patient after the first asymptomatic voiding. If there are gross hematuria and/or voiding difficulty, the patient remains at the hospital for observation for 2–3 hours.

Results of Transperineal Biopsy

Transperineal biopsy is effective in prostate cancer detection. In 129 patients with increased PSA (>4.0 ng/mL) and/or abnormal DRE, systematic transperineal sextant biopsy found cancer in 52 cases (40%).[7]

Of 300 selected patients with PSA levels of 2.5–20 ng/mL, TRUS-guided, 12-core systematic biopsy detected prostate cancer in 108 (36%). The cancer detection rate was 18.2% for PSA levels of 2.5–4.0, 31% for PSA of 4.01–10.0, and 50% for PSA of 10.01–20.0 ng/mL.[8] In other work from Japan, two additional cores from the transition zone (TZ) were added to the 12-core transperineal biopsy. In 289 patients with increased PSA and/or positive DRE, prostate cancer detection rate was 36% (105/289).[9]

Ficarra and coworkers[10] performed 14-core transperineal prostate biopsy in 480 patients with PSA between 2.5 and 20 ng/mL. Overall cancer detection rate was 42%. They evaluated results according to the number of cores and prostate gland volume. For prostate volume <30 cc, the cancer detection rate was the same for 8-core and 14-core biopsy. For prostate volume 30–50 cc, cancer detection rate was the same for 12- and 14-core biopsy. For prostate volume >50 cc, even with 14-core biopsy, the cancer detection rate was low (24%). The authors concluded that transperineal biopsy protocols should include different numbers of cores according to prostate volume. In another study,[11] 122 patients with abnormal DRE and PSA >10 ng/mL underwent 12-core transperineal biopsy. The 6- and the 12-core (which included two transition zone cores) biopsy protocols were compared. Cancer diagnosis was obtained in 88 of 122 (72.1%) and in 92 of 122 (75.4%) patients with 6- and 12-core biopsy, respectively. The authors concluded that in selected men with a PSA >10 ng/mL and a positive DRE, a six-core transperineal biopsy can be a reasonable approach. However, the population they studied is very selected and at extremely high risk for prostate cancer. We reviewed our experience, and in a similar population with positive DRE and PSA >10 ng/mL, cancer detection rate with 12-core transperineal biopsy was 85.4% (88/103).

Complication rates of transperineal prostate biopsy are low. We performed transperineal biopsy in 988 patients with increased PSA (>4.0 ng/mL). Transient and mild hematuria at initial voiding, lasting 1–8 days, occurred in 192 cases (19.8%), mild hemospermia lasting up to 3 months occurred in 589 cases (59.6%), moderate perineal discomfort in 28 cases (2.8%), genitourinary infection in 6 cases (0.7%), acute urinary retention requiring catheterization in 4 cases. There was no need for hospitalization, and no major complication occurred. Hematuria usually occurs when the needle is passed through the urethra.

Comparison of Transperineal and Transrectal Prostate Biopsy

Few papers have compared the efficacy of the transperineal to the transrectal approach in prostate cancer detection. Simulated transrectal and transperineal sextant biopsies were performed on 40 radical prostatectomy specimens in a multicenter study.[12] The cancer detection rate was 82% (33/40) and 72% (29/40) for the transperineal and transrectal approach, respectively (p = 0.14). Transperineal biopsy missed either very small cancers (<2 mm) or prostatic base tumors.

In a prospective study,[13] 107 patients with increased PSA (>4 ng/mL, median 8.2 ng/mL) underwent both sextant transrectal and sextant transperineal prostate biopsy. The combined technique diagnosed prostate cancer in 43 patients (40%). Cancer detection rate was 38% (41/107) and 30% (33/107) for transperineal and transrectal biopsy, respectively. The transperineal approach detected 41 of 43 cancers (95%) and the transrectal approach detected 34 of 43 cancers (79%) (p = 0.0238).

Another prospective study[14] failed to find a significant difference in prostate cancer detection between transperineal and transrectal biopsy. Four hundred two patients underwent simultaneous six-core transperineal and six-core transrectal biopsies for increased PSA levels (>4.0 ng/mL) and/or abnormal DRE. Overall cancer detection rate was 48.5% (195/402). For transperineal and transrectal approaches, cancer detection rates were 41.3% and 40%, respectively. However, one bias is that two of the six cores of the transperineal biopsy were taken from the TZ, where cancer rarely

TABLE 14.1. Cancer detection rate with six-core prostate biopsy for prostate-specific antigen >4.0 ng/mL.

Author	Year	No. of patients	Technique	Detection rate (%)
Cooner et al.[15]	1990	602	Sextant	35
Brawer et al.[16]	1992	187	Sextant	31
Catalona et al.[17]	1993	112	Sextant	33
Reissigl et al.[18]	1995	778	Sextant	25
Bangma et al.[19]	1997	512	Sextant	29
Rietbergen et al.[20]	1999	1176	Sextant	30
Babaian et al.[21]	2000	315	Sextant	23
Emiliozzi et al.[13]	2003	107	Sextant	34
Tanaka et al.[22]	1998	442	**Sextant transperineal**	**48**
Emiliozzi et al.[13]	2003	107	**Sextant transperineal**	**41**

occurs. Therefore, two of six transperineal cores were less likely to find cancer. The authors concluded that the combined technique with both six-core transperineal and transrectal biopsy was very effective for prostate cancer diagnosis.

It is difficult to compare literature series from different institutions. The characteristics of the population studied and local factors may contribute to largely dissimilar results. For example, different median age, median prostate size, and positive DRE rate, can all lead to diverging conclusions. We chose papers that selectively studied a population undergoing biopsy for increased PSA (>4.0 ng/mL) or in the "gray zone" of PSA 4–10 ng/mL.

When six-core biopsy techniques are evaluated (Table 14.1), a transperineal procedure, with all the given possible biases, seems superior to traditional transrectal sextant biopsy for prostate cancer detection. The advantage of transperineal biopsy is less clear when a more specific population with PSA between 4.0 and 10.0 ng/mL is evaluated (Table 14.2).

TABLE 14.2. Cancer detection rate with six-core prostate biopsy for prostate-specific antigen 4.0–10.0 ng/mL.

Author	Year	No. of patients	Technique	Detection rate (%)
Cooner et al.[15]	1990	366	Sextant	20
Brawer et al.[16]	1992	87	Sextant	26
Bazinet et al.[23]	1994	264	Sextant	31
Schmid et al.[24]	1996	153	Sextant	29
Babaian et al.[21]	2000	196	Sextant	19
Canto et al.[25]	2004	350	Sextant	30
Yamamoto et al.[8]	2004	237	Sextant	20
Maffezzini et al.[26]	2005	466	Sextant	36
Tanaka et al.[22]	1998	486	**Sextant transperineal**	**48**
Ito et al.[27]	2002	100	**Sextant transperineal**	**31**
Emiliozzi et al.[13]	2003	70	**Sextant transperineal**	**30**

TABLE 14.3. Cancer detection rate with extended-needle prostate biopsy for prostate-specific antigen >4.0 ng/mL.

Author	Year	No. of patients	Technique	Detection rate (%)
Ravery et al.[28]	1999	131	Sextant + 4 on the same plane	42
Eskew et al.[29]	1997	102	Sextant + 5 region (13–18 cores)	41
Presti et al.[30]	2000	400	Sextant + 4 lateral	46
Babaian et al.[21]	2000	315	11-cores (sextant + 2 TZ +1 midgland + 2 lateral horns)	33
Siu et al.[31]	2005	293	>10 (sextant + lateral base + 1 lateral apex + 2 anterior horns)	50
Present report	2006	988	Transperineal "fan" 12 cores	47

TZ = transition zone.

When the results of extended-needle biopsy for prostate cancer detection are evaluated (Tables 14.3 and 14.4), apparently there is no significant difference in positive biopsy rate between the transperineal and transrectal approach for patients with PSA above 4.0 ng/mL and with PSA between 4.0 and 10.0 ng/mL. Several prospective trials have shown that increasing the number of cores improves cancer detection rate with both transrectal and transperineal prostate biopsy.[21,35–38]

It is reasonable to assume that an increased number of cores reduces the variation of cancer detection rate for different protocols and techniques. Probably, most extended-needle biopsy techniques have similar efficacy, regardless of the core scheme and of the approach—transperineal or transrectal.

Transperineal cores are obtained on a longitudinal plane which is parallel to the rectum and which passes through the posterior and lateral peripheral

TABLE 14.4. Cancer detection rate with extended prostate biopsy for prostate-specific antigen 4.0–10.0 ng/mL.

Author	Year	No. of patients	Technique	Detection rate (%)
Ravery et al.[28]	1999	70	Sextant + 4 on the same plane	24
Eskew et al.[29]	1997	64	Sextant + 5 region (13–18 cores)	36
Babaian et al.[21]	2000	196	Sextant + 2 TZ + 1 midgland + 2 lateral horns	30
Canto et al.[25]	2004	350	Sextant + 6 lateral	41
Pelzer et al.[32]	2005	1250	Sextant + 2 lateral apex + 2 TZ	27
Jones et al.[33]	2006	40	Sextant + 2 mid lateral + 2 base lateral	47
Ito et al.[27]	2002	100	**Transperineal 8–20 cores**	**46**
Yamamoto et al.[34]	2005	300	**Transperineal 12 cores**	**31**
Present report	2006	622	**Transperineal "fan" 12 cores**	**45**

TZ = transition zone.

area of the prostate, where most cancers are found. However, every part of the prostate can be easily reached with the transperineal approach. With a fan technique, a significant part of any single core comes from the apical area, where most cancer starts at the early phase.[39] Transperineal cores are taken exclusively from the peripheral area and they might be more likely to detect cancer, and to find higher quantity of cancer in the specimen. With transrectal biopsy, the cores are taken along an oblique axis crossing the prostate. Especially in large prostates, a part of the core could pass through the adenoma, where the chance of cancer detection is usually lower. With the transrectal approach, it is easy to target the area desired, along the needle marker. Nevertheless, sometimes not all the prostatic areas can be reached straightforwardly, because of the obligatory passage of the needle through the channel of the probe.

Typically with a fan transperineal technique, the TZ is not biopsied. The incidence of cancer exclusively in the TZ is expected to be low. In 1990, for specimens from radical prostatectomy, TZ cancer incidence was 11%.[40] When further TZ cores are added to extended-needle biopsy protocols, additional cancer detection rate exclusively attributable to TZ biopsy is 1.5–7%[41–43]. Recently, the addition of two TZ cores to a standard 12-core transperineal biopsy, especially in large glands, has been proposed.[10]

In another study, 247 men underwent 12-core transperineal prostate biopsy, with an original protocol including four TZ cores.[6] Cancer detection rate was 40% (98/247). The additional TZ cores improved cancer detection rates, particularly in patients with PSA levels <10 ng/mL, in patients with negative DRE and/or TRUS. However, at radical prostatectomy, only three cases had cancer only in the TZ. Although TZ cancer is usually an indolent tumor, in a subset of men, it can show aggressive behavior with Gleason pattern 4/5.[44]

We do not regularly include the TZ in our first set of transperineal biopsy, unless a hypoechoic lesion is clearly visible inside the adenoma or in the anterior portion of the prostate. In such cases, we add two further cores from the TZ, including the suspicious area. In our experience, 38 of 989 patients (3.8%) undergoing 12-core transperineal prostate biopsy had a hypoechoic area in such location. Of these 38 patients, cancer was found in 19 (50%). In nine cases, the TZ biopsy was negative, in 10 cases positive. However, in just three patients, the tumor was detected only in the TZ biopsy (3/38 = 7.8%).

In repeated biopsies, we routinely include cores from the TZ. In 80 repeated biopsies performed for persistently increased PSA, a cancer was found in the TZ in only six patients (7.5%).

Transperineal biopsy is more difficult to perform. Maintaining both probe and needle parallel while pointing at a given area of the prostate may not be easy, especially at the beginning, and some learning skill is necessary in the first 20–30 procedures. Transrectal biopsy, on the contrary, is quite easy to perform, because of the insertion of the needle in a channel, with the path of the needle shown on the screen by a needle marker.

Transperineal prostate biopsy requires local anesthesia. In more than 1500 transperineal biopsies, we have never experienced severe side effects or major complications of local anesthesia. The anesthesia is usually well accepted by the patients, and most men who underwent a previous transrectal biopsy without local anesthesia express a preference for the transperineal approach with anesthesia.

Although local anesthesia is not strictly needed for transrectal biopsy, most recent reports on transrectal biopsy agree that any form of anesthesia, including a local one, provides to the patient a better acceptance and tolerability of the procedure.[45–47]

Because the rectum is not traversed, the transperineal biopsy might provide a better approach in patients with severe rectocolitis. Likewise, transperineal biopsy does not require antibiotic coverage. We evaluated 920 procedures performed with the same technique by the same urologist (P.E.) at two institutions. The material used for the biopsy was the same, including the same ultrasound machine. At one institution (n = 550), oral antibiotic with a fluoroquinolone was provided the day before, the same day, and the day after the procedure. At the other institution (n = 370), no antibiotic was administered. Infective complication rates (urinary infection or fever) were 2/370 = 0.5% and 4/550 = 0.7% for patients without and with antibiotic coverage, respectively (p = 0.7301).

Transperineal Saturation Biopsy

Transperineal "saturation biopsy" has been proposed to detect prostate cancer in patients with previous negative prostate biopsy, but with high prostate cancer suspicion (such as men with increasing or persistently high PSA). The procedure is performed with the transperineal approach, through a grid such as the one used for brachytherapy seeds implant. All the cores are obtained by inserting the needle along parallel lines crossing the perineum and the prostate, according to the scheme of the grid. The technique was introduced in 2001 by Igel and coworkers.[48] Inclusion criteria were the following: PSA ≥10 ng/mL, PSA velocity of ≥0.75 ng/mL per year, or a diagnosis of prostatic intraepithelial neoplasia and/or atypical small cell acinar proliferation in previous biopsy. In 88 patients meeting these criteria, cancer was found in 38 (43%). A group of patients required general anesthesia. From 12 to 29 cores (median 17 cores) per biopsy were needed to diagnose prostatic cancer. Most cases (76%) had cancer in the TZ. The prevalent Gleason sum was 6. Urinary retention occurred in two cases (3%).

In a recent study,[49] 210 patients with at least one negative transrectal prostate biopsy (81% had undergone two or more biopsies) underwent transperineal saturation biopsy. The inclusion criteria were the same as those described in the article by Igel et al. The average number of cores was 21[12–41]. Cancer detection rate was 37% (78/210), including 36 patients with cancer only from the TZ, and Gleason score was 6 in the majority of patients. Acute urinary retention occurred in 11% of cases. Pathologic stage T2 was found in 27 of 30 patients (90%) undergoing radical prostatectomy.

In 128 patients who had already undergone one or more negative prostate biopsies, a systemic ultrasound-guided biopsy with a transperineal template, 22-core protocol was performed.[50] Cancer detection rate was 22.7%.

Crawford and coworkers[51] conducted a three-dimensional computer simulation of 106 prostate cancers (20 obtained by radical prostatectomy for T1c cancer; 86 autopsy specimens). A transperineal biopsy with a "grid" size of 5 or 10 mm was reproduced on the computer. Twelve to one hundred eight simulated cores were studied, according to prostate volume. Cancer detection rates for 5- and 10-mm grids were 86% versus 61% (autopsy) and 100% versus 95% (prostatectomy), respectively. Although the 5-mm grid found more cancer in the autopsy specimen, only 37% of the autopsy cancers were clinically significant. The 5-mm grid diagnosed 53% of all the insignificant tumors. However, the 5-mm grid could detect more tumors with a high Gleason pattern ($p > 0.001$).

The high incidence of cancer detected by transperineal saturation biopsy could be attributed to the increased number of cores, rather than to the technique itself. Stewart et al.[52] performed saturation needle biopsy with the transrectal approach in 224 patients with previous negative biopsies and persistently elevated PSA or previous prostatic intraepithelial neoplasia and/or atypical small cell acinar proliferation diagnosis. Median PSA was 8.7 ng/mL. The mean number of cores obtained was 23^{14-45}. General anesthesia was required. Cancer detection rate was 34% (77/224), similar to the one obtained by the transperineal saturation biopsy technique. After radical prostatectomy, organ-confined disease and Gleason score of 6–7 were found in 92% and in 88% of cases, respectively. Rabets et al.[53] performed office saturation transrectal biopsy and diagnosed 34 cancers (27%) in 117 patients at high risk for prostate cancer, as described before, and with previously negative biopsy.

Demura et al.[54] proposed a transperineal template biopsy as the first approach to diagnose prostate cancer. In a recent study, 312 patients with increased PSA and/or positive DRE underwent saturation transperineal biopsy. With a median of 19 cores per biopsy, the cancer detection rate was 51% (159/312). The procedure morbidity was low: urinary retention in six patients (2%), and long-lasting hematuria with perineal pain in one patient. The authors suggested that the transperineal approach could detect more nonpalpable tumors located in the anterior zone of the prostate.

Transperineal saturation biopsy can be a viable option in patients with persistently high or increasing PSA, with previously negative one or more biopsies. However, such an extensive biopsy may not be necessary as the first approach, because current protocols of extended-needle biopsy with 10–12 cores obtain a high cancer-detection rate (Tables 14.3 and 14.4).

TABLE 14.5. Advantages and disadvantages of transperineal biopsy.

Pros
    Every area of the prostate can be easily reached
    Cores obtained only from peripheral area if desired
    No passage through the rectal wall
    No antibiotic coverage needed in most cases
    Low complication rate
Cons
    Local anesthesia always required
    Learning curve
    Slightly longer procedure compared with transrectal approach

Conclusions

Transperineal prostate biopsy is effective for prostate cancer detection, with low morbidity. Although the procedure is technically more demanding compared with the transrectal approach, possible advantages include obtaining cores easily from any part of the prostate gland, and avoiding antibiotic coverage. In patients with severe inflammatory disease of the rectum, the transperineal technique might offer additional benefit (Table 14.5).

With six-core techniques, the cancer detection rate might be higher with transperineal than with transrectal biopsy. However, with extended-needle biopsy protocols, there are probably no significant differences in prostate cancer diagnosis between the transperineal and transrectal approaches. Transperineal template saturation biopsy can be a viable option in patients with persistently high PSA and one or more previous negative biopsies. In these patients, prostate cancer detection rate between 23%–40% can be expected.

As an alternative to the transrectal approach, transperineal prostate biopsy can be a valuable option in the urologist armamentarium.

References

1. Peck S. Transperineal needle biopsy of the prostate. J Urol 1972;107(6): 1025–7.
2. Webb JA, Shanmuganathan K, McLean A. Complications of ultrasound-guided transperineal prostate biopsy. A prospective study. Br J Urol 1993;72(5 Pt 2): 775–7.
3. Hodge KK, McNeal JE, Terris MK, Stamey TA. Random systematic versus directed ultrasound guided transrectal core biopsies of the prostate. J Urol 1989;142(1):71–4.
4. Emiliozzi P, Longhi S, Scarpone P, Pansadoro A, DePaula F, Pansadoro V. The value of a single biopsy with 12 transperineal cores for detecting prostate cancer in patients with elevated prostate specific antigen. J Urol 2001;166(3):845–50.

5. Shandera KC, Thibault G P, Deshon JE Jr. Variability in patient preparation for prostate biopsy among American urologists. Urology 1998;52(4): 644–6.

6. Takenaka A, Hara R, Hyodo Y, et al. Transperineal extended biopsy improves the clinically significant prostate cancer detection rate: a comparative study of 6 and 12 biopsy cores. Int J Urol 2006;13(1):10–14.

7. Ishidoya S, Ogata Y, Inaba Y, et al. Screening of prostate cancer with PSA and transperineal six sextant biopsy. Nippon Hinyokika Gakkai Zasshi 1999;90(5): 579–85.

8. Yamamoto S, Ito T, Aizawa T, et al. Does transrectal ultrasound guided eight-core prostate biopsy improve cancer detection rates in patients with prostate-specific antigen levels of 4.1–10 ng/mL? Int J Urol 2004;11(6):386–91.

9. Kawakami S, Kihara K, Fujii Y, Masuda H, Kobayashi T, Kageyama Y. Transrectal ultrasound-guided transperineal 14-core systematic biopsy detects apico-anterior cancer foci of T1c prostate cancer. Int J Urol 2004;11(8):613–18.

10. Ficarra V, Novella G, Novara G, Galfano A, Pea M, Martignoni G, Artibani W. The potential impact of prostate volume in the planning of optimal number of cores in the systematic transperineal prostate biopsy. Eur Urol 2005;48(6): 932–7.

11. Luciani LG, De Giorgi G, Valotto C, Zanin M, Bierti S, Zattoni F. Role of transperineal six-core prostate biopsy in patients with prostate-specific antigen level greater than 10 ng/mL and abnormal digital rectal examination findings. Urology 2006;67(3):555–8.

12. Vis AN, Boerma MO, Ciatto S, Hoedemaker RF, Schroder FH, van der Kwast TH. Detection of prostate cancer: a comparative study of the diagnostic efficacy of sextant transrectal versus sextant transperineal biopsy. Urology 2000;56 (4):617–21.

13. Emiliozzi P, Corsetti A, Tassi B, Federico G, Martini M, Pansadoro V. Best approach for prostate cancer detection: a prospective study on transperineal versus transrectal six-core prostate biopsy. Urology 2003;61(5):961–6.

14. Watanabe M, Hayashi T, Tsushima T, Irie S, Kaneshige T, Kumon H. Extensive biopsy using a combined transperineal and transrectal approach to improve prostate cancer detection. Int J Urol 2005;12(11):959–63.

15. Cooner WH, Mosley BR, Rutherford CL Jr, et al. Prostate cancer detection in a clinical urological practice by ultrasonography, digital rectal examination and prostate specific antigen. J Urol 1990;143(6):1146–52.

16. Brawer MK, Chetner MP, Beatie J, Buchner DM, Vessella RL, Lange PH. Screening for prostatic carcinoma with prostate specific antigen. J Urol 1992;147:841–5.

17. Catalona WJ, Smith DS, Ratliff TL, Basler JW. Detection of organ-confined prostate cancer is increased through prostate-specific antigen-based screening. JAMA 199325;270(8):948–54.

18. Reissigl A, Pointner J, Horninger W, et al. Comparison of different prostate-specific antigen cutpoints for early detection of prostate cancer: results of a large screening study. Urology 1995;46(5):662–5.

19. Bangma CH, Rietbergen JB, Kranse R, Blijenberg BG, Petterson K, Schroder FH. The free-to-total prostate specific antigen ratio improves the specificity of prostate specific antigen in screening for prostate cancer in the general population. J Urol 1997;157(6):2191–6.

20. Rietbergen JB, Hoedemaeker RF, Kruger AE, Kirkels WJ, Schroder FH. The changing pattern of prostate cancer at the time of diagnosis: characteristics of screen detected prostate cancer in a population based screening study. J Urol 1999;161(4):1192–8.

21. Babaian RJ, Toi A, Kamoi K, et al. A comparative analysis of sextant and an extended 11-core multisite directed biopsy strategy. J Urol 2000;163(1):152–7.

22. Tanaka H, Shinkai M, Jo Y, Matsuki T. Transrectal ultrasound guided transperineal systematic prostate biopsy. Nippon Rinsho 1998;56(8):2067–71.

23. Bazinet M, Meshref AW, Trudel C, et al. Prospective evaluation of prostate-specific antigen density and systematic biopsies for early detection of prostatic carcinoma. Urology 1994;43(1):44–51.

24. Schmid HP, Ravery V, Billebaud T, et al. Early detection of prostate cancer in men with prostatism and intermediate prostate-specific antigen levels. Urology 1996;47(5):699–703.

25. Canto EI, Singh H, Shariat SF, et al. Effects of systematic 12-core biopsy on the performance of percent free prostate specific antigen for prostate cancer detection. J Urol 2004;172(3):900–4.

26. Maffezzini M, Gavazzi L, Calcagno T, Capponi G, Bandelloni R. Still a place for the classical systematic sextant technique? Cancer detection rates and complications in 1025 consecutive prostatic biopsies. Arch Ital Urol Androl 2005;77(2):106–8.

27. Ito K, Ohi M, Yamamoto T, et al. The diagnostic accuracy of the age-adjusted and prostate volume-adjusted biopsy method in males with prostate specific antigen levels of 4.1–10.0 ng/mL. Cancer 2002;95(10):2112–19.

28. Ravery V, Billebaud T, Toublanc M, et al. Diagnostic value of ten systematic TRUS-guided prostate biopsies. Eur Urol 1999;35(4):298–303.

29. Eskew LA, Bare RL, McCullough DL. Systematic 5 region prostate biopsy is superior to sextant method for diagnosing carcinoma of the prostate. J Urol 1997;157(1):199–202.

30. Presti JC Jr, Chang JJ, Bhargava V, Shinohara K. The optimal systematic prostate biopsy scheme should include 8 rather than 6 biopsies: results of a prospective clinical trial. J Urol 2000;163(1):163–6.

31. Siu W, Dunn RL, Shah RB, Wei JT. Use of extended pattern technique for initial prostate biopsy. J Urol 2005;174(2):505–9.

32. Pelzer AE, Volgger H, Bektic J, et al. The effect of percentage free prostate-specific antigen (PSA) level on the prostate cancer detection rate in a screening population with low PSA levels. BJU Int 2005;96(7):995–8.

33. Jones JS, Patel A, Schoenfield L, Rabets JC, Zippe CD, Magi-Galluzzi C. Saturation technique does not improve cancer detection as an initial prostate biopsy strategy. J Urol 2006;175(2):485–8.

34. Yamamoto S, Kin U, Nakamura K, et al. Transperineal ultrasound-guided 12-core systematic biopsy of the prostate for patients with a prostate-specific antigen level of 2.5–20 ng/mL in Japan. Int J Clin Oncol 2005;10(2):117–21.

35. Eskicorapci SY, Baydar DE, Akbal C, et al. An extended 10-core transrectal ultrasonography guided prostate biopsy protocol improves the detection of prostate cancer. Eur Urol 2004;45(4):444–8.

36. Durkan GC, Sheikh N, Johnson P, Hildreth AJ, Greene DR. Improving prostate cancer detection with an extended-core transrectal ultrasonography-guided prostate biopsy protocol. BJU Int 2002;89(1):33–9.

37. O'Connell MJ, Smith CS, Fitzpatrick PE, et al. Transrectal ultrasound-guided biopsy of the prostate gland: value of 12 versus 6 cores. Abdom Imaging 2004;29(1):132–6.

38. Emiliozzi P, Scarpone P, DePaula F, et al. The incidence of prostate cancer in men with prostate specific antigen greater than 4.0 ng/mL: a randomized study of 6 versus 12 core transperineal prostate biopsy. J Urol 2004;171(1): 197–9.

39. Kabalin JN, McNeal JE, Price HM, Freiha FS, Stamey TA. Unsuspected adenocarcinoma of the prostate in patients undergoing cystoprostatectomy for other causes: incidence, histology and morphometric observations. J Urol 1989;141: 1091–4.

40. Steuber T, Karakiewicz PI, Augustin H, et al. Transition zone cancers undermine the predictive accuracy of Partin table stage predictions. J Urol 2005; 173(3):737–41.

41. Liu IJ, Macy M, Lai YH, Terris MK. Critical evaluation of the current indications for transition zone biopsies. Urology 2001;57(6):1117–20.

42. Deliveliotis C, Varkarakis J, Albanis S, Argyropoulos V, Skolarikos A. Biopsies of the transitional zone of the prostate. Should it be done on a routine basis, when and why? Urol Int 2002;68(2):113–17.

43. Miyake H, Kurahashi T, Muramaki M, Yamanak K, Hara I. Significance of routine transition zone biopsies in Japanese men undergoing transrectal ultrasound-guided prostate biopsies. Int J Urol 2005;12(11):964–8.

44. Shannon BA, McNeal JE, Cohen RJ. Transition zone carcinoma of the prostate gland: a common indolent tumour type that occasionally manifests aggressive behaviour. Pathology 2003;35(6):467–71.

45. Obek C, Ozkan B, Tunc B, Can G, Yalcin V, Solok V. Comparison of 3 different methods of anesthesia before transrectal prostate biopsy: a prospective randomized trial. J Urol 2004;172(2):502–5.

46. Aus G, Damber JE, Hugosson J. Prostate biopsy and anaesthesia: an overview. Scand J Urol Nephrol 2005;39(2):124–9.

47. Autorino R, De Sio M, Di Lorenzo G, et al. How to decrease pain during transrectal ultrasound guided prostate biopsy: a look at the literature. J Urol 2005;174(6):2091–7.

48. Igel TC, Knight MK, Young PR, et al. Systematic transperineal ultrasound guided template biopsy of the prostate in patients at high risk. J Urol 2001; 165(5):1575–9.

49. Pinkstaff DM, Igel TC, Petrou SP, Broderick GA, Wehle MJ, Young PR. Systematic transperineal ultrasound-guided template biopsy of the prostate: three-year experience. Urology 2005;65(4):735–9.

50. Satoh T, Matsumoto K, Fujita T, et al. Cancer core distribution in patients diagnosed by extended transperineal prostate biopsy. Urology 2005;66(1): 114–18.

51. Crawford ED, Wilson SS, Torkko KC, et al. Clinical staging of prostate cancer: a computer-simulated study of transperineal prostate biopsy. BJU Int 2005;96(7):999–1004.

52. Stewart CS, Leibovich BC, Weaver AL, Lieber MM. Prostate cancer diagnosis using a saturation needle biopsy technique after previous negative sextant biopsies. J Urol 2001;166(1):86–91.

53. Rabets JC, Jones JS, Patel A, Zippe CD. Prostate cancer detection with office based saturation biopsy in a repeat biopsy population. J Urol 2004;172(1): 94–7.
54. Demura T, Hioka T, Furuno T, et al. Differences in tumor core distribution between palpable and nonpalpable prostate tumors in patients diagnosed using extensive transperineal ultrasound-guided template prostate biopsy. Cancer 2005;103(9):1826–32.

15
Repeat Prostate Biopsies and the Vienna Nomograms

Bob Djavan and Sibylle Marihart

Abstract

Based on the Vienna nomograms, repeat prostate biopsy is indicated in patients with negative initial findings who have high-grade prostatic intraepithelial neoplasia, continue to have increasing abnormal prostate-specific antigen levels, or prostate volumes >45 cc and/or transition zone volumes >25 cc. The Vienna nomograms evaluate the minimum number of cores based on patient's age and prostate gland volume required to ensure 90% certainty of cancer detection. The authors found that more than six biopsy cores are needed and that biopsies should be directed more laterally. Location and density measurements suggest that repeat biopsy should be directed in a more apico-dorsal location which is rather spared during initial biopsy. Current data suggest that cancers detected on repeat biopsy have a similar stage and grade distribution and total prostate-specific antigen values compared with cancers found on initial biopsy. Patients younger than 60 years of age need to be counseled regarding higher pain and discomfort during repeat biopsy. Local or topical anesthesia should be offered.

Keywords: nomograms, biopsy strategy, repeat biopsy

The widespread use of measurement of prostate-specific antigen (PSA) for prostate cancer screening has led to a dramatic increase in the number of men undergoing prostate biopsy guided by transrectal ultrasound (TRUS). Systematic parasagittal sextant biopsies have been widely adopted as the standard protocol for prostate biopsy. Significant numbers of men undergo repeat biopsy because of clinical indications [abnormal digital rectal exami-

From: *Current Clinical Urology: Prostate Biopsy: Indications, Techniques, and Complications*
Edited by J.S. Jones © Humana Press, Totowa, NJ

nation (DRE), elevated PSA] or atypical findings on the initial biopsy, or because it is well known that prostate cancer is often multifocal.[1] Frequently, urologists are faced with the dilemma of treating a patient with a high index of suspicion of prostate cancer, but an initial set of negative biopsies.

In recent studies, cancer detection rate on repeat prostate biopsy was found to be between 10% and 20%. If cancer is still present in 1/10 to 1/5 of patients with a negative initial biopsy, one has to reevaluate the biopsy policy. However, the question is when to stop repeat prostate biopsy. The answer to this dilemma lies in a prospective evaluation of cancers detected on repeat biopsy. If cancers detected on repeat biopsy have "significant" features or similar features to cancers detected on initial biopsy, then repeat biopsy should be advocated and balanced against biopsy-related costs and patient morbidity.

A number of diagnostic dilemmas arise regarding repeat biopsies:

- Should lesion-directed or random biopsies be performed?
- How many biopsy cores should be obtained for optimal diagnostic yield, to reduce the incidence of false-negative biopsies?
- What areas of the prostate should be biopsied to give the best diagnostic results?
- If the initial biopsy fails to detect cancer, which patients should undergo repeat biopsy? And how often should it be repeated?
- What role do PSA and PSA parameters such as PSA density (PSAD), PSA-transition zone (TZ), PSA velocity, and percent free PSA (%fPSA) have in the outcome of repeat biopsy?
- Are cancers detected on multiple repeat biopsies clinically "significant" and thus deserve therapy?

The Impact of Prostate Volume

The impact of prostate volume in the decision of prostate biopsy technique and when to perform a repeat prostate biopsy is still a matter of debate. Given that sextant prostatic systematic biopsies sample only about 90 mm of prostate tissue (6 × 15 mm cores), increased prostatic volume may significantly reduce the chance of detecting cancer.[2–4]

Because of the wide variation in gland sizes and shapes, it seems logical that in smaller glands the prostate biopsy leads to a more extensive sampling, and in larger prostates a less-extensive or suboptimal sampling, with accompanying significant differences in biopsy yields.[5,6] Several groups have proposed new biopsy strategies, often increasing the number of biopsies and the sectors to be sampled or performing biopsies more laterally, but controversial data have been reported about the real advantage of these new techniques.[7–10] Concerned by the fact that the original sextant method may not include adequate sampling of the prostate, Norberg et al.[11] found in a prospective study including 512 patients that the standard method left 15% of cancers undetected as compared with the results of a more extensive procedure using 8–10 biopsies.

Recently, the influence of the total and TZ prostate volumes on prostate cancer detection was prospectively analyzed in 1018 men using two successive sets of sextant biopsies plus two TZ biopsies.[12] Compared with patients diagnosed with cancer of the prostate (CaP) after the first set of biopsies, patients diagnosed after the second set had larger total prostate and TZ volumes (43.1 ± 13.0 vs. 32.5 ± 10.6 cc, $p < 0.0001$ and 20.5 ± 8.3 vs. 12.8 ± 6.0 cc, $p < 0.0001$). Receiver operating characteristic (ROC) curves showed that total and TZ volumes of 45 and 22.5 cc, respectively, provided the best combination of sensitivity and specificity for discriminating between patients diagnosed with CaP after the first set from those diagnosed after a second set. In patients with total prostate volume >45 cc and TZ > 22.5 cc, a single set of sextant biopsies was not sufficient to rule out CaP, and a repeat biopsy was to be considered in case of a negative first biopsy.

Evaluating the variation of cancer detection in relation to prostate size, through random systematic sextant biopsies, Uzzo et al.[13] found 23% of the patients had cancer and a large prostate ≥ 50 cc compared with 38% in patients with smaller prostates ($p < 0.01$). This group concluded that significant sampling errors may occur in men with large glands, suggesting the need for repeat biopsies.

One of the central difficulties elucidating the relationship of prostate size and biopsy yield is the fact that prostates without cancer are virtually unavailable for pathologic analysis. Chen and colleagues[14] approached this problem by developing a novel computer simulation that allowed comparison of biopsy results for given prostate and cancer volumes. The authors first evaluated 180 whole-mount radical prostatectomy specimens. The prostates were weighed, step-sectioned, and digitized for computer modeling. Tumor volumes were calculated and compared with prostate volumes. Overall, 607 tumors in 180 prostates were quantified. Computer-simulated biopsy runs were performed on the digitized prostates. Sextant biopsies in glands weighing ≤ 50 g and glands >50 g were positive in 67% and 48% of cases, respectively. Small-volume cancers were more prevalent in larger prostates. The authors concluded that biopsy rates in large glands were lower than in small glands because biopsy of larger glands is often driven by elevations of PSA that may be produced by benign prostate tissue. They argued that if sampling error were the primary reason for the consistent finding of lower biopsy yields in larger prostates, larger-volume cancers would preferentially be found in large prostates. Chen and associates recommended against obtaining extra biopsies solely because of larger prostate size, arguing that this would likely detect a disproportionate number of small-volume cancers. The question of optimal biopsy sites and number of cores (independent of prostate volume) is still unanswered. Chen et al., following a stochastic computer-simulation model, developed a 10-core biopsy scheme incorporating the midline peripheral zone (PZ), inferior portion of the anterior horn of the PZ, significantly improving cancer detection to 96% and thus recommending the sampling of these zones in the repeat biopsy strategy after previously negative biopsies.[14] Eskew et al.[8] have recommended the use of a five-region sampling technique to improve the cancer detection rate because the 11-core technique increased the percentage of prostate cancer detected from 26% to 40% compared with the usual sextant biopsies.

The importance of the total volume on prostate cancer yielded by sextant biopsies is generally accepted. The importance of the TZ was less investigated.[15] Many authors have already stressed the importance of the TZ and especially of the TZ density for predicting prostate cancer in men with serum PSA levels <10 ng/mL.[16,17]

Levine et al.[18] have used two consecutive sets of TRUS-guided sextant biopsies for improving prostate cancer detection. These two sets were performed during the same session. Prostate cancer was detected in 43%, 27%, and 24% of men with prostate volumes <30, 30–50, and >50 cc, respectively. Analyzing the second set of biopsies, performed in the same session, the probability of detecting a prostate cancer was approximately twofold greater in men with large prostates compared with men with smaller- and intermediate-sized prostates.

Djavan et al.[16] and Letran et al.[19] suggested that the total and PZ volumes significantly affected the biopsy yield only when both were above the 75th percentile.

Interestingly, the debate over the need of more lateral biopsies is open. When tumor foci from the 40 cases in which sextant biopsies did not reliably detect tumor were mapped, Chen et al.[14] found that the foci were distributed in areas not biopsied by the sextant method, namely, the TZ, midline PZ, and inferior portion of the anterior horn of the PZ. A 10-core biopsy scheme incorporating these areas as well as the posterolateral prostate reliably detected cancer in 141 of 147 patients (96%) with total tumor volumes >0.5 cc.

A systematic five-region biopsy technique had been proposed whereby, in addition to random sextant biopsies, two sets of lateral PZ and three midline biopsies were obtained.[8] Twelve to 15 cores were taken when the prostate volume was <50 cc and up to 18 cores if the volume was >50 cc. An improvement in diagnostic yield of 35% over the systematic sextant biopsy method alone was noted, with 83% of the additional tumors identified having a Gleason score of six or more.[8] Levine and coworkers[18] noted that cancer detection rates could be increased by 30% by performing two consecutive sets of sextant biopsies at a single office visit.

Creating an accurate model for prostate biopsy requires the ability to determine prostate gland volume and the minimum number of cores required to detect cancers with a high degree of certainty. Clinically, patient's age is the major determinant of life-threatening tumor volume at

TABLE 15.1. Djavan-Vienna nomogram: number of cores per biopsy to ensure 90% certainty of cancer detection as a function of prostate gland size and age.

	Vienna nomogram			
	Age (years)			
Size (cc)	<50	50–60	60–70	>70
20–29	8	8	8	6
30–39	12	10	8	6
40–49	14	12	10	8
50–59	16	14	12	10
60–69	—	16	14	12
>70	—	18	16	14

Source: Djavan et al.[16]

diagnosis. Subsequently, Vashi et al.[20] and Djavan et al.[16] proposed a nomogram concerning the number of cores for biopsy required to ensure a 90% certainty of cancer detection as a function of prostate gland size and life-threatening volume. The Vienna nomogram was based on patient's age and gland volume (Table 15.1). The authors evaluated the minimum number of cores needed to accurately detect cancer. This model was based on the finding of the European Prostate Cancer Detection Study and a three-dimensional model of virtual biopsies taken from a prostatectomy specimen.

- Increasing (>6) biopsy cores are needed.
- Biopsies should be directed more laterally (PZ).
- Repeat biopsies should be performed when initial biopsy shows no prostate cancer in total prostate volumes >45 cc and/or TZ volumes >25 cc.
- There is a significant sampling error in larger prostate glands (>50 cc), therefore a repeat biopsy is needed if initial biopsy yield showed no prostate cancer.
- Small-volume cancers are more frequent in larger prostates.
- Performing two sets of sextant biopsy in patients with larger prostates (>50 cc) yields a twofold-higher probability of detecting prostate cancer.

The Impact of Prostate-Specific Antigen Derivatives

As we know from PSA-based screening studies, approximately 9% of all asymptomatic men will have elevated serum PSA values but only about a third will have cancer detected on initial biopsy.[21,22] The question is whether the 66% of men with an initially negative prostate biopsy have an elevated serum PSA value because of benign prostatic hyperplasia, prostatitis, or undetected cancer in their PZ or TZ of the prostate. Keetch and Catalona[23] have previously shown that cancer detection rates at biopsies two or three were 19% and 8%, respectively. However, their patients underwent serial biopsies of the PZ only.

In a recent study, the ability of %fPSA, PSAD, and PSA-TZ to increase the sensitivity and specificity of PSA screening was evaluated prospectively.[24] Of the 1051 men with a total PSA level of 4–10 ng/mL, the initial biopsy was positive for CaP in 22% (231/1051) of the subjects. All 820 subjects diagnosed with benign prostatic hyperplasia after the initial biopsy underwent a repeat prostatic biopsy 6 weeks later. CaP was detected in 10% (83/820) of these subjects. Compared with the 231 subjects in whom CaP was detected from the initial biopsy, both total prostate volume and TZ volume were significantly higher (p < 0.001) in the 83 subjects with CaP detected in the repeat biopsy sample. The majority of cancers (84%) were detected in the PZ, compared with 16% detected in the TZ. Total PSA, PSAD, and PSA-TZ were all significantly higher in subjects diagnosed with CaP at initial and repeat biopsy (p < 0.01).

Based on the results of a previous study,[16] cut-off values improving specificity with a sufficiently high level of cancer detection (sensitivity) were selected. At a cut-off of 30% and 0.26 ng/mL/cc, respectively, %fPSA and PSA-TZ were the most accurate predictors of a positive repeat biopsy result. Although a similar number of unnecessary repeat biopsies would have been eliminated by either %fPSA or PSA-TZ (approximately 50%), CaP detection was much lower for PSA-TZ (78%) compared with %fPSA (90%).

In both the overall group (initial biopsy results plus repeat biopsy results) and the repeat biopsy group, %fPSA and PSA-TZ were the best predictors of CaP (r = 0.2150, p < 0.001). The respective area under the curves (AUCs) for %fPSA and PSA-TZ were 74.2% and 82.7% in the overall group, and 74.5% and 69.1% in the repeat biopsy group (p < 0.001). Although Zlotta et al.[25] previously reported that measurement of the TZ volume is accurate and reproducible, all TRUS measurements are operator dependent and, therefore, subject to possible variability. Furthermore, the measurement of the TZ in small or large prostates sometimes might be difficult. It was reported previously that PSA-TZ was not a significant predictor of biopsy results when the total prostate volume was <30 cc.[16]

In a multicenter study of 773 men with a total PSA level between 4 and 10 ng/mL (379 with CaP and 394 with benign prostatic hyperplasia), a %free PSA cut-off of 25% had a sensitivity of 95% and a specificity of 20%.[26] Another multicenter study of 317 men with a total PSA level between 4.0 to 10.0 ng/mL found that a %free PSA cut-off of 26% detected 95% of subjects with CaP and eliminated 29% of negative biopsies.[27] In another study of 308 volunteers with an elevated total PSA level (2.5–10.0 ng/mL), a %fPSA cut-off of <20% would have eliminated 45.5% of negative biopsies. When %fPSA was combined with a PSA-TZ density cut-off of >0.22 ng/mL/cc, 54.2% of negative biopsies could have been avoided.[28]

Although some previous studies focused on repeat-biopsy results, most have been retrospective trials conducted in relatively small patient populations.[23,29-38] In one study of 193 men with a negative initial biopsy, 51 (26%) were found to have CaP on repeat biopsy. Total PSA and volume-referenced PSA had the highest sensitivity. Another retrospective study in 51 men with a total serum PSA level of 2–15 ng/mL demonstrated a lower median %fPSA value in patients with a positive repeat biopsy compared with those with a negative biopsy (15% vs. 19%, respectively; p = 0.05).[30] A %fPSA cut-off of 22% yielded a sensitivity of 95% and a specificity of 44% for predicting repeat biopsy results. In a prospective study of 67 men with persistent total PSA elevations and normal DRE, a low %fPSA (<10%) was a powerful predictor of CaP, even after two negative biopsies. The AUC of the ROC curve was 0.93 for %fPSA, compared with 0.69, 0.66, and 0.51 for free PSAD, PSAD, and total PSA, respectively.[31] In another study that used %fPSA to predict repeat biopsy results, CaP was detected in 20 (20%) of 99 men with a total PSA level between 4.1 and 10.0 ng/mL and an initial biopsy that was negative for CaP.[33] Percent free PSA cut-offs of 28% and 30% had a sensitivity of 90% and 95%, respectively, and a specificity of 13% and 12%, respectively. For PSAD cut-offs of 0.10 and 0.08 ng/mL/cc, the respective sensitivities were 90% and 95%, and the respective specificities were 31% and 12%.

In three of the previous studies, the positive repeat biopsy rate was 17% after an interval of 14.7 months between the first and second biopsies,[29] 29% after an interval of 19.1 months,[30] and 30% after 12.8 month.[32]

- PSA, PSA-TZ, and PSAD were significantly higher in patients detected for prostate cancer in the second prostate biopsy.
- %free PSA (cut-off 30%) was better than PSA-TZ (cut-off 0.26 ng/mL/cc) for prostate cancer detection in repeat biopsy.
- Using %free PSA, PSAD, PSA-TZ leads to higher specificity at 95% sensitivity for first prostate biopsy and increases sensitivity and specificity in repeat prostate biopsy.

Pathologic Features of Prostate Biopsy: When to Stop?

Little was reported on the differences in pathologic stage, grade, and cancer behavior of cancers detected on initial and repeat prostate biopsy. Although optimal predictors of cancer detection on repeat biopsy are crucial, one can spare or delay a repeat biopsy if cancers detected are "insignificant." Certainly, the dilemma of CaP is that only a small portion of men with untreated cancer will die from it, especially if these are small in volume, well differentiated, and detected on repeat biopsy.

In a recent study, Djavan et al.[24] showed that cancers detected on initial (n = 231) and repeat biopsy (n = 83), 148/231 (64%) and 56/83 (67.5%), respectively, were clinically localized disease, and patients were offered radical prostatectomy or radiation therapy. Watchful waiting was not offered as a primary option. Therefore, 10/148 (6.7%) and 3/56 (5.3%), respectively, opted for radiation therapy, and 138/148 (93.2%) and 53/56 (94.6%), respectively, underwent radical retropubic prostatectomy. All specimens underwent histopathologic evaluation by a single pathologist. Overall, 58.0% and 60.9% had organ-confined disease in both groups, respectively. No differences were noted with respect to organ confinement (p = 0.15), extracapsular extension (p = 0.22), and seminal vesical invasion (p = 0.28). Positive margins were noted in 23% and 18%, respectively (p = 0.23). No differences were noted between both cancer groups (initial vs. repeat) in the biopsy Gleason score (6.0 vs. 5.7; p = 0.252) as well as in Gleason score of the surgical specimen (5.3 vs. 4.9; p = 0.358). The same accounted for the % Gleason grade 4/5 (31.1% vs. 29.8%; p = 0.10). In contrast, cancers detected on initial biopsy expressed a higher rate of multifocality (p = 0.009), whereas overall cancer volume was identical (p = 0.271) in both groups.[24]

Recently, Stamey et al.[39] challenged the "traditional" predictors of cancer progression such as stage, capsular penetration, and surgical margins. In a retrospective analysis of 379 men treated by radical prostatectomy only, eight morphologic variables were analyzed and associated with cancer progression, defined by an increasing PSA level (≥0.07 ng/mL). They identified % Gleason score 4/5, cancer volume, positive lymph node findings, and intraprostatic vascular invasions as independent predictors of cancer progression.[39]

In contrast, cancers detected on initial biopsy expressed a higher rate of multifocality (p = 0.0009), whereas overall cancer volume was identical (p = 0.271) in both groups. Based on these findings, Djavan et al.[24] concluded that cancers detected on repeat biopsy exhibit similar characteristics as cancers detected initially. Thus, repeat biopsies do detect significant cancers and a repeat biopsy policy should be advocated in case of a negative initial biopsy. This conclusion, however, is limited to cases in which initial and repeat biopsies are performed in a similar manner as was done in the current study. If the biopsy technique is modified, cancers detected may differ and the conclusion may differ as well.

Recently, Djavan et al.[24] presented the results of a prospective study of the pathologic features found in the first, second, third, and fourth prostate biopsy. Of those with benign prostatic tissue on the first, second, and third biopsy, 820/829, 737/756, and 94/101, respectively, agreed to undergo repeat biopsy. Cancer detection rates on first, second, third, and fourth biopsy were 22% (231/1051), 10% (83/820), 5% (36/737), and 4% (4/94), respectively. Overall, of patients with clinically localized disease (67% of cancers detected), 86% underwent radical prostatectomy and 14% opted for watchful waiting or radiation therapy. Of cancers detected on initial (n = 231), repeat (n = 83), third (n = 36), and fourth biopsy (n = 4), 148/231

(64%), 56/83 (67.5%), 33/36 (91.6%), and 4/4 (100%) had a clinically local-ized disease, respectively, and were offered radical prostatectomy or radia-tion therapy. Watchful waiting was not offered as a primary option. Therefore, 10/148 (6.7%), 3/56 (5.3%), 1/33 (3%), and 0/4 (0%), respec-tively, opted for radiation therapy, and 138/148 (93.3%), 53/56 (94.7%), 32/33 (97%), and 4/4 (100%), respectively, underwent radical retropubic prostatectomy. All specimens underwent histopathologic evaluation by a single pathologist at each institution. Overall, 58.0%, 60.9%, 86.3%, and 100% had organ-confined disease on first, repeat, third, and fourth biopsy, respectively. No differences were noted with respect to organ confinement (p = 0.15), extracapsular extension (p = 0.22), and seminal vesical invasion (p = 0.28) between first and repeat biopsy, whereas the same parameters were significantly different (higher values for organ confinement and lower for all other parameters) for cancers on third versus first biopsy (p = 0.001, p = 0.02, p = 0.01, respectively) as well as cancers on fourth versus first biopsy (p = 0.001, p = 0.01, p = 0.001, respectively). Positive margins were noted in 23%, 18% (p = 0.23), 8% (p = 0.03), and 0% respectively. No dif-ferences were noted between cancers detected on initial versus repeat biopsy in the biopsy Gleason score (6.0 vs. 5.7; p = 0.252) as well as in Gleason score of the surgical specimen (5.3 vs. 4.9; p = 0.358). The same accounted for the % Gleason grade 4/5 (31.1% vs. 29.8%; p = 0.10). Cancers detected on initial biopsy expressed a higher rate of multifocality (p = 0.009), whereas overall cancer volume was identical (p = 0.271) on first and second biopsy. In contrast, cancers detected on third and fourth biopsy had a significantly lower biopsy Gleason score (4.6, p = 0.02 and 4.4, p = 0.01), Gleason score of the specimen (4.2, p = 0.001 and 4.0, p = 0.001), grade 4/5 cancer (8.2%, p = 0.02 and 0%), rate of multifocality (p = 0.009 and p = 0.008), cancer volume (0.83 cc, p = 0.001 and 0.79 cc, p = 0.001), and stage (p = 0.001 and p = 0.001), respectively, compared with cancers detected on first biopsy (Table 15.2).

- Cancers detected after second prostate biopsy have significantly lower Gleason score, Gleason 4/5 grade, multifocality, cancer volume, and pathologic stage. Therefore, these prostate cancers can be called "insig-nificant." However, based on these findings, a systematic prostate biopsy after a second repeat biopsy is not needed.

TABLE 15.2. Cancer characteristics and grading of prostate cancers detected on first through fourth biopsy (Bx).

	First Bx	Second Bx	p value*	Third Bx	p value*	Fourth Bx	p value*
Gleason score Bx	6.0 ± 0.7	5.7 ± 0.5	0.25	4.6 ± 0.4	0.02	4.4 ± 0.7	0.01
Gleason score RPE	5.3 ± 0.5	4.9 ± 0.8	0.36	4.2 ± 0.3	0.001	4.0 ± 0.4	0.001
% Grade 4/5	31.1	29.8	0.1	8.2	0.02	0	—
Multifocality	2.6 ± 0.4	1.8 ± 0.2	0.009	1.6 ± 0.4	0.009	1.9 ± 0.1	0.008
Cancer volume	4.2 ± 0.7	4.9 ± 0.8	0.27	0.83 ± 0.5	0.001	0.79 ± 0.4	0.001

Biopsy (Repeat) Techniques

After the introduction of the widely practiced technique of random systematic sextant prostatic biopsies by the Stanford group in 1989,[40] the optimal biopsy technique is a matter of debate. In a study of 273 men with suspected prostate cancer, whereas sextant biopsies alone detected 82% of cancers and lateral PZ biopsies alone detected 70% of cancers, when both techniques were combined, the cancer detection rate increased to 96%. A cancer detection rate of 59% was achieved if only hypoechoic lesions were targeted for biopsy. The authors concluded that combining both systematic sextant and lateral PZ biopsies would detect the majority of prostate cancers and eliminate the need for lesion-directed biopsies.[10]

Perhaps the most sensible approach to this issue is that proposed by Presti and coworkers,[41] who performed lateral PZ biopsies of the base (two) and midgland (two) in addition to routine sextant biopsies in 483 consecutive men referred for biopsy with an abnormal DRE and/or an increased serum PSA. Two hundred two cancers (42%) were detected, the majority (96%) by the combination of lateral PZ and sextant biopsies. Of the eight "missed" cancers, five were detected by lesion-directed biopsies. Furthermore, three cancers were found in the TZ of prostates >50 cc. If midlobar base biopsies were omitted from the protocol, the resultant eight-biopsy PZ regimen detected 95% of tumors. The systematic sextant biopsy method, practiced for a decade now, is inadequate and more extensive biopsy protocols obtaining a minimum of eight tissue cores, particularly from the lateral PZs, should be performed.

The detailed maps of consecutive radical prostatectomies have shown that prostate cancers expand mostly in the transverse direction across the posterior surface of the capsule, followed by the cephalocaudal direction.[2] Directing the biopsies more lateral to the mid-parasagittal plane might enable sampling of the large group of cancers located more laterally in the PZ.[2]

The posterior and posterolateral border of compressed fibromuscular tissues caused by the expansion of TZ hyperplastic nodules, observed on TRUS, serves as an excellent marker for placement of PZ biopsies where more than 70% of cancers originate.[2] Using a three-dimensional, computer-assisted prostate biopsy simulator and mounted step-sectional radical prostatectomy specimens, Bauer et al.[9] found that all the biopsy protocols that use laterally placed biopsies based on the 5-region anatomic model are superior to the routinely used sextant prostate biopsy technique.[9]

Although the majority of tumors arise in the PZ, up to 24% of prostate cancers originate in the TZ.[42] Other studies have reported rates significantly lower than this. Of 847 men who underwent TRUS-guided systematic sextant and TZ biopsies, only 8 patients (2.9%) (4.1% of only state T1c considered) had solitary TZ tumors.[43] Terris et al.[44] noted that patients undergoing routine TZ biopsies in addition to sextant biopsies had positive biopsies involving the TZ alone in 1.8% of cases. In a similar study, isolated TZ cancer was found in only 2.6% of men biopsied.[45] The Johns Hopkins

group performed repeat sextant and TZ biopsies in 193 radical prostatectomy specimens. They found that the TZ biopsy by itself was positive in
only 2.1% of cases, concluding that routine TZ biopsies are not justified in
light of such low detection rates.[46]

The low diagnostic yield of systematic TZ biopsy at the time of initial
biopsy argues strongly against its routine use for detection of early-stage
prostate cancer. However, performing TZ biopsies as part of a protocol of
repeat systematic biopsies in selected men with prior negative biopsies may
sometimes provide important additional information to that obtained by
repeating sextant biopsies alone.

To evaluate cancer location on initial and repeat biopsy in the European
Prostate Cancer Detection Study, all cancers were entered in a three-
dimensional spatial model and areas of highest cancer density were measured by means of a computer-based three-dimensional image reconstruction.[9]
Whereas cancers detected on initial biopsy are distributed homogeneously
over the entire prostate, cancers on repeat biopsy are found in a more
apico-dorsal location. A comparison of tumor density between both groups
shows significant differences in apical tumor density ($p = 0.001$), in dorsal
tumor density ($p = 0.02$), and especially in apico-dorsal tumor density
($p < 0.001$).

This may explain the lower cancer detection rate on repeat biopsies
(biopsies are rarely directed apico-dorsally) as well as the fact that these
cancers are frequently missed on initial biopsy. Thus, upon repeat biopsy,
the biopsy technique should be modified and needles should be directed to
a more apico-dorsal location.[9]

- A minimum of eight prostate cores (particularly from the lateral PZ) is
  needed.
- Impact of systematic TZ biopsies is still unclear.
- Repeat prostate biopsies should be directed more apico-dorsally.

Prostatic Intraepithelial Neoplasia/Atypia and Prostate Biopsy

High-grade prostatic intraepithelial neoplasia (PIN) is most likely a precursor of prostate cancer and is frequently associated with it, whereas a direct
link between low-grade PIN and cancer has not been established. The clinical evolution of isolated high-grade PIN has been the object of much
concern because of the possibility of undiagnosed prostate cancer or the
evolution of this premalignant lesion in invasive carcinoma.

High-grade PIN has been identified in approximately 4%–14% of prostate needle biopsies.[47–49] In an evaluation of pathology trends in 62,537
initial prostate needle core biopsies submitted by office-based urologists,
processed at a single pathology laboratory, isolated high-grade PIN was
diagnosed in 4.1% of the biopsies, a number which probably reflects the

real incidence of this entity in general practice as opposed to reference centers.[47]

According to Raviv et al.[50,51] and Zlotta et al.,[52] who analyzed 93 patients with a diagnosis of isolated PIN without concurrent carcinoma, cancer detection rate on repeat biopsy or operated specimen increased with PIN grades. In each PSA subgroup (0–4, 4.1–10, >10 ng/mL), the subsequent cancer detection rate was higher for high-grade PIN than for low-grade PIN. Nearly 50% of patients with isolated high-grade PIN were found to have prostate cancer on repeat biopsy, whereas only 13% of patients with low-grade PIN did so.

Weinstein and Epstein[53] noted that serum PSA levels were elevated in 90% of patients with high-grade PIN and cancer compared with 50% of those with PIN without associated cancer at the time of initial diagnosis, suggesting that serum PSA may be useful in distinguishing patients with PIN who will have cancer detected on repeat biopsy.

In the study by Raviv et al.,[50,51] the group of patients that later developed cancer had significantly higher PSA levels compared with patients without later cancer found on repeat biopsy. In high-grade PIN, the incidence of later cancer was 33% and 62% when PSA was <4 ng/mL or >10 ng/mL, respectively.[51] Therefore, all subgroups of patients with high-grade PIN, but especially those with elevated PSA, should undergo repeat biopsy. Low-grade PIN was associated with subsequent cancer in 42.8% of cases when PSA was >10 ng/mL, in 10.7% when PSA was between 4–10 ng/mL, and in none of the cases when PSA was ≤4 ng/mL.[51] Low grade should cause no further action unless other factors such as an elevated PSA increase the suspicion of prostate cancer and should prompt repeat biopsies. The high detection rate of later cancer when PSA is >10 ng/mL in low-grade PIN is similar to the report by Cooner et al.[54] on the detection of prostate cancer without reference to PIN. When PSA is >10 ng/mL, at whatever PIN grade, it seems clear that the high detection rate is more reflective of the undetected presence of cancer rather than the presence of PIN.

Most experts agree that high-grade PIN is clearly a preneoplastic lesion because it fulfills all requirements for such a lesion. Thus, high-grade PIN, especially when associated with high PSA or abnormal DRE or TRUS, should be taken as a signal of high to extremely high probability of prostate cancer and repeat biopsies should be performed.[52]

- High-grade PIN in first prostate biopsy requires repeat biopsy.

Morbidity of First and Repeat Prostate Biopsy

Generally, TRUS-guided biopsies are considered safe and are frequently performed in an outpatient setting. Djavan et al.[24] found only two major complications in 1871 biopsies performed. In contrast, minor complications were frequent, with 69.7% of all patients experiencing at least one complication. Although these complications generally do not need intervention (neither conservative nor surgical), patients need to be adequately informed.

When evaluating 81 patients undergoing TRUS-guided biopsy, Irani et al.[55] reported a mean visual analog pain scale score of 3. Nineteen percent of patients refused a repeat biopsy without some sort of anesthesia, and the authors questioned the safety and morbidity of repeat biopsies.[55] Except for moderate to severe vasovagal episodes (2.8% vs. 1.4%, p = 0.03), no differences were noted in pain apprehension (visual analog pain scale score 2.4 vs. 2.6, p = 0.09) and patient discomfort (moderate to severe in 8% vs. 11%, p = 0.29) during first and repeat biopsy, respectively.[24] In contrast, in a series reported by Collins et al.[56] and Clements et al.,[57] 22% and 30% of patients, respectively, considered the procedure significantly painful. Djavan et al.[24] found an age-dependent pattern in pain apprehension, with the younger patient (age <60 years) reporting a higher discomfort rate. Seventy-eight percent of patients younger than 60 years reported significant discomfort compared with 33%, 11%, and 8% for those in the age ranges 60–69, 70–80, and >80 years, respectively. Thus, younger patients need to be counseled adequately and local or topical anesthesia used. Rodriguez and Terris[58] also reported a higher discomfort rate in the younger age group.

A review of the literature shows that the majority of the studies evaluated infectious and bleeding complications only at first biopsy. Several studies demonstrated a significant decrease in infectious complications when prophylactic antibiotics were used.[24,58–62] Thompson et al.[63] reported asymptomatic bacteremia, frequently with *Bacteroides* species and *Enterococcus*. Symptomatic infections were most frequently caused by *Escherichia coli* and *Enterococcus*, suggesting the use of fluoroquinolones and metronidazole for antibiotic prophylaxis.[59,63–65]

Sieber et al.,[66] in a retrospective review of 4439 patients, reported an infection rate of 0.1%. Infectious complications are rare, and when needed, oral therapy is sufficient. Thus, cost issues need to be considered when selecting the type of antibiotic prophylaxis to be used.

Urinary tract infection with fever was seen in 2.1% and 1.9% (p = 0.02) of patients at first and repeat biopsy, respectively.[24] In one case (0.1%), a patient had to be admitted for prolepsis and was managed with intravenous antibiotics and discharged on day 6. In the immediate postbiopsy period, rectal bleeding (2.1% vs. 2.4%, p = 0.13), mild hematuria (62% vs. 57%, p = 0.06), and severe hematuria (0.7% vs. 0.5%, p = 0.09) were reported for the first and repeat biopsy, respectively. Delayed hemorrhagic morbidity included hematospermia (9.8% vs. 10.2%, p = 0.1) and recurrent mild hematuria (15.9% vs. 16.6%, p = 0.06), respectively. Again, no difference was noted between first and repeat biopsy. The rate of persistent hematuria was lower than previously reported (30%–50%).[58] This may be attributable to the fact that we routinely performed sextant biopsies and two additional TZ biopsies, whereas others had various numbers and sites of biopsy cores.

Hematospermia was obviously reported for those patients who had ejaculation before the biopsy procedure (n = 671). The lower rate in our population (compared with 59% reported in the literature) was similar to that reported by Rodriguez and Terris.[58]

TRUS-guided biopsy of the prostate is generally well tolerated with minor pain and morbidity. Repeat biopsies can be performed 6 weeks later with no significant difference in pain apprehension, or infectious or hemorrhagic complications.

- The morbidity of prostate biopsy in general is very low.
- Prophylactic antibiotic decreases morbidity.
- A systematic repeat biopsy has no increased morbidity.
- Patients younger than 60 years need to be counseled about a higher pain and discomfort level during repeat biopsy, and local or topical anesthesia should be provided if desired.

Summary

It seems that traditional sextant biopsies might become obsolete in future designed trials because a body of evidence supports the finding that this technique is far from optimal in patients with large prostates. Whether the future lies in performing biopsies more laterally, increasing the number of biopsies to 10, 12, 15, or even 18, or simply repeating the sextant biopsy scheme still needs to be verified. Current data suggest that cancers detected on repeat biopsy have a similar stage and grade distribution and total PSA values compared with cancers found on initial biopsy. Moreover, specific biologic determinants such as % Gleason grade 4/5, Gleason score, and cancer volume were identical in both groups, suggesting similar biologic properties and at least identical characteristics, thus supporting a repeat biopsy policy. Location and density measurements of cancers detected suggest that cancers missed on initial biopsy and subsequently detected on repeat biopsy are located in a more apico-dorsal location. Repeat biopsies should thus be directed to this rather spared area to improve cancer detection rates.

However, cancers detected on third and fourth systematic biopsy show characteristics of "insignificant" cancers. Therefore, a systematic repeat biopsy after the second biopsy in a PSA range of 2.5–10 ng/mL is not indicated, and PSA-based watchful waiting should be advocated.

Percent free PSA and PSA-TZ are the best markers for repeat prostate biopsy to increase sensitivity and specificity. In patients whose prostate cancer was detected on repeat biopsy, PSAD and PSA-TZ were higher. In all patients with high-grade PIN, a repeat biopsy should be performed.

Repeat biopsies performed as early as 6 weeks after the initial biopsy were generally well tolerated with minor pain and morbidity. Vasovagal episodes were more frequent after first biopsy. Antibiotic prophylaxis seems to be warranted and limited to 4 days at least. Patients younger than 60 years need to be counseled about a higher pain and discomfort level during repeat biopsy, and local or topical anesthesia provided if desired.

References

1. Djavan B, Susani M, Bursa B, Basharkhah A, Simak R, Marberger M. Predictability and significance of multifocal prostate cancer in the radical prostatectomy specimen. Tech Urol 1999;5(3):139–42.
2. Stamey TA. Making the most out of six systematic sextant biopsies. Urology 1995;45(1):2–12.
3. Billebaud T, Villers A, Astier L, et al. Advantage of systematic random ultrasound-guided biopsies, measurement of serum specific antigen levels and determination of prostate volume in the early diagnosis of prostate cancer. Eur Urol 1992;21:6–14.
4. Vashi AR, Wojno KJ, Gillespie B, Oesterling JE. A model for the number of cores per prostate biopsy based on patient age and prostate gland volume. J Urol 1998;159:920–4.
5. Karakiewicz PI, Aprikian AG, Meshref AW, Bazinet M. Computer-assisted comparative analysis of four-sector and six section biopsies of the prostate. Urology 1996;48:747–50.
6. Karakiewicz PI, Hanley JA, Bazinet M. Three-dimensional computer-assisted analysis of sector biopsy of the prostate. Urology 1998;52:208–12.
7. Ravery V, Billeband T, Toublanc M, et al. Diagnostic value of the systematic TRUS-guided prostate biopsies. Eur Urol 1999;35:298–303.
8. Eskew AL, Bare RL, McCullongh DL. Systematic 5-region prostate biopsy is superior to sextant method for diagnosing carcinoma of the prostate. J Urol 1997;157:199–202.
9. Bauer JJ, Zeng J, Weir J, et al. Three-dimensional computer-simulated prostate models: lateral prostate biopsies increase the detection rate of prostate cancer. Urology 1999;53:961–7.
10. Chang JJ, Shinohara K, Bhargava V, Presti JC Jr. Prospective evaluation of lateral biopsies of the peripheral zone for prostate cancer detection. J Urol 1998;160:2111–14.
11. Norberg M, Egevad L, Holmberg L, Sparen P, Norlen BJ, Busch C. The sextant protocol for ultrasound-guided core biopsies of the prostate underestimates the presence of cancer. Urology 1997;50:562–6.
12. Djavan B, Zlotta AR, Ekane S, et al. Is one set of sextant biopsies enough to rule out prostate cancer? Influence of transition and total prostate volumes on prostate cancer yield. Eur Urol 2000;38(2):218–24.
13. Uzzo RG, Wei JT, Waldbaum RS, Perlmutter AP, Byrne JC, Vaughan ED. The influence of prostatic size on cancer detection. Urology 1995;46:831–6.
14. Chen ME, Troncoso P, Johnston DA, Tang K, Babaian RJ. Optimization of prostate biopsy strategy using computer based analysis. J Urol 1997;158:2168–75.
15. Djavan B, Zlotta AR, Remzi M, et al. Total and transition zone prostate volume and age: how do they affect the utility of PSA based diagnostic parameters for early prostate cancer detection? Urology 1999;54(5):846–52.

16. Djavan B, Zlotta AR, Byttebier G, et al. Prostate specific antigen density of the TZ for early detection of prostate cancer. J Urol 1998;160(2):411–18.

17. Zlotta AR, Djavan B, Marberger M, Schulmann CC. Prostate specific antigen density of the transition zone: a new effective parameter for prostate cancer prediction. J Urol 1997;157:1315–21.

18. Levine MA, Ittman M, Melamed J, Lepor H. Two consecutive sets of transrectal ultrasound guided sextant biopsies of the prostate for the detection of prostate cancer. J Urol 1998;159:471–6.

19. Letran JL, Meyer GE, Loberiza FR, Brawer MK. The effect of prostate volume on the yield of needle biopsy. J Urol 1998;160(5):1718–21.

20. Vashi AR, Wojno KJ, Gillespie B, Oesterling JE. A model for the number of cores per prostate biopsy based on patient age and prostate gland volume. J Urol 1998;159:920–4.

21. Catalona WJ, Smith DS, Ratliff TD, et al. Measurement of prostate specific antigen in serum as a screening test for prostate cancer. New Engl J Med 1991;324:1156–61.

22. Brawer MK, Chetner MP, Beatie J, Buchner DM, Vessella RL, Lange PH. Screening for prostatic carcinoma with prostate specific antigen. J Urol 1992;147(2):841–5.

23. Keetch DW, Catalona WJ. Prostatic TZ biopsies in men with previous negative biopsies and persistently elevated serum prostate specific antigen values. J Urol 1995;154:1795–7.

24. Djavan B, Zlotta AR, Remzi M, et al. Optimal predictors of prostate cancer in repeat prostate biopsy: a prospective study in 1051 men. J Urol 2000;163(4):1144–8.

25. Zlotta AR, Djavan B, Roumeguere T, Marberger M, Schulmann CC. Transition zone volume on transrectal ultrasonography is more accurate and reproducible than the total prostate volume. Br J Urol 1997;Suppl 80:A926.

26. Catalona WJ, Partin AW, Slawin KM, et al. Use of the percentage of free prostate-specific antigen to enhance differentiation of prostate cancer from benign prostatic disease. JAMA 1998;279:1542–7.

27. Chan DW, Sokoll LJ, Partin AW, et al. The use of %free PSA to predict prostate cancer probabilities: an eleven center prospective study using an automated immunoassay system in a population with nonsuspicious DRE. J Urol 1999;161(Suppl 4):A353.

28. Horninger W, Reissigl A, Klocker H, et al. Improvement of specificity in PSA-based screening by using PSA transition zone density and percent free PSA in addition to total PSA levels. Prostate 1998;37:133–9.

29. Ukimura O, Durrani O, Babaian J. Role of PSA and its indices in determining the need for repeat prostate biopsies. Urology 1997;50:66–72.

30. Letran JL, Blasé AB, Loberiza FR, et al. Repeat ultrasound guided prostate needle biopsy: use of free to total PSA ratio in predicting prostatic carcinoma. J Urol 1998;60:426–9.

31. Morgan TO, McLeod DG, Leifer ES, Murphy GP, Moul JW. Prospective use of free prostate-specific antigen to avoid repeat prostate biopsies in men with elevated total prostate-specific antigen. Urology 1996;48:76–80.

32. Fleshner NE, O'Sullivan M, Fair WR. Prevalence and predictors of a positive repeat transrectal ultrasound guided needle biopsy of the prostate. J Urol 1997;158:505–9.

33. Catalona WJ, Beiser JA, Smith DS. Serum free prostate specific antigen and prostate specific antigen density measurements for predicting cancer in men with prior negative prostatic biopsies. J Urol 1997;158:2162–7.

34. Keetch DW, McMurtry JM, Smith DS, Andriole GL, Catalona WJ. Prostate specific antigen density versus prostate specific antigen slope as predictors of prostate cancer in men with initially negative prostatic biopsies. J Urol 1996;156:428–31.

35. Rietbergen JBW, Boeken Kruger AE, Hoedemaeker RF, Bangma CH, Kirkels WJ, Schröder FH. Repeat screening for prostate cancer after 1-year followup in 984 biopsied men: clinical and pathological features of detected cancer. J Urol 1998;160:2121–5.

36. Durkan GC, Greene DR. Elevated serum prostate specific antigen levels in conjunction with an initial prostatic biopsy negative for carcinoma: who should undergo a repeat biopsy? BJU Int 1999;83:34–8.

37. Noguchi M, Yahara J, Koga H, Nakashima O, Noda S. Necessity of repeat biopsies in men for suspected prostate cancer. Int J Urol 1999;6:7–12.

38. Keetch DW, Catalona WJ, Smith DS. Serial prostatic biopsies in men with persistently elevated serum prostate specific antigen values. J Urol 1994;151: 1571–4.

39. Stamey TA, McNeal JE, Yemoto CM, Sigal BM, Johnstone IM. Biological determinants of cancer progression in men with prostate cancer. JAMA 1999;281:1395–400.

40. Hodge KK, McNeal JE, Terris MK, et al. Random systematic versus directed ultrasound guided transrectal core biopsies of the prostate. J Urol 1989;142: 71–4.

41. Presti JR, Chang JJ, Bhargava V, Shinohara K. The optimal systematic prostate biopsy scheme should include 8 rather than 6 biopsies: results of a prospective clinical trial. J Urol 2000;163:163–7.

42. McNeal JE, Redwine EA, Freiha FS, Stamey TA. Zonal distribution of prostatic adenocarcinoma: correlation with histologic pattern and direction of spread. Am J Surg Pathol 1988;12:897–906.

43. Bazinet M, Karakiewicz PI, Aprikian AG, et al. Value of systematic TZ biopsies in the early detection of prostate cancer. J Urol 1996;155:605–6.

44. Terris MK, Pham TQ, Issa MM, Kabalin JN. Routine TZ and seminal vesicle biopsies in all patients undergoing transrectal ultrasound guided prostate biopsies are not indicated. J Urol 1997;157:204–6.

45. Morote J, Lopes M, Encabo G, de Torres I. Value of routine TZ biopsies in patients undergoing ultrasound-guided sextant biopsies for the first time. Eur Urol 1999;35:294–7.

46. Epstein JI, Walsh PC, Sauvageot J, Carter HB. Use of repeat sextant and transition zone biopsies for assessing extent of prostate cancer. J Urol 1997;158: 1886–90.

47. Orozco R, O'Dowd GJ, Kunnel B, et al. Observations on pathology trends in 62,537 prostate biopsies obtained from urology private practices in the United States. Urology 1998;51:186–95.

48. Bostwick DG, Qian J, Frankel K. The incidence of high grade prostatic intraepithelial neoplasia in needle biopsies. J Urol 1995;154:1791–4.

49. Green J, Feneley MR, Young M, Peeling B, Kirby R, Parkinson C. The prevalence of prostatic intraepithelial neoplasia (PIN) in biopsies from hospital

practice and pilot screening: clinical implications. J Urol 1996;155(Suppl): A1260.

50. Raviv G, Janssen TH, Zlotta AR, Descamps F, Verhest A, Schulman CC. Prostatic intraepithelial neoplasia: influence of clinical and pathological data on the detection of invasive prostate cancer, in patients initially diagnosed on previous needle biopsy. J Urol 1996;156:1050–5.

51. Raviv G, Zlotta AR, Janssen TH, Descamps F, Verhest A, Schulman CC. Does prostate-specific antigen and prostate-specific antigen density enhance the detection of prostate cancer in patients initially diagnosed to have prostatic intraepithelial neoplasia? Cancer 1996;77:2103–8.

52. Zlotta AR, Raviv G, Schulman CC. Clinical prognostic criteria for later diagnosis of prostate carcinoma in patients with initial isolated prostatic intraepithelial neoplasia. Eur Urol 1996;30:249–55.

53. Weinstein MH, Epstein JI. Significance of high grade prostatic intraepithelial neoplasia on needle biopsy. Hum Pathol 1993;24:624–9.

54. Cooner WH, Mosley BR, Rutherford CL, et al. Prostate cancer detection in a clinical urological practice by ultrasonography, digital rectal examination and prostate specific antigen. J Urol 1990;143:1146–52.

55. Irani J, Fournier F, Bon D, et al. Patient tolerance of transrectal ultrasound-guided biopsy of the prostate. Br J Urol 1997;79(4):608–10.

56. Collins GN, Lloyd SN, Hehir M, et al. Multiple transrectal ultrasound-guided prostatic biopsies: true morbidity and patient acceptance. Br J Urol 1993;71: 460–3.

57. Clements R, Aideyan OU, Griffiths GJ, et al. Side effects and patient acceptability of transrectal biopsy of the prostate. Clin Radiol 1993;47:125–6.

58. Rodriguez LV, Terris MK. Risks and complications of transrectal ultrasound guided prostate needle biopsy: a prospective study and review of the literature. J Urol 1998;160:2115–20.

59. Crawford ED, Haynes AL Jr, Story MW, et al. Prevention of urinary tract infection and sepsis following transrectal prostatic biopsy. J Urol 1982;127: 449–51.

60. Davison P, Malament M. Urinary contamination as a result of transrectal biopsy of the prostate. J Urol 1971;105:545–6.

61. Fawcett DP, Eykyn S, Bultidue MI. Urinary tract infection following transrectal biopsy of the prostate. Br J Urol 1975;47:679–81.

62. Ashby EC, Rees M, Dowding CH. Prophylaxis against systemic infection after transrectal biopsy for suspected prostatic carcinoma. Br Med J 1978;2:1263–4.

63. Thompson PM, Talbot RW, Packham DA, et al. Transrectal biopsy of the prostate and bacteremia. Br J Surg 1980;67:127–8.

64. Thompson PM, Prior JP, Williams JP, et al. The problem of infection after prostatic biopsy: the case for the transperineal approach. Br J Urol 1982;54: 736.

65. Gustafsson O, Norming U, Nyman CR, et al. Complications following combined transrectal aspiration and core biopsy of the prostate. Scand J Urol Nephrol 1990;24:249–51.

66. Sieber PR, Rommel FM, Agusta VE, et al. Antibiotic prophylaxis in ultrasound guided transrectal prostate biopsy. J Urol 1997;157:2199–200.

16
Saturation Biopsy for Detection and Characterization of Prostate Cancer

J. Stephen Jones

Abstract

Saturation biopsy can be defined as a multicore biopsy strategy obtaining 20 or greater cores. Initial reports were from operating rooms, anesthetic-based series, but it has become clear that the procedure can be safely and efficiently performed in the office setting using periprostatic block. The rationale, detection rates, and implications for both screening and management are discussed.

Keywords: saturation biopsy, prostate biopsy, repeat biopsy, parasagittal, repeat biopsy

Systematic ultrasound-guided transrectal prostate biopsy became the mainstay for the diagnosis of prostate cancer after the landmark report of Hodge and Stamey in 1989.[1] Their initial biopsy scheme included six evenly distributed parasagittal cores—a number chosen based on Dr. Stamey's observation that six cores detected most of the large palpable tumors that they were seeing clinically before the prostate-specific antigen (PSA) era (personal communication, November 2004).

Subsequent studies have demonstrated that a traditional sextant technique misses substantial numbers of cancers and that additional sampling of the lateral and apical peripheral zone tissue increases the diagnostic yield.[2,3] Even when obtaining 10–14 cores, the false-negative rate remains substantial.[4] As a result, "saturation" biopsy has been adopted in several centers, resulting in cancer detection rates approaching one third when extended biopsy schemes of 14–45 cores were used even after multiple negative biopsies.[5,6] This procedure was initially performed in the operating room under general or regional anesthesia, although the Cleveland Clinic has demonstrated that office-based biopsy is appropriate and well tolerated.[7]

From: *Current Clinical Urology: Prostate Biopsy: Indications, Techniques, and Complications*
Edited by J.S. Jones © Humana Press, Totowa, NJ

What Is "Saturation" Biopsy?

The initial report was published by Borboroglu et al.,[5] but the term "saturation biopsy" was coined by Stewart et al.[6] to describe the multicore technique that they had developed almost simultaneously in the late 1990s. The studies obtained a mean of 22.5 and 23 cores, respectively. When Jones et al.[7] explored the concept in the office setting using local anesthesia beginning in 2002, it was determined that a 24-core template would qualify using either benchmark for "saturation," so used that threshold as the definition. However, subsequent studies have shown that the additional value of obtaining more than 20 cores may be limited, so most recent studies use this minimum as the definition of saturation technique.

Rationale for Saturation Biopsy

Many urologists initially were concerned regarding the morbidity such an aggressive biopsy strategy would entail when Hodge and Stamey proposed the sextant biopsy. Such concerns were soon proven needless, as their sextant or six-core technique tested in 136 patients became the standard of care almost immediately. Systematic biopsy was shown to be associated with acceptable complication risk and morbidity that patients usually accepted based on the inability to anesthetize the prostate during that era. Although the six cores described by Stamey were originally feared to be excessive, even more aggressive strategies previously believed unthinkable (8–14 cores) were soon demonstrated to involve no increased morbidity compared with the sextant technique,[8,9] and have become the new standard of care. The advent of periprostatic block[10] allowed these schemes to be tolerated routinely.

Nevertheless, even after extensive biopsy strategies using 12–14 cores, many patients continue to demonstrate findings creating suspicion of undiagnosed malignancy. The yield of a second biopsy is significant as outlined by Djavan and Marihart in Chapter 15. However, after two negative biopsies, repeat sextant or even extended biopsy is unlikely to find malignancy. Of those infrequent cancers identified using traditional biopsy templates after two routine 6- to 12-core biopsies, the vast majority are clinically insignificant as described by Djavan and Marihart. In contrast, saturation biopsy has been shown in several series to identify substantial risk of high-grade cancers even after multiple routine biopsies.[6,11–14]

This scenario evokes a concept inaccurately attributed in various sources to Mark Twain, Benjamin Franklin, or Albert Einstein, although its origin is actually in the writings of the 17th century poet, John Dryden: It is unreasonable (Dryden would suggest "insane") to do the same thing over and over again, and expect different results. If no cancer is identified in the parasagittal cores once, twice, or more, it probably means that cancer does not exist in that location. It should be obvious that an infinite number of cores in that location will still fail to find what is not there. As a result, we do not repeat the initial strategy, but use a different scheme both numerically and geometrically in order to find cancer where it may have been previously overlooked. This has led to saturation biopsy.

History

Even in patients with multiple previous negative biopsies, approximately one third of the time cancer was found when extended biopsy schemes of 14–45 cores were used in the initial studies.[5,6] This indicates that the risk of undiagnosed malignancy is substantial even after multiple biopsies, so a high index of suspicion is appropriate in determining surveillance strategies for these patients. Because most of these biopsies involved at least quadruple the number of cores described by Stamey, these early saturation biopsies were performed under systemic or regional anesthesia.

Based on the effectiveness of pain prevention using periprostatic block, we began performing saturation biopsy in the office on patients requiring repeat biopsy, and demonstrated that it was as well tolerated as routine biopsy. Complication rates were no higher than for routine biopsy, and cancer was identified in almost 30% of patients. Importantly, most of these patients had undergone extended 8- to 12-core previous biopsy instead of traditional sextant biopsy of the previous reports.[11]

The description of periprostatic nerve block was vital to creating widespread acceptance of multicore biopsy strategies.[10] With the adequate anesthesia it affords, the number of cores has little impact on pain experience. This has allowed "saturation" prostate biopsy to become a routine approach for all repeat biopsies in our patients.

Techniques

The original reports of saturation biopsy involved multiple random needle passes performed in the operating room. The use of a brachytherapy stepper in order to map the prostate through a transperineal approach has also been proposed, but data to support its advantages are unclear.[12] This approach also requires anesthetic-based operating room utilization.

We originally used a 24-core transrectal template as shown in Figure 16.1, with cores concentrated laterally and apically based on the preponderance of cancer in these locations. This focus is especially important during repeat biopsy after extended schemes, as shown by Hong et al.[15] In early evaluation of the site of positive cores, it soon became clear that the lateral sectors (dark shading) were the site of all tumors in this repeat biopsy population, but further breakdown by apex, midgland, and base were not informative.

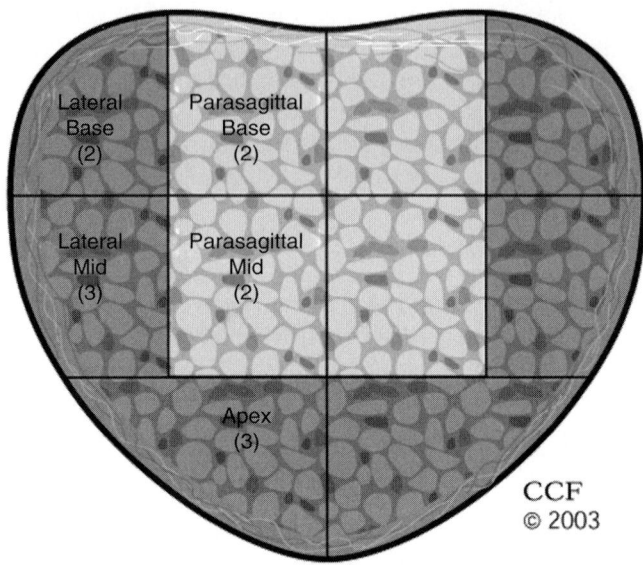

FIGURE 16.1. Initial saturation biopsy template showing sectors and number of cores obtained from each. Note that the darkly shaded sectors are regarded as lateral biopsies, and that the entire apex is considered lateral based on its composition of peripheral zone tissue alone.

Based on the knowledge that cancers occur primarily in the peripheral zone, and that all apical tissue is peripheral zone tissue, all tissue removed from the apical sector is considered a lateral core. No tumors were identified as a unique finding in the medial cores, although some patients with positive lateral cores will have cancer extending into the areas biopsied by medial cores. As a result, we reduced sampling from two cores to one core per medial sector (midgland and base), resulting in a 20-core template for patients undergoing repeat biopsy (Figure 16.2).[16]

To avoid repeat biopsy of the same site, the examiner should be observant of the hyperechoic linear signs on ultrasound that occur as a result of the interface of tissue with blood and the needle tract. With experience, it is possible to determine the site of biopsies taken earlier in the session in order to truly distribute sampling (Figure 16.3).

It is also important to perform the biopsy in areas likely to harbor cancer undiagnosed during previous biopsy sessions. Hong et al.[15] have shown that the apex is the most likely site for this to occur, so focus of at least three cores is made at that level. Unlike other levels where transition zone tissue is identified, apical tissue is comprised entirely of peripheral zone tissue, which is much more likely than transition zone tissue to contain cancer (Figures 16.4 and 16.5).

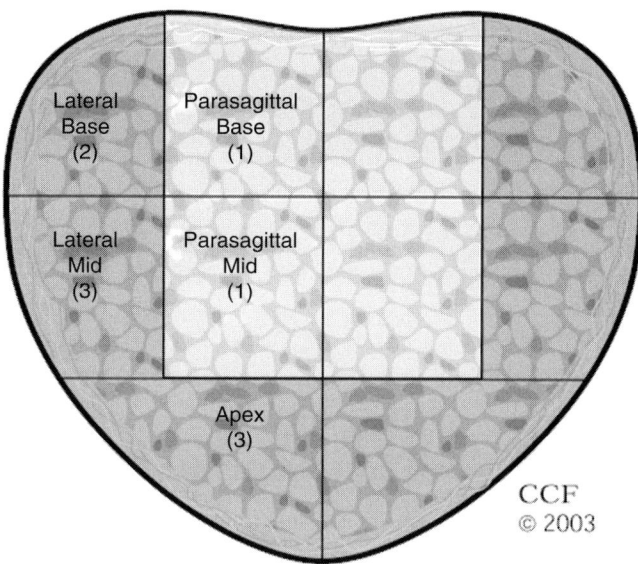

FIGURE 16.2. Current Cleveland Clinic saturation biopsy template showing reduced sampling in the medial sectors, which are almost never the site of unique positive cores in the absence of positive lateral cores.

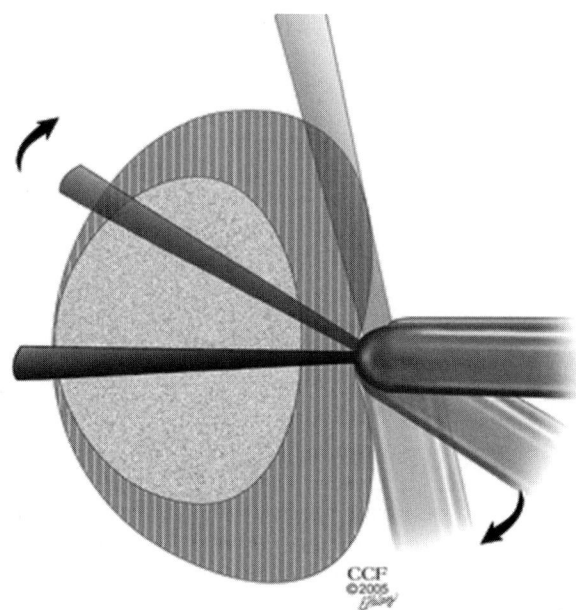

FIGURE 16.3. The biopsy guide shows the direction of previous needle tracks obtained earlier during this biopsy session. Observation of the previous hyperechoic (white) tracks allows the physician to avoid repeat biopsy in the same site, increasing the detection of cancer in other, unbiopsied locations.

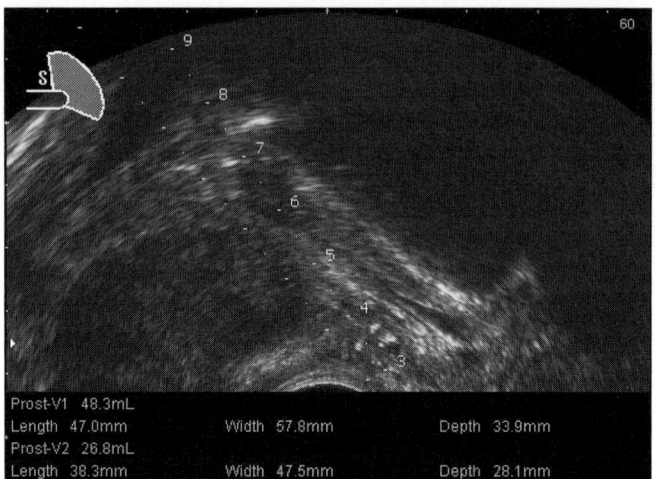

FIGURE 16.4. Transition zone tissue is unlikely to harbor cancer, so apical biopsy is often positive because it is entirely comprised of peripheral zone tissue. The "anterior horn" of peripheral zone tissue can be seen to the right of the more heterogeneous transition zone tissue.

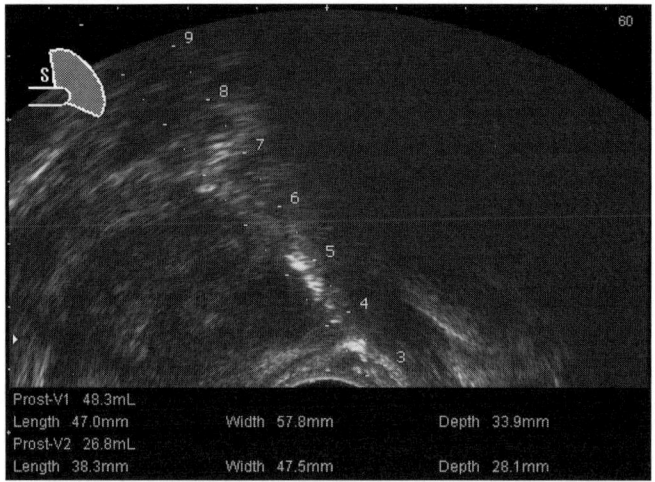

FIGURE 16.5. The needle has been placed caudal (to the right) to the transition zone in the "anterior horn" of peripheral zone tissue that wraps around the transition zone. These anterior biopsies are the most likely place for cancer to have gone undiagnosed during previous biopsy sessions.

Results

Operating room–based saturation strategy has been reported to yield a 30% (57 patients)[5] to 34% (224 patients)[6] positive biopsy rate. Those studies obtained a mean of 22.5 and 23 cores, respectively. These data must be interpreted with the understanding that all patients had previously undergone sextant biopsies alone, which are known to be an inadequate biopsy strategy. There was no clear trend toward decreasing positivity with the number of previous biopsies in the larger study, where the mean number of previous sextant biopsies was 1.8.

To date, we have successfully performed office-based saturation biopsy obtaining 20–24 cores in hundreds of patients using periprostatic block without increased complications. No analgesics, sedatives, or other pain control has been given beyond the periprostatic block. In this nonrandomized series, we have found the cancer detection rate to be almost 30%. Interestingly, in our initial series, we detected significant cancer in the majority of patients who were evaluated previously with a single sextant biopsy, although the number of such patients who have had only a sextant biopsy is diminishing greatly.[11]

Walz et al.[13] identified cancer in 41% of 161 patients undergoing repeat saturation biopsy obtaining a mean of 24 cores. A French study reported 303 patients biopsied for 21 cores under local anesthesia. This again confirmed the safety of this approach compared with operating room–based saturation biopsy, with complication rates at levels expected of even sextant biopsy. The 78 patients undergoing a second biopsy were found to have cancer in 25.6%, whereas only 1 of 37 patients who had undergone more than one prior biopsy was found to have cancer. Again, medial cores were of little additional value.[14]

A report of 210 men biopsied transperineally using a brachytherapy template obtaining a mean of 21 cores identified cancer in 37% of men, 81% of whom were undergoing their second or greater biopsy. Urinary retention occurred in 11%, suggesting this more involved technique offers no improvement in detection rate but a potentially higher complication rate.[12]

In contrast, Fleshner and Klotz[17] found little value for saturation biopsy in 37 patients who had undergone multiple previous negative biopsies. Their study obtaining 24 peripheral zone cores, 6–12 transition zone cores, and two lateral lobe transurethral samples under general or regional anesthesia is sometimes misinterpreted as proving that saturation biopsy has no benefit. On the contrary, their study shows that in the selected population of men who have undergone multiple (3–6) negative biopsies are unlikely to have significant cancer identified using saturation or any biopsy, with only 13.5% positive. Their report does not address saturation biopsy as the first repeat biopsy. Predictably, all cancers were identified in the peripheral zone biopsies.[17]

Although there is a clearly defined relationship between cancer detection and prostate size as defined in Chapter 15, it is unclear whether this should have an impact on the number of cores obtained during saturation biopsy. To date, no studies have been able to make a clear recommendation, so we use the number of 20 cores for the reasons stated above.

Saturation Biopsy as an Initial Biopsy Strategy

With our experience that cancer detection was improved with saturation biopsy as a repeat biopsy strategy,[11] we explored its use as an initial biopsy strategy in 139 patients in order to enhance cancer detection in a single setting. All patients tolerated complete biopsies obtaining the planned numbers of cores.

In contrast to our theory that this would increase cancer detection, we found that increasing the number of cores to 24 did not yield a higher detection rate. Cancer was detected in 62 of 139 patients (44.6%) who underwent saturation biopsy compared with 45 of 87 control patients (51.7%) who underwent 10-core biopsy (p > 0.9). Breakdown by PSA level failed to show benefit to the saturation technique for any degree of PSA elevation. Six of 21 men (28.6%) who had saturation biopsy and 7 of 18 (38.9%) who had 10-core biopsy with a PSA of 2.5–3.9 ng/dL had cancer. Forty-seven of 101 men (46.5%) who had saturation biopsy and 19 of 40 (47.5%) who had 10-core biopsy with a PSA between 4.0 and 9.9 ng/dL were found to have cancer. Therefore, 53 of 122 men (43.4%) who underwent saturation biopsy and 26 of 58 (44.8%) who underwent 10-core biopsy with PSA of 2.5–9.9 ng/dL were found to have cancer. None of the differences were statistically significant.[18]

In the French report of patients undergoing a 21-core strategy as their initial biopsy (n = 188), the detection rate was 39.3%, or similar to 10- to 12-core biopsy schemes.[14] The detection rates in both these reports are consistent with the multiple reports of approximately 40% detection rate for all schemes using 12 or more cores for initial diagnosis, so it is clear that saturation biopsy offers no advantage when used as an initial biopsy strategy.

Management of Suspicion of Prostate Cancer after Negative Saturation Biopsy

Djavan and others have demonstrated that repeat routine biopsy is unlikely to identify significant cancer in men who have undergone two negative saturation biopsies. The findings of high-grade prostatic intraepithelial neoplasia or atypical small acinar proliferation still carry the risk of cancer and must be addressed separately as described by Weizer et al. in Chapter 19.

In patients who have undergone repeat saturation biopsy (by definition at least their second biopsy overall), we have exceedingly rarely identified cancer in follow-up. Of cancer identified, none to date has been identified as metastatic, and the few patients with cancer (fewer than five) have had low-volume, low-grade, presumably clinically insignificant disease. Therefore, our threshold to repeat saturation biopsy is very high, and is usually only triggered by a severe increase in PSA.

Risk of Diagnosing Clinically Insignificant Cancer with Saturation Biopsy

There is no doubt regarding the potential of any biopsy scheme to detect clinically insignificant cancer. This risk has received significant attention when saturation biopsy is used based on the fear that this will be even more likely when more cores are obtained.

When Hodge and Stamey originally described the sextant biopsy, concern was expressed that it would identify undue numbers of clinically insignificant cancer. This concern was dismissed by studies showing that most tumors identified by a modest increase in PSA were indeed clinically significant.[19] In addition, a recent report from the CAPSure database determined that increasing the number of cores improved cancer detection, but failed to increase the risk of finding clinically insignificant cancer, so a downside was not identified.[20] However, as shown by Djavan and Marihart in Chapter 15 of this book, cancers identified on such schemes after a second negative biopsy are usually clinically insignificant, presumably because significant cancers in the areas normally biopsied should be identified during the first or second biopsies.

Patients with cancer at low risk of progression will theoretically be less likely to be treated aggressively with surgical intervention, so radical prostatectomy studies may underestimate this risk. Mindful of this, studies from Johns Hopkins Hospital have found that the risk of insignificant cancer even using any biopsy strategy is at least 16%, and that the risk of "truly minute" cancer is currently 5%.[21] There is no universally accepted definition of "clinically insignificant," but they reported that tumors were "insignificant" (confined tumor smaller than 0.2 cm^3 with a Gleason score of less than 7) in 17% and "minimal" (confined tumor 0.2 to less than 0.5 cm^3 with a Gleason score of less than 7) in 12% of 240 men who underwent radical prostatectomy, suggesting that more than one fourth of men who are treated with prostatectomy may be "overdiagnosed" using traditional biopsy strategies.[22]

Drawing the same conclusion for cancer identified during saturation biopsy is not automatically intuitive, because the cancers identified may be different than those identified using traditional templates. The original two saturation biopsy studies had conflicting conclusions on whether the risk of incidental cancer was higher. Borboroglu and colleagues[5] found that 12 of 13 patients who underwent radical prostatectomy had clinically significant cancer by traditional criteria. However, Stewart and colleagues[7] found that the risk of incidental cancer increased from 11.1% to 15.4% to 22.2% in patients with 1, 2, or 3 or more previous sextant biopsies, respectively; 30.6% of the tumors removed at prostatectomy were less than 0.5 cc. Of four patients who underwent prostatectomy in the series by Rabets et al.,[11] all were deemed clinically significant with volumes >0.5 cc and three of the four were Gleason 7. Of patients who underwent radical prostatectomy in the perineal saturation report, all had tumors >0.5 cc and 90% had stage pT2 disease.[12]

Upon examination of the specimen in men who underwent radical prostatectomy in our series using saturation for the initial biopsy, cancer was clinically significant by published definitions[23] in 16 of 19 patients (84.2%), which compares favorably with the risk of identifying clinically insignificant cancer during sextant biopsy as shown in the Johns Hopkins studies above.

The single patient in Fleshner and Klotz's small series of men who had undergone multiple (3–6) previous negative biopsies and underwent radical prostatectomy had extensive Gleason 7 cancer and multiple positive margins.

The concern of overdetection must be weighed against the risk of clinically significant malignancy being missed by inadequate biopsy strategies that have considerable false-negative rates. We believe the best approach to balance these risks at the current time involves the concept espoused by Carroll—"unlinking detection and treatment, as they are separate processes."[24] Many men with low-volume, low-grade disease may be managed expectantly, and treatment can be safely delayed until the time that clinical indicators such as sequential PSA, repeat biopsy, or physical examination indicate disease progression and the need for deferred intervention.[25] If this approach is accepted for men whose biopsies suggest clinically insignificant disease, careful observation will usually allow detection of progression while still curable as discussed below.

Saturation Biopsy in Management of Candidates for Active Surveillance for Prostate Cancer

Although initial efforts focused on the use of saturation biopsy to identify cancer in difficult to diagnose cases after previous negative biopsy, its use for quantification and qualification of prostate cancer may be as important. When we began using saturation biopsy for all repeat biopsies in 2002, we also began using the technique for patients who were managed with an active surveillance protocol. Patients with low risk of progression based on biopsy findings were recommended to have a repeat PSA and repeat saturation biopsy within 1 year of initial diagnosis if they chose active surveillance.

All patients were informed of the risks of observation, as well as other options the surgeon believed appropriate for the patient. These patients were managed the same as those routinely offered active surveillance, but with an emphasis on repeat assessment biopsy. This population has experienced cancer progression to higher grade or volume in fewer than 25% of cases, and has proceeded to therapy with curative intent in fewer than 10% of cases based on stable PSA levels, digital rectal examination findings, and biopsy findings. No patient has developed metastatic disease, but the follow-up is 4 years or less at this date.

Epstein et al.[21] performed saturation biopsy on pathologic specimens after radical prostatectomy on patients they determined would have been candidates for active surveillance based on favorable pathologic features. Their technique using a plastic template obtained an average of 44 cores from 103 ex vivo surgical specimens. Their full saturation scheme predicted insignificant cancer if the Gleason score was less than 7 with three or fewer positive cores, or if the maximum length of cancer in one core was less than 4.5 mm and the total millimeters of cancer for all cores failed to exceed 5.5 mm. These criteria for clinically significant cancer had a sensitivity of 71.9% and a specificity of 95.5%. An alternate scheme using only every other biopsy core was assessed. Half as many cores (mean 22 cores, or similar to most clinically utilized saturation schemes) could predict clinically insignificant cancer if the Gleason score was less than 7 and the total millimeters of cancer was less than 2.75, or if the total millimeters positive in all cores was less than 9.5 mm. This approach yielded the same sensitivity (71.9%) but an increased specificity of 97.1%, suggesting the 22-core scheme may be preferred to a more extensive scheme. This notably approximates the same technique we and the other groups referenced use in clinical practice.

Summary

Cancers missed on initial biopsy are almost without exception laterally based,[16] so focus should be on the lateral areas most likely to be positive in patients undergoing repeat biopsy. The apex is entirely composed of peripheral zone tissue and is the most likely site of undiagnosed malignancy. With the morbidity reportedly no higher than with published rates for sextant biopsy, there is little disincentive to increase the number of cores to 20–24 if cancer is suspected after negative biopsy. Counterintuitively, despite its tolerability, saturation biopsy does not seem to provide additional value during the initial biopsy, so should be reserved for repeat biopsy. The risk of significant undiagnosed cancer after a negative repeat saturation biopsy is very low, so is reserved for situations involving a high risk of undiagnosed malignancy such as rapidly increasing PSA and atypical small acinar proliferation. The role and appropriate number of cores for saturation biopsy continue to be defined, but we currently recommend 20 cores with emphasis on the lateral areas for any patient having a repeat biopsy.

References

1. Hodge KK, McNeal JE, Terris MK, et al. Random systematic versus directed ultrasound guided transrectal core biopsies of the prostate. J Urol 1989;142:71.
2. Keetch DW, Catalona WJ, Smith DS. Serial prostate biopsies in men with persistently elevated serum prostate specific antigen values. J Urol 1994;151: 1571.
3. Epstein JI, Walsh PC, Carter HB. Importance of posterolateral needle biopsies in the detection of prostate cancer. Urology 2001;57:1112.
4. Applewhite JC, Matagla BR, McCullough D. Results of the 5 region prostate biopsy method: the repeat biopsy population. J Urol 2002;168:500–3.
5. Borboroglu PG, Comer SW, Riffenburgh RH, Amling CL. Extensive repeat transrectal ultrasound guided prostate biopsy in patients with previous benign sextant biopsies. J Urol 2000;163:158–62.
6. Stewart CS, Leibovich BC, Weaver AL, Lieber MM. Prostate cancer diagnosis using a saturation needle biopsy technique after previous negative sextant biopsies. J Urol 2001;166:86–92.
7. Jones JS, Oder M, Zippe CD. Saturation biopsy with periprostatic block can be performed in office. J Urol 2002;168:2108–10.
8. Naughton CK, Ornstein DK, Smith DS, Catalona WJ. Pain and morbidity of transrectal ultrasound guided prostate biopsy: a prospective randomized trial of 6 versus 12 cores. J Urol 2000;163(1):168–71.
9. Chang SS, Alberts G, Wells N, Smith JA Jr, Cookson MS. Intrarectal lidocaine during transrectal prostate biopsy: results of a prospective double-blind randomized trial. J Urol 2001;166(6):2178–80.
10. Nash P, Bruce J, Indudhara R, et al. Transrectal ultrasound guided prostatic nerve blockade eases systemic needle biopsy of the prostate. J Urol 1996;155:607.
11. Rabets J, Jones JS, Patel A, Zippe CD. Prostate cancer detection with office-based saturation biopsy in a repeat biopsy population. J Urol 2004;172: 94–7.
12. Pinkstaff DM, Igel TC, Petrou SP, Broderick GA, Wehle MJ, Young PR. Systematic transperineal ultrasound-guided template biopsy of the prostate: three-year experience. Urology 2005;65(4):735–9.
13. Walz J, Graefen M, Chun FK, et al. High incidence of prostate cancer detected by saturation biopsy after previous negative biopsy series. Eur Urol 2006;50(3): 498–505.
14. de la Taille A, Antiphon P, Salomon L, et al. Prospective evaluation of a 21-sample needle biopsy procedure designed to improve the prostate cancer detection rate. Urology 2003;61(6):1181–6.
15. Hong YM, Lai FC, Chon CH, McNeal JE, Presti JC Jr. Impact of prior biopsy scheme on pathologic features of cancers detected on repeat biopsies. Urol Oncol 2004;22(1):7–10.
16. Patel A, Jones JS, Rabets J, DeOreo G, Klein E, Zippe CD. Parasagittal biopsies add minimal information in repeat saturation prostate biopsy. Urology 2004;63:1, 87–89.
17. Fleshner N, Klotz L. Role of "saturation biopsy" in the detection of prostate cancer among difficult diagnostic cases. Urology 2002;60(1):93–7.

18. Jones JS, Patel A, Schoenfield L, Rabets JC, Zippe CD, Magi-Galluzzi C. Saturation technique does not improve cancer detection as an initial prostate biopsy strategy. J Urol 2006;175(2):485–8.
19. Scaletscky R, Koch MO, Eckstein CW, Bicknell SL, Gray GF Jr, Smith JA Jr. Tumor volume and stage in carcinoma of the prostate detected by elevations in prostate specific antigen. J Urol 1994;152(1):129–31.
20. Meng MV, Elkin EP, DuChane J, Carroll PR. Impact of increased number of biopsies on the nature of prostate cancer identified. J Urol 2006;176(1):63–8.
21. Epstein JI, Walsh PC, Carmichael M, Brendler CB. Pathologic and clinical findings to predict tumor extent of nonpalpable (stage T1c) prostate cancer. JAMA 1994;271(5):368–74.
22. Carter HB, Sauvageot J, Walsh PC, Epstein JI. Prospective evaluation of men with stage T1C adenocarcinoma of the prostate. J Urol 1997;157(6):2206–9.
23. Jack GS, Cookson MS, Coffey CS, et al. Pathological parameters of radical prostatectomy for clinical stages T1c versus T2 prostate adenocarcinoma: decreased pathological stage and increased detection of transition zone tumors. J Urol 2002;168(2):519–24.
24. Carroll PR. Early stage prostate cancer—do we have a problem with over-detection, overtreatment or both? J Urol 2005;173(4):1061–2.
25. Patel MI, DeConcini DT, Lopez-Corona E, Ohori M, Wheeler T, Scardino PT. An analysis of men with clinically localized prostate cancer who deferred definitive therapy. J Urol 2004;171(4):1520–4.

17
Pathologic Implications of Prostate Biopsy

Ming Zhou and Cristina Magi-Galluzzi

Abstract

Information included in pathology reports has a critical role in patient management. Descriptions of samples positive for prostate cancer should include information on the location of relevant cores, histologic subtypes, and Gleason scoring although the calculation and interpretation of this scoring method is currently under debate. The amount of cancer found in the biopsy cores, extraprostatic extension, seminal vesicle invasion, and perineural invasion must be documented. High-grade prostatic intraepithelial neoplasia and atypical glands suspicious for prostate cancer should be reported because their presence is associated with prostate cancer detection on repeat biopsy. Emerging molecular prognostic markers are extremely promising for prostate cancer diagnosis. Whereas many types of molecular evaluation are already in widespread use, others require large, prospective studies to be validated for inclusion in routine practice.

Keywords: prostate biopsy, high-grade prostatic intraepithelial neoplasia, atypical small acinar proliferation (ATYP), atrophy

With widespread use of prostate-specific antigen (PSA) screening and digital rectal examination in an effort to detect early prostate cancer, there has been a dramatic increase in the number of men undergoing ultrasound-guided transrectal prostate biopsy. The pathologic diagnosis of prostate cancer in needle biopsy has been the subject of many excellent review articles and is beyond the scope of this review.[1-3] This article instead focuses on the contemporary issues in the laboratory processing of prostate biopsies and the information that should be included in prostate biopsy pathology

From: *Current Clinical Urology: Prostate Biopsy: Indications, Techniques, and Complications*
Edited by J.S. Jones © Humana Press, Totowa, NJ

reports. In addition, emerging molecular prognostic markers are reviewed.

Laboratory Processing of Prostate Needle Biopsy

Submission of Prostate Needle Biopsy Specimens

Currently, ultrasound-guided transrectal 18-gauge needle biopsy remains the principal mode of diagnosis of prostate adenocarcinoma. Although the biopsy schemes, including the standard sextant biopsy, and more recently extended biopsy and modified biopsy protocols, have been uniformly applied,[4] submission of the biopsy specimens, however, has been less standardized. Many urologists submit the biopsy core(s) from each anatomic site in separate containers to preserve the information of the core location. Some submit the biopsy cores from the right and left sides in two separate containers. Yet others place all the biopsy cores in a single container.

The distribution of prostate cancer, as indicated by the location(s) of the involved biopsy cores, provides important prognostic information. For example, cancer involving different anatomic sites may imply different risk for extraprostatic extension and positive surgical margins. The amount of cancer in the biopsies from the base and apex is reported to correlate with extraprostatic extension and positive surgical margins, respectively.[5] Gleason score 7–9 cancer in biopsies from the mid and base of the prostate gland has been associated with seminal vesicle invasion and lymph node metastasis.[6] Involvement of 50% or more of the biopsies from the base seems to predict the extraprostatic extension in the posterolateral region and neurovascular bundle invasion.[7]

Information on the cancer distribution in the prostate gland may also help in planning the field of brachytherapy, or may influence nerve- or bladder neck-sparing radical prostatectomy. Sanwick et al.[8] found that the nerve bundle could be safely preserved on the side of the prostate gland that harbored low- to intermediate-grade cancer provided at least three biopsy cores were taken from each side of the prostate gland.

Knowledge of the location of positive biopsy cores allows for a more focused rebiopsy strategy. If a prostate needle biopsy is diagnosed as "atypical glands, suspicious for prostate cancer (ATYP)," the patient carries approximately 40% risk of having cancer detected in subsequent biopsies, and rebiopsy is warranted.[9] However, rebiopsy should focus predominantly on the site where the ATYP diagnosis was initially obtained.[10] For example, if the biopsy from the right mid has atypical glands, then three cores should be taken from this site, two cores each from the adjacent sites, including right apex, right base and left mid, and one core each from other sites, including the left apex and left base.

Therefore, the locations of positive biopsy cores are potentially important pathologic parameters that should be reported by pathologists. Pathologists will be able to provide such information only if the anatomic locations of the biopsy cores are provided by urologists. Urologists are encouraged to provide such information by separately submitting biopsy cores from different anatomic locations.

One reason why urologists hesitate to submit needle biopsy specimens in separate containers is that it may lead to higher pathology charges. If this is an issue, it is important for urologists and pathologists to devise an alternative specimen submission strategy that will preserve the biopsy location information. Biopsy cores from several different sites can be submitted in the same cassette after being inked in different colors. Although this strategy may be helpful, we are not in favor of placing all the cores from the same biopsy session in one cassette. When multiple tissue cores are submitted in a single cassette, it is difficult to embed them in the same plane of section. As a result, the surface representation of the biopsy cores and the possibility of detecting cancer decrease.[11] Moreover, the presence of multiple, tangled-up tissue cores on a slide makes complete visualization of all the cores difficult, increasing the risk that the pathologist will not screen all the tissue present on the slide and miss important diagnostic features. For these reasons, embedding individual biopsy cores is appropriate. In our laboratory, a maximum of two cores are placed in each cassette even when multiple cores are submitted in a single container.

Fixation of Prostate Biopsy

Delayed fixation of a prostate biopsy may result in autolytic changes that significantly alter the morphology of benign and malignant prostate glands. Rather than waiting until the end of a biopsy session, prostate cores should be placed in the fixative solution immediately after each core is obtained.

The most frequently used fixative is 10% neutral buffered formalin. Other fixatives include Bouin solution, Hollandes, alcohol-based fixative, and other commercial preparations. Formalin is the preferred fixative for prostate biopsies for several reasons. Most of the histologic diagnostic criteria are derived based on formalin-fixed tissue sections.[1-3] Other fixatives may alter (enhance or diminish) certain histologic features of prostate biopsies that are important for diagnosis. For example, prominent nucleoli are an important histologic feature, the presence of which may help establish a diagnosis of prostate cancer. Prominent nucleoli are also the single most important histologic feature for high-grade prostatic intraepithelial neoplasia (HGPIN).[12] However, the nucleolar prominence depends very much on a number of factors, including tissue fixatives. Alcohol-based fixatives often obscure the nuclear details and therefore hinder the recognition of nucleoli. Some fixatives, such as Hollandes, provide superior nuclear details, enhancing nucleoli even in benign prostatic glands.[13] Therefore,

HGPIN may be overdiagnosed in Hollandes fixed prostate biopsies. These morphologic differences induced by fixatives are often minimal and do not affect significantly the pathologic interpretation of prostate biopsies. However, pathologists should be aware of them to avoid diagnostic pitfalls.

Another reason why formalin has become the preferred fixative in pathology laboratories is its compatibility with immunohistochemical and nucleic acid–based molecular tests.[14,15] In contrast, other fixatives, Hollandes in particular, are known to affect molecular studies, and are therefore less desirable because many of these immunohistochemical and molecular tests may supplement the histologic evaluations of the prostate biopsies.

Other factors include environmental and health considerations. Both Bouin and Hollandes solutions contain picric acid, a very volatile chemical and neurotoxin. Therefore, these fixatives are losing favor in most pathology laboratories.

Prostate biopsies should be fixed in formalin for 4–8 hours. Adequate fixation minimizes the tissue fragmentation and augments the nuclear details.[16] However, prolonged fixation may result in ablation of antigenicity of certain proteins and hamper immunohistochemical staining, and therefore should be avoided.[17]

Interpretation and Reporting of Prostate Needle Biopsies

Examination of prostate biopsy cores yields a wealth of information that may be clinically significant. Foremost, it generates a pathologic diagnosis. There are several diagnostic categories (Table 17.1), including benign HGPIN, ATYP, prostate adenocarcinoma, and other uncommon-to-rare entities. The information relating to prognostic and therapeutic implications should also be sought and included in the report. Such information will invariably remain to some extent in a state of flux as more clinical, pathologic, molecular, and genetic data become available and integrated into the diagnosis and clinical management of prostate cancer. Recently, several organizations and authorities have put forth recommendations for the minimum data sets for reporting of prostate biopsies.[17a]

Update on Gleason Grading of Prostate Cancer

Histologic grade has been recognized for years as a powerful predictor of the biologic behavior of prostate cancer. The Gleason grading system, spearheaded by Donald Gleason through the Veterans Administration Cooperative Urological Research Group, is universally adopted and endorsed by the World Health Organization as the grading system in the United States and worldwide.[18] The Gleason grading system assigns histo-

TABLE 17.1. Diagnostic categories in prostate needle biopsy.

Benign
• Benign prostatic tissue

High-grade prostatic intraepithelial neoplasia

Atypical glands, suspicious for prostate cancer

Adenocarcinoma of the prostate
• Location and distribution of cancer
• Histologic type
• Gleason score
• Cancer extent
• Extraprostatic extension
• Seminal vesicle invasion
• Lymphovascular invasion
• Perineural invasion
• Therapy-related changes

Epithelial tumor other than adenocarcinoma of the prostate
• Basal cell adenoma
• Basal cell carcinoma
• Urothelial carcinoma
• Small cell carcinoma

Prostatic stroma tumor
• Stromal tumor of uncertain malignant potential
• Stromal sarcoma

Other rare tumors, including neuroendocrine, mesenchymal, hematolymphoid, and metastatic tumors

Source: Adapted from Amin et al.[17a]

logic patterns from 1 to 5 based on degree of architectural differentiation of cancer glands, with 1 being well-differentiated and 5 undifferentiated. A Gleason score or sum is obtained by adding the most prevalent and second most prevalent patterns. If the tumor has only one pattern, the pattern is doubled to obtain the Gleason score (i.e., for a tumor composed solely of pattern 3, the Gleason score is 3 + 3 = 6).

The Gleason score of prostate cancer on needle biopsy is one of the most important prognostic factors, because it correlates with pathologic parameters (tumor volume, extraprostatic extension, seminal vesicle invasion, surgical margin status) in radical prostatectomy, PSA failure, lymph node status, local and distant metastases, regardless of therapy.[19-26] Gleason scores can be segregated into biologically meaningful score groupings based on their behavior. Gleason scores 2–4 tumors are considered as well-differentiated, 5–6 as moderately differentiated, 7 as moderately to poorly differentiated, and 8–10 as poorly differentiated. It is important to distinguish between Gleason scores 5–6 and Gleason score 7, because Gleason score 7 tumors have a significantly worse prognosis and patients may be managed differently.[27,28]

The diagnosis and management of prostate cancer have evolved significantly since the initial inception of the Gleason grading system in late 1960. Widespread PSA screening results in detection of earlier-stage cancer. The use of ultrasound-guided transrectal 18-gauge needle biopsy and systemic biopsy templates allows more extensive sampling of the prostate gland.[29] Immunostain for basal cell markers helps the identification of some benign entities, such as adenosis (atypical adenomatous hyperplasia) that was erroneously classified as low-grade cancer in the past.[30] Finally, several morphologic variants of prostate cancer have been described, the grading of which has been controversial and inconsistent among pathologists. For these reasons, the application of the Gleason grading system has varied considerably among pathologists in present-day practice. Therefore, a consensus conference on Gleason grading of prostatic adeno-carcinoma was recently convened by the International Society of Urologic Pathology to achieve consensus in controversial areas, although many of the proposed changes have already been adopted by pathologists and clinicians.[31]

The schematic diagram of the modified Gleason grading system is shown in Figure 17.1. The consensus recommends that a Gleason score 2–4 should not be diagnosed on prostate needle biopsies for several reasons.[32] Most cases that were diagnosed as Gleason score $1 + 1 = 2$ in the past would be referred to as adenosis today. Low-grade cancer (Gleason score 2–4) is predominantly seen in the transition zone and rarely encountered in the peripheral zone of the prostate, which is sampled by transrectal needle biopsies. Many Gleason score 2–4 prostate cancers erroneously diagnosed on needle biopsies are actually pathologically aggressive tumors with extra-prostatic extension; therefore, labeling these cases with a Gleason score 2–4 may mislead clinicians and patients to falsely believe the disease is an indolent one. Finally, Gleason score 2–4 cancer on needle biopsy is poorly reproducible, even among expert genitourinary pathologists.[33,34]

It is not uncommon that the secondary pattern constitutes <5% of the tumor. In the setting of high-grade cancer, one should ignore such minor lower-grade pattern if it occupies <5% of the tumor area. For example, a needle biopsy specimen extensively involved by cancer with 98% Gleason pattern 4 and 2% Gleason pattern 3 should be diagnosed as Gleason score $4 + 4 = 8$, not $4 + 3 = 7$. In contrast, if such minor secondary pattern is of higher grade, it should then be included in the final Gleason score. For example, a cancer containing 98% Gleason pattern 3 and 2% Gleason pattern 5 should be graded as Gleason score $3 + 5 = 8$.

Another important change is the recognition of the tertiary pattern on needle biopsy.[31] It is recommended that when the tertiary pattern is the highest grade, the final Gleason score should be derived from the most prevalent pattern and the worst pattern. For instance, a biopsy containing primary pattern 3, secondary pattern 4, and tertiary pattern 5 should be graded as Gleason score $3 + 5 = 8$.

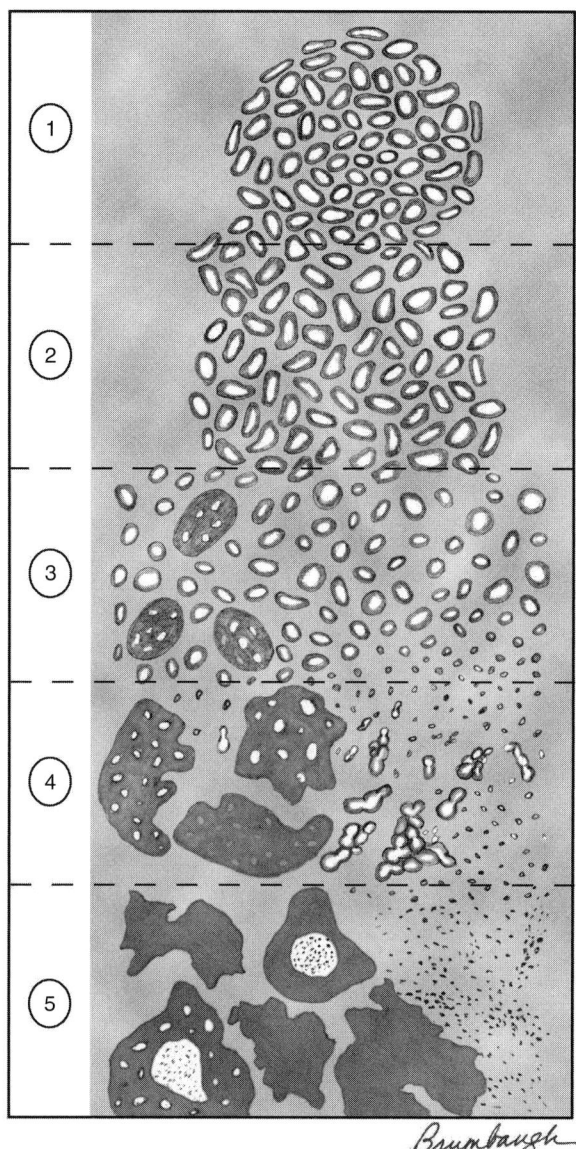

FIGURE 17.1. Modified Gleason grading system. Similar to the initial system, the modified Gleason grading system categorizes prostate adenocarcinoma into five patterns (patterns 1–5) based on the architectural differentiation with several modifications. Notably, the definition of cribriform pattern 3 is much stricter. Poorly formed glands with ill-defined lumina are graded as pattern 4.

Prostate biopsy with different cores showing different Gleason grade are not uncommon. Each core should be given a separate grade if the anatomic location is known. One has the option to also give an overall score to the case. However, if multiple cores are placed in one container without location designation, one could grade each core separately, or give an overall grade to each container.

Histologic Variants of Prostate Cancer

The majority of prostate cancers detected on needle biopsy are the so-called conventional acinar adenocarcinoma, although several morphologic variants and variations of acinar adenocarcinoma are occasionally encountered. Some histologic variants of acinar adenocarcinoma of the prostate, including atrophic cancer, foamy gland carcinoma, and pseudohyperplastic cancer,[35–37] may pose diagnostic difficulty, but are similar to acinar cancer clinically; therefore, they need not to be mentioned in the report and the Gleason grading should be based solely on the architecture of the epithelial component. However, other histologic subtypes, including ductal adenocarcinoma, mucinous (colloid) adenocarcinoma, sarcomatoid carcinoma, adenosquamous carcinoma, basaloid carcinoma, urothelial carcinoma, and small cell carcinoma, are known to have important and unique diagnostic, prognostic, and therapeutic implications, and therefore should be specified in the report.[38–43] Small cell carcinoma, basaloid and urothelial carcinoma of the prostate should not be assigned a Gleason grade.

Correlation of Biopsy Gleason Score with Radical Prostatectomy Gleason Score

Several recent studies have correlated needle biopsy Gleason score with that found on radical prostatectomy specimens.[44–46] In a large study performed at the Johns Hopkins Hospital, a Gleason score of 5–6 on biopsy corresponded to the same score in the radical prostatectomy in 64% of the cases.[45] With a Gleason score ≥7 on biopsy, the radical prostatectomy score was the same in 87.5% of the cases. In general, adverse findings on needle biopsy accurately predict adverse findings on radical prostatectomy specimen whereas favorable findings on needle biopsy do not necessarily predict favorable findings on prostatectomy specimen.

Three major factors account for the discrepancy between biopsy and radical prostatectomy grade. The first major source of discrepancy is interobserver variability among pathologists evaluating biopsy specimens. As discussed above, there is a marked tendency for pathologists to undergrade prostate cancer of limited extent on needle biopsy. Another source of discrepancy between biopsy and radical prostatectomy Gleason scores is the presence of tumors that are borderline between two grades. The final major source of discrepancy reflects the heterogeneous nature of prostate cancer and the inherent limitation of prostate needle biopsy which samples only a very small fraction of the prostate gland. When there is a high-grade component present within the radical prostatectomy specimen that is not sampled by needle biopsy, a discrepancy results. This typically occurs when a tumor on needle biopsy is graded as Gleason score 3 + 3 = 6, yet the corresponding radical prostatectomy also has Gleason pattern 4 which was not sampled on the biopsy and results in an undergrading of the biopsy (3 + 3 = 6) compared with the prostatectomy specimen (3 + 4 = 7). Extended needle biopsy schemes, entailing taking more than 10–12 cores per biopsy session, as opposed to sextant biopsy, improve correlation between biopsy and radical prostatectomy Gleason scores.[47]

Use of Gleason Score in Nomograms

The importance of grade is evidenced by the use of various nomograms to predict final pathologic stage on radical prostatectomy, and disease progression after treatment (radiation or radical prostatectomy).[26,48–50] These nomograms use preoperative parameters such as Gleason score on biopsy, clinical stage, serum PSA, and in more recent studies, the extent of cancer on biopsy to predict the risk of extraprostatic disease, seminal vesicle invasion, and lymph node metastases. Therefore, they are often used by clinicians to counsel patients as to what treatments are available. Obviously, the validity of these tables in part rests on accurate Gleason grading.

Quantification of Amount of Cancer on Needle Biopsy

Multiple methods of quantifying the amount of cancer found on needle biopsy have been developed and studied, including measurement of the: 1) number of positive cores, 2) total millimeters of cancer among all cores, 3) percentage of each core occupied by cancer, 4) greatest percentage of tumor involving any single core, and 5) total percent of cancer in the entire specimen. There are multiple studies claiming superiority of one technique over the other, although there is no one method clearly shown to be superior to the others.

Numerous studies show a correlation between the number of positive cores and various prognostic variables, including risk of extraprostatic extension of cancer found at radical prostatectomy. These studies have shown that the involvement of multiple biopsy cores on systematic prostate biopsy is a powerful predictor of adverse pathologic findings at radical prostatectomy. The converse is not true, however, with prostate cancer limited to even one or two cores on needle biopsy offering no guarantee of favorable findings at final surgical staging. Extraprostatic extension was found in 7%–47% of cases which only had one or two biopsy cores positive for cancer.[5,51–55] The number of cores containing prostate cancer also correlates with the presence of seminal vesicle invasion,[54–56] lymph node metastases,[57] radical prostatectomy tumor volume,[54,58] positive surgical margins,[59,60] and postprostatectomy cancer progression.[53,55,61]

The other widely used method of quantifying the amount of cancer on needle biopsy is measurement of the percentage of each biopsy core containing cancer, which is correlated with the likelihood of extraprostatic extension,[5,56,62–66] seminal vesicle invasion,[62] and positive surgical margins.[56] However, multiple studies have demonstrated that a limited total extent (<3 mm) of cancer on all biopsy cores in a set does not necessarily predict "insignificant" amounts of tumor in the entire prostate.[28,63,67–70] One feasible and rational approach would be to have pathologists report the number of cores containing cancer, as well as one other system quantifying tumor extent. Several recent studies found that both the number of cores positive for cancer, and total percentage of core length involved by cancer, independently predict extraprostatic extension, and positive surgical margins.[71,72] At the Cleveland Clinic, the number of cores containing cancer is reported, along with the percentage of cancer present on each involved core.

Extraprostatic Extension and Seminal Vesicle Invasion

The presence of cancer glands in extraprostatic tissue and seminal vesicle indicates non–organ-confined disease. Prostatic biopsy may occasionally contain, and urologists may also target, seminal vesicles or extraprostatic tissue. Because the presence of fat within the prostate gland is exceedingly rare, finding cancer cells within fat on prostate needle biopsy can be safely interpreted as extraprostatic extension[73] (Figure 17.2). However, distinction

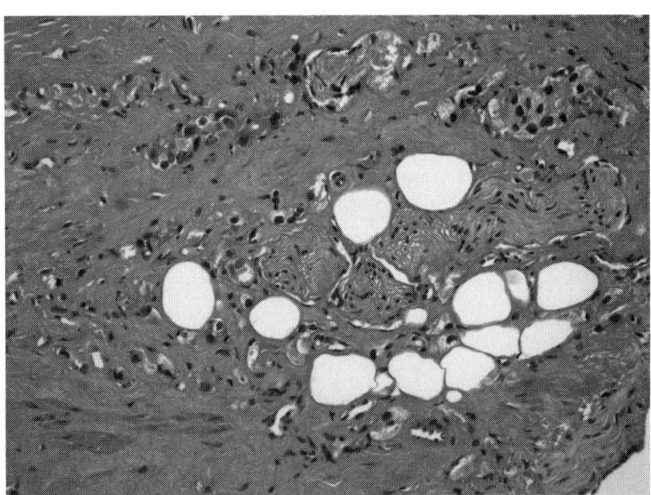

FIGURE 17.2. Extraprostatic extension. Cancer cells are adjacent to fat cells and large nerve fibers, indicative of extraprostatic spread of cancer cells.

between seminal vesicle and ejaculatory duct, an intraprostatic structure, is not always possible. Therefore, the diagnostic term "prostate cancer involving seminal vesicle/ejaculatory duct structure" may be used. However, finding cancer cells invading the "seminal vesicle/ejaculatory duct structure" is an adverse pathologic feature. We recently studied 72 radical prostatectomy specimens with involvement of the intraprostatic ejaculatory ducts and found that the majority of cases also had extraprostatic extension (97%) and seminal vesicles invasion (87%) (Zhou et al., manuscript in preparation). These cases all had other adverse pathologic features, including Gleason score ≥7 (98%), tumor volume >2 cc (79%), and positive pelvic lymph nodes (22%).

Urologists may also biopsy the neurovascular bundle, extraprostatic tissue, and seminal vesicles for "preoperative pathologic staging".[53,74] If the biopsy is positive for cancer, it should be specified in the biopsy report whether the intended tissues are present. For example, if a biopsy of "seminal vesicles" is positive for cancer, yet seminal vesicle tissue is not present in the biopsy, one should then specify that the seminal vesicle tissue is not present in the biopsy to avoid misinterpretation of the seminal vesicle as positive for cancer.

Perineural Invasion

Perineural invasion is defined as the presence of prostate cancer tracking along or around a nerve (Figure 17.3). Because perineural invasion has been demonstrated to be one of the major mechanisms of extension of

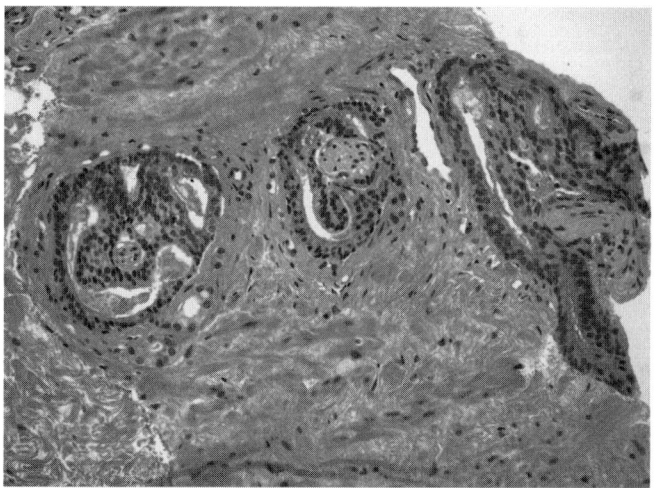

FIGURE 17.3. Perineural invasion is defined as tight, circumferential or near-circumferential encircling of a nerve fiber by cancer cells.

prostate cancer from the prostatic parenchyma to the periprostatic soft tissue, perineural invasion extensive enough to be sampled on needle biopsy may signal an increased risk of extraprostatic extension of cancer.[75] The absence of perineural invasion on biopsy, however, does not indicate organ-confined disease in radical prostatectomy.

The reported positive predictive value of biopsy perineural invasion for extraprostatic cancer extension at radical prostatectomy ranges from 38% to 93%.[76] No clear consensus exists on whether perineural invasion on needle biopsy provides independent prediction of extraprostatic extension beyond that provided by biopsy Gleason score and preoperative serum PSA level. The presence of perineural invasion on needle biopsy has also recently been shown to independently predict lymph node metastases and postoperative cancer progression.[77,78] When perineural invasion is seen on biopsy, the urologist should consider excising the neurovascular bundle on that side.[79] Some of the radiation oncology studies have found that peri-neural invasion is an independent risk factor for adverse outcome after external-beam radiation therapy, and in patients with a high Gleason score and perineural invasion, adjuvant hormonal therapy or dose escalation (brachytherapy) have been advocated.[80–84] However, our recent study sug-gested that perineural invasion on needle biopsy does not predict biochemi-cal failure after low-dose brachytherapy.[85] Other pathologic features of perineural invasion, including multifocality and largest diameter of peri-neural invasion, may help improve the prognostic significance of perineural invasion.[86]

Prostatic Intraepithelial Neoplasia

Prostatic intraepithelial neoplasia (PIN) is the preferred diagnostic term for a putative premalignant proliferation of atypical epithelial cells within the preexisting prostatic ducts and acini.[87] In other words, PIN glands archi-tecturally resemble benign glands but are lined with cytologically malignant cells (Figure 17.4). PIN can only be diagnosed by histologic examination of prostatic tissue, because there are no specific clinical or radiologic findings. It does not increase serum PSA level.

Based on the severity of architectural and cytologic atypia, PIN can be categorized into low and high grade, with much more pronounced atypia in the latter. Low-grade PIN (LGPIN) should not be diagnosed on prostate biopsy for several reasons. First, finding LGPIN on needle biopsy is not associated with increased risk for detecting cancer on subsequent biopsies, as is HGPIN. If the first biopsy shows LGPIN and patients undergo repeat biopsy, cancer would be found in approximately 18% of the patients. However, if the first biopsy shows benign prostatic tissue and patients undergo repeat biopsy, prostate cancer would be found in 18.7% of the patients. Therefore, finding LGPIN is not associated with increased risk for cancer detected in subsequent biopsies.[88–92] Furthermore, there is poor diag-

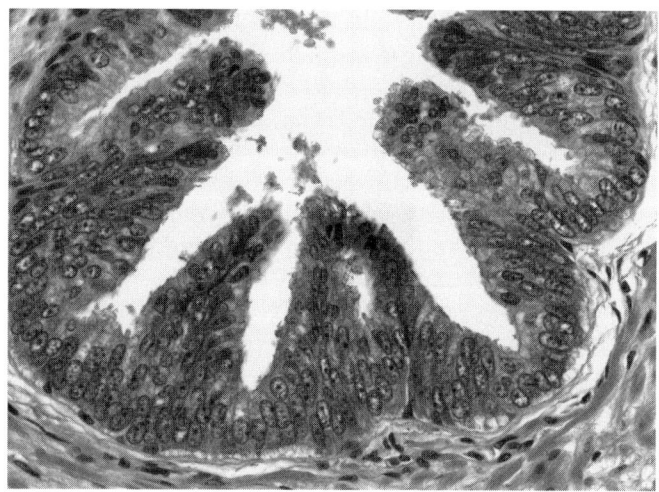

FIGURE 17.4. High-grade prostatic intraepithelial neoplasia (HGPIN). The HGPIN gland has a benign architecture with an irregular luminal border and papillary infolding. However, the gland is lined with cytologically malignant cells with nuclear stratification, enlarged nuclei, coarse chromatin, and prominent nucleoli.

nostic reproducibility for LGPIN even among expert urologic pathologists.[93]

The incidence of HGPIN on prostate needle biopsies varies remarkably in the literature from 0% to 24.6% with a mean of 7.7%.[9] There seems to be no correlation between the incidence and the setting of pathology practice, time and extent of prostate sampling. Rather, such variation in incidence is likely the result of lack of clearly defined diagnostic criteria and technical factors in prostate biopsy processing.

The importance of recognizing HGPIN on needle biopsy is its association with prostate cancer on subsequent repeat biopsy.[9] In studies performed in early 1990, the average risk of cancer associated with HGPIN was nearly 50%. Such risk, however, has decreased dramatically in recent studies. In the studies published since 2000, the mean cancer risk is 23.5%, similar to the cancer risk of 22.7% associated with the initial benign diagnosis published in the studies during the same period of time. A plausible explanation is that the extended biopsy scheme used increasingly in recent years improves cancer detection on the initial biopsy, and therefore may reduce cancer detection on subsequent biopsies.[94] These findings seem to cast doubt on the previously held notion that HGPIN is a significant risk factor for cancer detected on subsequent biopsy and patients with such a diagnosis should undergo repeat biopsy. However, one should not rush to such conclusion, because two recent studies found that cancer risk after initial HGPIN diagnosis was significantly higher than after a benign diagnosis.[47,95]

Our recommendation is that HGPIN should still be considered as a risk factor for detecting cancer on subsequent prostate biopsies, and therefore should be diagnosed and reported until new data and consensus emerge.

Many studies have also examined whether clinical and other histologic factors may help predict which men are at higher risk for cancer after a biopsy diagnosis of HGPIN. However, no clinical parameters, including serum PSA level, PSA velocity and density, or free to total PSA ratio, and digital rectal examination and transrectal ultrasound results, predict which men will have cancer after an initial HGPIN diagnosis.[9] It is controversial whether the number of cores with HGPIN can predict the risk of cancer. Most studies found no association, although a few studies found that the cancer risk was significantly higher when more than two cores were involved with HGPIN compared with when only one core was involved.[96–98] In general, different architectural patterns of HGPIN do not differ significantly in cancer risk. A few recent studies also fail to demonstrate the value of molecular markers in stratifying the cancer risk associated with HGPIN.[9]

There is no consensus regarding when and how often repeat biopsy should be performed after an HGPIN diagnosis. Most studies recommend repeat biopsy at 3–6 or 6–12 months, or at 36 months.[89,99,100] Without a clear guideline, such recommendation should be individualized and based on clinical parameters, and the preference of patient and physician. Because the prostate lobe contralateral to the site where the initial HGPIN was diagnosed also carries considerable risk for cancer, albeit not as high as the site where HGPIN was diagnosed,[101–104] the rebiopsy should sample the entire gland, with an emphasis on the area where PIN was initially found.

Atypical Glands Suspicious for Prostate Cancer

ATYP is a diagnostic term used by pathologists to describe a gland or a focus of glands suspicious for prostate cancer, but lacking sufficient architectural and/or cytologic atypia to establish a definitive diagnosis. Unlike prostate cancer or HGPIN, ATYP is not a diagnostic entity. Rather, it encompasses benign lesions that exhibit architectural and cytologic atypia, and undersampled small foci of cancer. Many terms have been used in the past, including atypia, atypical hyperplasia, borderline lesion, lesion of uncertain significance, or atypical small acinar proliferation (ASAP). However, many of these terms have been used to describe other morphologic entities. For example, atypical hyperplasia was used for HGPIN. ASAP has been widely used, although it is not an accurate term because many atypical glands are not small. In addition, some urologists mistake ASAP with HGPIN.[105] For these reasons, we advocate the use of the descriptive terminology "atypical glands suspicious for prostate cancer," or ATYP.

The incidence of ATYP on prostate biopsies varies depending on patient population and pathologist's experience. With better-defined diagnostic criteria for limited cancer in prostate biopsy and immunohistochemical markers, one would expect more atypical diagnosis to be resolved and therefore a reduction of the incidence. On average, ATYP is found in 4.4% (range 0.7%–23.4%) of prostate biopsies.[9]

Similar to HGPIN, the clinical significance of recognizing ATYP on needle biopsies is its association with prostate cancer on repeat biopsies.[10,19,95,106,107] Unlike HGPIN, the cancer risk associated with ATYP has held steadily from early 1990 to present.[107] On average, 40% (17%–70%) of men with ATYP on initial biopsy would be found to have cancer on subsequent biopsies. Similar to HGPIN, no clinical parameters, including serum PSA, transrectal ultrasound, or digital rectal examination, predict which patients with an ATYP diagnosis will be found to have cancer on repeat biopsy.[9]

Several studies found that after an initial ATYP diagnosis, cancer was detected at the same site as the initial ATYP diagnosis in approximately 50% of cases, and at the same site or in the adjacent sextant sites in 71%–85% of cases, and in the contralateral site only in 17%–27% of cases.[10,101,104,108] Based on these data, a rational approach for rebiopsy after initial ATYP diagnosis should include a collection of three cores from the site of the initial ATYP biopsy, two cores each from adjacent sites, and one core each elsewhere.[10] Because of the high risk of cancer on rebiopsy after an ATYP diagnosis, patients should be advised to undergo rebiopsy as soon as possible, typically within 3–6 months after the initial biopsy.

Emerging Molecular Prognostic Markers

The advent of gene-expression profiling and tissue microarray promises rapid identification and validation of prognostic markers for prostate cancer, and there has been an exponential increase in the literature of the number of markers that are of potential prognostic significance. These markers include genes that are involved in almost every aspect of cell proliferation, apoptosis, differentiation, and cell–cell and cell–stroma interaction. Most of the studies used tissues from radical prostatectomy specimens with only a few studies examining the utility of these markers on prostate needle biopsies. One study found that a low p27 labeling index (<45%) in cancer correlated with PSA recurrence after radical prostatectomy.[109] Interestingly, another study showed that a low p27 labeling (<50%) on prostate biopsy actually predicted localized disease at radical prostatectomy, although a high p27 labeling (>50%) poorly predicted prostate cancer of favorable pathologic features.[110]

One study has demonstrated that proliferation status of cancer on biopsy as measured by Ki-67 and percentage of cells in S-phase and G_2M correlated better than biopsy grade with PSA failure after radical prostatectomy.[111] In a recent study of molecular markers predicting PSA failure after radiotherapy, a Ki-67 index >3.5% on prostate biopsy correlated with PSA failure both in univariate and multivariate analysis, independently of pretreatment PSA, clinical stage, and biopsy Gleason score. In a separate work, needle biopsy p53 expression and Gleason score were independent predictors of biochemical relapse after radical prostatectomy.[112,113] The use of multiple biomarkers may be advantageous over a single marker in that different markers may work synergistically. Pollack et al.[114] examined the expression of Bcl-2 and Bax in patients with prostate cancer treated with radiotherapy. Although Bcl-2 and Bax both correlated with biochemical recurrence after radiotherapy, combining both markers stratified patients into more-precise prognostic groups.

Methylation of the promoter region of the glutathione *S*-transferase-p1 (*GSTP1*) gene is the most common epigenetic change in prostate cancer.[115,116] The quantitative *GSTP1* methylation assay, a recently developed methylation-specific and polymerase chain reaction–based technique, allows accurate discrimination of benign prostate tissue and prostate cancer, even on small, formalin-fixed prostate needle biopsies.[117,118] We also found quantitative *GSTP1* methylation levels to correlate with prostate cancer Gleason score and tumor volume, with higher *GSTP1* methylation level in prostate cancer with higher Gleason score and larger tumor volume, suggesting that quantitative *GSTP1* methylation levels may be of prognostic significance.[119]

Although offering promise that new molecular markers applied to needle biopsy will be able to enhance our prognostication for prostate cancer, further studies, especially prospective ones, are needed before these techniques can be considered part of routine clinical practice.

Second-Opinion Pathology Review of Prostate Biopsies

Second-opinion pathology review should be sought in two settings. The prostate biopsy should be reviewed for the presence of cancer and Gleason score before definitive treatment, either radical prostatectomy or radiation therapy, takes place. In most cases, both the diagnosis and the Gleason score are confirmed. However, such review led to reclassification of cancer to benign in 1.3% of cases before radical prostatectomy,[120] and change in Gleason score, and subsequently clinical management in 10% of cases that were being considered for radiation therapy.[121] The cost of the second-opinion pathology review, including pathology- and repeat biopsy-related charges, would amount to only 50% of the expenses should patients have undergone surgery with a false cancer diagnosis, not including lost wage, morbidity, and potential litigation.[120]

Such second-opinion pathology review may also be of benefit when the prostate biopsy carries a difficult diagnosis, such as a minute focus of cancer or ATYP. In a study by Chan and Epstein[122] of consultation cases initiated by patients and/or urologists, the majority of cancer, HGPIN and benign diagnoses, were confirmed. In contrast, ATYP diagnosis was changed either to benign or cancer in almost two thirds of cases.

Conclusion

Pathologic evaluation of prostate cancer in needle biopsy generates a wealth of information, some of which has been validated by many studies, whereas other information has uncertain prognostic significance. This review has detailed the information that has critical roles in patient management; therefore, it should be included in pathology reports. Recent advances in molecular biology of prostate carcinogenesis have discovered many molecular markers for prostate cancer. Whereas several are extremely promising in the diagnosis of prostate cancer, other prognostic markers are not ready to be included in routine practice until they are validated by large, prospective studies.

References

1. Bostwick DG, Iczkowski KA. Minimal criteria for the diagnosis of prostate cancer on needle biopsy. Ann Diagn Pathol 1997;1(2):104–29.
2. Epstein JI. Diagnosis and reporting of limited adenocarcinoma of the prostate on needle biopsy. Mod Pathol 2004;17(3):307–15.
3. Thorson P, Humphrey PA. Minimal adenocarcinoma in prostate needle biopsy tissue. Am J Clin Pathol 2000;114(6):896–909.
4. Eichler K, Hempel S, Wilby J, Myers L, Bachmann LM, Kleijnen J. Diagnostic value of systematic biopsy methods in the investigation of prostate cancer: a systematic review. J Urol 2006;175(5):1605–12.
5. Badalament RA, Miller MC, Peller PA, et al. An algorithm for predicting nonorgan confined prostate cancer using the results obtained from sextant core biopsies with prostate specific antigen level. J Urol 1996;156(4):1375–80.
6. Calvanese CB, Kahane H, Carlson GD, Campagna RL, Narayan P, Tewari A. Presurgical staging of prostate cancer. Infect Urol 1999;12(1):22–8.
7. Naya Y, Slaton JW, Troncoso P, Okihara K, Babaian RJ. Tumor length and location of cancer on biopsy predict for side specific extraprostatic cancer extension. J Urol 2004;171(3):1093–7.
8. Sanwick JM, Dalkin BL, Nagle RB. Accuracy of prostate needle biopsy in predicting extracapsular tumor extension at radical retropubic prostatectomy: application in selecting patients for nerve-sparing surgery. Urology 1998;52(5): 814–18; discussion 818–19.
9. Epstein JI, Herawi M. Prostate needle biopsies containing prostatic intraepithelial neoplasia or atypical foci suspicious for carcinoma: implications for patient care. J Urol 2006;175(3 Pt 1):820–34.
10. Allen EA, Kahane H, Epstein JI. Repeat biopsy strategies for men with atypical diagnoses on initial prostate needle biopsy. Urology 1998;52(5):803–7.
11. Kao J, Upton M, Zhang P, Rosen S. Individual prostate biopsy core embedding facilitates maximal tissue representation. J Urol 2002;168(2):496–9.
12. Epstein JI, Grignon DJ, Humphrey PA, McNeal JE, Sesterhenn IA, Troncoso P, Wheeler TM. Interobserver reproducibility in the diagnosis of prostatic intraepithelial neoplasia. Am J Surg Pathol 1995;19(8):873–86.

13. Murphy WM, Ramsey J, Soloway MS. A better nuclear fixative for diagnostic bladder and prostate biopsies. J Urol Pathol 1993;1:79–87.
14. Nuovo GJ, Richart RM. Buffered formalin is the superior fixative for the detection of HPV DNA by in situ hybridization analysis. Am J Pathol 1989;134(4):837–42.
15. Glickman JN, Ormsby AH, Gramlich TL, Goldblum JR, Odze RD. Interinstitutional variability and effect of tissue fixative on the interpretation of a Barrett cytokeratin 7/20 immunoreactivity pattern in Barrett esophagus. Hum Pathol 2005;36(1):58–65.
16. Delahunt B, Nacey JN. Broadsheet number 45: thin core biopsy of prostate. The Royal College of Pathologists of Australia. Pathology 1998;30(3): 247–56.
17. Varma M, Linden MD, Amin MB. Effect of formalin fixation and epitope retrieval techniques on antibody 34betaE12 immunostaining of prostatic tissues. Mod Pathol 1999;12(5):472–8.
17a. Amin M, Boccon-Gibod L, Egevad L, et al. Prognostic and predictive factors and reporting of prostate carcinoma in prostate needle biopsy specimens. Scand J Urol Nephrol Suppl 2005;(216):20–33.
18. Gleason DF, Mellinger GT. Prediction of prognosis for prostatic adenocarcinoma by combined histological grading and clinical staging. J Urol 1974; 111(1):58–64.
19. Yang XJ, Lecksell K, Potter SR, Epstein JI. Significance of small foci of Gleason score 7 or greater prostate cancer on needle biopsy. Urology 1999;54(3):528–32.
20. Holmberg L, Bill-Axelson A, Helgesen F, et al. A randomized trial comparing radical prostatectomy with watchful waiting in early prostate cancer. N Engl J Med 2002;347(11):781–9.
21. Ohori M, Kattan MW, Koh H, et al. Predicting the presence and side of extracapsular extension: a nomogram for staging prostate cancer. J Urol 2004;171(5): 1844–9; discussion 1849.
22. Gancarczyk KJ, Wu H, McLeod DG, et al. Using the percentage of biopsy cores positive for cancer, pretreatment PSA, and highest biopsy Gleason sum to predict pathologic stage after radical prostatectomy: the Center for Prostate Disease Research nomograms. Urology 2003;61(3):589–95.
23. D'Amico AV, Whittington R, Malkowicz SB, et al. Combined modality staging of prostate carcinoma and its utility in predicting pathologic stage and postoperative prostate specific antigen failure. Urology 1997;49(3A Suppl):23–30.
24. Pisansky TM, Kahn MJ, Rasp GM, Cha SS, Haddock MG, Bostwick DG. A multiple prognostic index predictive of disease outcome after irradiation for clinically localized prostate carcinoma. Cancer 1997;79(2):337–44.
25. Kattan MW, Eastham JA, Wheeler TM, et al. Counseling men with prostate cancer: a nomogram for predicting the presence of small, moderately differentiated, confined tumors. J Urol 2003;170(5):1792–7.
26. Partin AW, Kattan MW, Subong EN, et al. Combination of prostate-specific antigen, clinical stage, and Gleason score to predict pathological stage of localized prostate cancer. A multi-institutional update. JAMA 1997;277(18): 1445–51.
27. McNeal JE, Villers AA, Redwine EA, Freiha FS, Stamey TA. Histologic differentiation, cancer volume, and pelvic lymph node metastasis in adenocarcinoma of the prostate. Cancer 1990;66(6):1225–33.

28. Epstein JI, Partin AW, Sauvageot J, Walsh PC. Prediction of progression following radical prostatectomy. A multivariate analysis of 721 men with long-term follow-up. Am J Surg Pathol 1996;20(3):286–92.
29. Hodge KK, McNeal JE, Terris MK, Stamey TA. Random systematic versus directed ultrasound guided transrectal core biopsies of the prostate. J Urol 1989;142(1):71–4; discussion 74–5.
30. Gaudin PB, Epstein JI. Adenosis of the prostate. Histologic features in transurethral resection specimens. Am J Surg Pathol 1994;18(9):863–70.
31. Epstein JI, Allsbrook WC Jr, Amin MB, Egevad LL. The 2005 International Society of Urological Pathology (ISUP) Consensus Conference on Gleason Grading of Prostatic Carcinoma. Am J Surg Pathol 2005;29(9):1228–42.
32. Epstein JI. Gleason score 2–4 adenocarcinoma of the prostate on needle biopsy: a diagnosis that should not be made. Am J Surg Pathol 2000;24(4):477–8.
33. Fleshner NE, Cookson MS, Soloway SM, Fair WR. Repeat transrectal ultrasound-guided prostate biopsy: a strategy to improve the reliability of needle biopsy grading in patients with well-differentiated prostate cancer. Urology 1998;52(4):659–62.
34. Allsbrook WC Jr, Mangold KA, Johnson MH, Lane RB, Lane CG, Epstein JI. Interobserver reproducibility of Gleason grading of prostatic carcinoma: general pathologist. Hum Pathol 2001;32(1):81–8.
35. Humphrey PA, Kaleem Z, Swanson PE, Vollmer RT. Pseudohyperplastic prostatic adenocarcinoma. Am J Surg Pathol 1998;22(10):1239–46.
36. Nelson RS, Epstein JI. Prostatic carcinoma with abundant xanthomatous cytoplasm. Foamy gland carcinoma. Am J Surg Pathol 1996;20(4):419–26.
37. Cina SJ, Epstein JI. Adenocarcinoma of the prostate with atrophic features. Am J Surg Pathol 1997;21(3):289–95.
38. Shannon RL, Ro JY, Grignon DJ, et al. Sarcomatoid carcinoma of the prostate. A clinicopathologic study of 12 patients. Cancer 1992;69(11):2676–82.
39. Parwani AV, Kronz JD, Genega EM, Gaudin P, Chang S, Epstein JI. Prostate carcinoma with squamous differentiation: an analysis of 33 cases. Am J Surg Pathol 2004;28(5):651–7.
40. Oesterling JE, Hauzeur CG, Farrow GM. Small cell anaplastic carcinoma of the prostate: a clinical, pathological and immunohistological study of 27 patients. J Urol 1992;147(3 Pt 2):804–7.
41. Brinker DA, Potter SR, Epstein JI. Ductal adenocarcinoma of the prostate diagnosed on needle biopsy: correlation with clinical and radical prostatectomy findings and progression. Am J Surg Pathol 1999;23(12):1471–9.
42. Grignon DJ. Unusual subtypes of prostate cancer. Mod Pathol 2004;17(3):316–27.
43. Randolph TL, Amin MB, Ro JY, Ayala AG. Histologic variants of adenocarcinoma and other carcinomas of prostate: pathologic criteria and clinical significance. Mod Pathol 1997;10(6):612–29.
44. Spires SE, Cibull ML, Wood DP Jr, Miller S, Spires SM, Banks ER. Gleason histologic grading in prostatic carcinoma. Correlation of 18-gauge core biopsy with prostatectomy. Arch Pathol Lab Med 1994;118(7):705–8.
45. Steinberg DM, Sauvageot J, Piantadosi S, Epstein JI. Correlation of prostate needle biopsy and radical prostatectomy Gleason grade in academic and community settings. Am J Surg Pathol 1997;21(5):566–76.
46. Bostwick DG. Gleason grading of prostatic needle biopsies. Correlation with grade in 316 matched prostatectomies. Am J Surg Pathol 1994;18(8):796–803.

47. San Francisco IF, DeWolf WC, Rosen S, Upton M, Olumi AF. Extended prostate needle biopsy improves concordance of Gleason grading between prostate needle biopsy and radical prostatectomy. J Urol 2003;169(1):136–40.
48. D'Amico AV, Whittington R, Malkowicz SB, et al. Combination of the preoperative PSA level, biopsy Gleason score, percentage of positive biopsies, and MRI T-stage to predict early PSA failure in men with clinically localized prostate cancer. Urology 2000;55(4):572–7.
49. Kattan MW, Eastham JA, Stapleton AM, Wheeler TM, Scardino PT. A preoperative nomogram for disease recurrence following radical prostatectomy for prostate cancer. J Natl Cancer Inst 1998;90(10):766–71.
50. Narayan P, Gajendran V, Taylor SP, et al. The role of transrectal ultrasound-guided biopsy-based staging, preoperative serum prostate-specific antigen, and biopsy Gleason score in prediction of final pathologic diagnosis in prostate cancer. Urology 1995;46(2):205–12.
51. Sebo TJ, Cheville JC, Riehle DL, et al. Predicting prostate carcinoma volume and stage at radical prostatectomy by assessing needle biopsy specimens for percent surface area and cores positive for carcinoma, perineural invasion, Gleason score, DNA ploidy and proliferation, and preoperative serum prostate specific antigen: a report of 454 cases. Cancer 2001;91(11):2196–204.
52. Wills ML, Sauvageot J, Partin AW, Gurganus R, Epstein JI. Ability of sextant biopsies to predict radical prostatectomy stage. Urology 1998;51(5):759–64.
53. Ravery V, Boccon-Gibod LA, Dauge-Geffroy MC, et al. Systematic biopsies accurately predict extracapsular extension of prostate cancer and persistent/recurrent detectable PSA after radical prostatectomy. Urology 1994;44(3):371–6.
54. Peller PA, Young DC, Marmaduke DP, Marsh WL, Badalament RA. Sextant prostate biopsies. A histopathologic correlation with radical prostatectomy specimens. Cancer 1995;75(2):530–8.
55. Huland H, Graefen M, Haese A, et al. Prediction of tumor heterogeneity in localized prostate cancer. Urol Clin North Am 2002;29(1):213–22.
56. Terris MK, Haney DJ, Johnstone IM, McNeal JE, Stamey TA. Prediction of prostate cancer volume using prostate-specific antigen levels, transrectal ultrasound, and systematic sextant biopsies. Urology 1995;45(1):75–80.
57. Conrad S, Graefen M, Pichlmeier U, et al. Prospective validation of an algorithm with systematic sextant biopsy to predict pelvic lymph node metastasis in patients with clinically localized prostatic carcinoma. J Urol 2002;167(2 Pt 1):521–5.
58. Lewis JS Jr, Vollmer RT, Humphrey PA. Carcinoma extent in prostate needle biopsy tissue in the prediction of whole gland tumor volume in a screening population. Am J Clin Pathol 2002;118(3):442–50.
59. Ackerman DA, Barry JM, Wicklund RA, Olson N, Lowe BA. Analysis of risk factors associated with prostate cancer extension to the surgical margin and pelvic node metastasis at radical prostatectomy. J Urol 1993;150(6):1845–50.
60. Tigrani VS, Bhargava V, Shinohara K, Presti JC Jr. Number of positive systematic sextant biopsies predicts surgical margin status at radical prostatectomy. Urology 1999;54(4):689–93.
61. Presti JC Jr, Shinohara K, Bacchetti P, Tigrani V, Bhargava V. Positive fraction of systematic biopsies predicts risk of relapse after radical prostatectomy. Urology 1998;52(6):1079–84.

62. Bostwick DG, Qian J, Bergstralh E, et al. Prediction of capsular perforation and seminal vesicle invasion in prostate cancer. J Urol 1996;155(4):1361–7.

63. Cupp MR, Bostwick DG, Myers RP, Oesterling JE. The volume of prostate cancer in the biopsy specimen cannot reliably predict the quantity of cancer in the radical prostatectomy specimen on an individual basis. J Urol 1995;153(5):1543–8.

64. Ravery V, Chastang C, Toublanc M, Boccon-Gibod L, Delmas V. Percentage of cancer on biopsy cores accurately predicts extracapsular extension and biochemical relapse after radical prostatectomy for T1-T2 prostate cancer. Eur Urol 2000;37(4):449–55.

65. Ukimura O, Troncoso P, Ramirez EI, Babaian RJ. Prostate cancer staging: correlation between ultrasound determined tumor contact length and pathologically confirmed extraprostatic extension. J Urol 1998;159(4):1251–9.

66. Rubin MA, Bassily N, Sanda M, Montie J, Strawderman MS, Wojno K. Relationship and significance of greatest percentage of tumor and perineural invasion on needle biopsy in prostatic adenocarcinoma. Am J Surg Pathol 2000;24(2):183–9.

67. Bruce RG, Rankin WR, Cibull ML, Rayens MK, Banks ER, Wood DP Jr. Single focus of adenocarcinoma in the prostate biopsy specimen is not predictive of the pathologic stage of disease. Urology 1996;48(1):75–9.

68. Dietrick DD, McNeal JE, Stamey TA. Core cancer length in ultrasound-guided systematic sextant biopsies: a preoperative evaluation of prostate cancer volume. Urology 1995;45(6):987–92.

69. Wang X, Brannigan RE, Rademaker AW, McVary KT, Oyasu R. One core positive prostate biopsy is a poor predictor of cancer volume in the radical prostatectomy specimen. J Urol 1997;158(4):1431–5.

70. Weldon VE, Tavel FR, Neuwirth H, Cohen R. Failure of focal prostate cancer on biopsy to predict focal prostate cancer: the importance of prevalence. J Urol 1995;154(3):1074–7.

71. Bismar TA, Lewis JS Jr, Vollmer RT, Humphrey PA. Multiple measures of carcinoma extent versus perineural invasion in prostate needle biopsy tissue in prediction of pathologic stage in a screening population. Am J Surg Pathol 2003;27(4):432–40.

72. Freedland SJ, Aronson WJ, Csathy GS, et al. Comparison of percentage of total prostate needle biopsy tissue with cancer to percentage of cores with cancer for predicting PSA recurrence after radical prostatectomy: results from the SEARCH database. Urology 2003;61(4):742–7.

73. Cohen RJ, Stables S. Intraprostatic fat. Hum Pathol 1998;29(4):424–5.

74. Debras B, Guillonneau B, Bougaran J, Chambon E, Vallancien G. Prognostic significance of seminal vesicle invasion on the radical prostatectomy specimen. Rationale for seminal vesicle biopsies. Eur Urol 1998;33(3):271–7.

75. Villers A, McNeal JE, Redwine EA, Freiha FS, Stamey TA. The role of perineural space invasion in the local spread of prostatic adenocarcinoma. J Urol 1989;142(3):763–8.

76. Zhou M, Epstein JI. The reporting of prostate cancer on needle biopsy: prognostic and therapeutic implications and the utility of diagnostic markers. Pathology 2003;35(6):472–9.

77. de la Taille A, Rubin MA, Bagiella E, et al. Can perineural invasion on prostate needle biopsy predict prostate specific antigen recurrence after radical prostatectomy? J Urol 1999;162(1):103–6.

78. Stone NN, Stock RG, Parikh D, Yeghiayan P, Unger P. Perineural invasion and seminal vesicle involvement predict pelvic lymph node metastasis in men with localized carcinoma of the prostate. J Urol 1998;160(5):1722–6.

79. Holmes GF, Walsh PC, Pound CR, Epstein JI. Excision of the neurovascular bundle at radical prostatectomy in cases with perineural invasion on needle biopsy. Urology 1999;53(4):752–6.

80. Bonin SR, Hanlon AL, Lee WR, Movsas B, al-Saleem TI, Hanks GE. Evidence of increased failure in the treatment of prostate carcinoma patients who have perineural invasion treated with three-dimensional conformal radiation therapy. Cancer 1997;79(1):75–80.

81. Quinn DI, Henshall SM, Brenner PC, et al. Prognostic significance of preoperative factors in localized prostate carcinoma treated with radical prostatectomy: importance of percentage of biopsies that contain tumor and the presence of biopsy perineural invasion. Cancer 2003;97(8):1884–93.

82. Beard CJ, Chen MH, Cote K, et al. Perineural invasion is associated with increased relapse after external beam radiotherapy for men with low-risk prostate cancer and may be a marker for occult, high-grade cancer. Int J Radiat Oncol Biol Phys 2004;58(1):19–24.

83. Beard C, Schultz D, Loffredo M, et al. Perineural invasion associated with increased cancer-specific mortality after external beam radiation therapy for men with low- and intermediate-risk prostate cancer. Int J Radiat Oncol Biol Phys 2006;66(2):403–7.

84. D'Amico AV, Whittington R, Malkowicz SB, et al. Clinical utility of the percentage of positive prostate biopsies in defining biochemical outcome after radical prostatectomy for patients with clinically localized prostate cancer. J Clin Oncol 2000;18(6):1164–72.

85. Weight CJ, Ciezki JP, Reddy CA, Zhou M, Klein EA. Perineural invasion on prostate needle biopsy does not predict biochemical failure following brachytherapy for prostate cancer. Int J Radiat Oncol Biol Phys 2006;65(2):347–50.

86. Maru N, Ohori M, Kattan MW, Scardino PT, Wheeler TM. Prognostic significance of the diameter of perineural invasion in radical prostatectomy specimens. Hum Pathol 2001;32(8):828–33.

87. Bostwick DG, Qian J. High-grade prostatic intraepithelial neoplasia. Mod Pathol 2004;17(3):360–79.

88. Goeman L, Joniau S, Ponette D, et al. Is low-grade prostatic intraepithelial neoplasia a risk factor for cancer? Prostate Cancer Prostatic Dis 2003;6(4):305–10.

89. Aboseif S, Shinohara K, Weidner N, Narayan P, Carroll PR. The significance of prostatic intra-epithelial neoplasia. Br J Urol 1995;76(3):355–9.

90. Langer JE, Rovner ES, Coleman BG, et al. Strategy for repeat biopsy of patients with prostatic intraepithelial neoplasia detected by prostate needle biopsy. J Urol 1996;155(1):228–31.

91. Raviv G, Janssen T, Zlotta AR, Descamps F, Verhest A, Schulman CC. Prostatic intraepithelial neoplasia: influence of clinical and pathological data on the detection of prostate cancer. J Urol 1996;156(3):1050–4; discussion 1054–5.

92. Shepherd D, Keetch DW, Humphrey PA, Smith DS, Stahl D. Repeat biopsy strategy in men with isolated prostatic intraepithelial neoplasia on prostate needle biopsy. J Urol 1996;156(2 Pt 1):460–2; discussion 462–3.

93. Epstein JI, Grignon DJ, Humphrey PA, et al. Interobserver reproducibility in the diagnosis of prostatic intraepithelial neoplasia. Am J Surg Pathol 1995;19(8):873–86.

94. Babaian RJ, Toi A, Kamoi K, et al. A comparative analysis of sextant and an extended 11-core multisite directed biopsy strategy. J Urol 2000;163(1): 152–7.

95. Fowler JE Jr, Bigler SA, Miles D, Yalkut DA. Predictors of first repeat biopsy cancer detection with suspected local stage prostate cancer. J Urol 2000;163(3):813–8.

96. Kronz JD, Allan CH, Shaikh AA, Epstein JI. Predicting cancer following a diagnosis of high-grade prostatic intraepithelial neoplasia on needle biopsy: data on men with more than one follow-up biopsy. Am J Surg Pathol 2001;25(8):1079–85.

97. Roscigno M, Scattoni V, Freschi M, et al. Monofocal and plurifocal high-grade prostatic intraepithelial neoplasia on extended prostate biopsies: factors predicting cancer detection on extended repeat biopsy. Urology 2004;63(6): 1105–10.

98. Abdel-Khalek M, El-Baz M, Ibrahiem el-H. Predictors of prostate cancer on extended biopsy in patients with high-grade prostatic intraepithelial neoplasia: a multivariate analysis model. BJU Int 2004;94(4):528–33.

99. Lefkowitz GK, Taneja SS, Brown J, Melamed J, Lepor H. Followup interval prostate biopsy 3 years after diagnosis of high grade prostatic intraepithelial neoplasia is associated with high likelihood of prostate cancer, independent of change in prostate specific antigen levels. J Urol 2002;168(4 Pt 1):1415–18.

100. Maatman TJ, Papp SR, Carothers GG, Shockley KF. The critical role of patient follow-up after receiving a diagnosis of prostatic intraepithelial neoplasia. Prostate Cancer Prostatic Dis 2001;4(1):63–6.

101. Park S, Shinohara K, Grossfeld GD, Carroll PR. Prostate cancer detection in men with prior high grade prostatic intraepithelial neoplasia or atypical prostate biopsy. J Urol 2001;165(5):1409–14.

102. Naya Y, Ayala AG, Tamboli P, Babaian RJ. Can the number of cores with high-grade prostate intraepithelial neoplasia predict cancer in men who undergo repeat biopsy? Urology 2004;63(3):503–8.

103. Kamoi K, Troncoso P, Babaian RJ. Strategy for repeat biopsy in patients with high grade prostatic intraepithelial neoplasia. J Urol 2000;163(3):819–23.

104. Borboroglu PG, Sur RL, Roberts JL, Amling CL. Repeat biopsy strategy in patients with atypical small acinar proliferation or high grade prostatic intraepithelial neoplasia on initial prostate needle biopsy. J Urol 2001;166(3): 866–70.

105. Rubin MA, Bismar TA, Curtis S, Montie JE. Prostate needle biopsy reporting: how are the surgical members of the Society of Urologic Oncology using pathology reports to guide treatment of prostate cancer patients? Am J Surg Pathol 2004;28(7):946–52.

106. Veltri RW, Miller MC, Mangold LA, O'Dowd GJ, Epstein JI, Partin AW. Prediction of pathological stage in patients with clinical stage T1c prostate cancer: the new challenge. J Urol 2002;168(1):100–4.

107. Schlesinger C, Bostwick DG, Iczkowski KA. High-grade prostatic intraepithelial neoplasia and atypical small acinar proliferation: predictive value for cancer in current practice. Am J Surg Pathol 2005;29(9):1201–7.
108. Iczkowski KA, Bassler TJ, Schwob VS, et al. Diagnosis of "suspicious for malignancy" in prostate biopsies: predictive value for cancer. Urology 1998; 51(5):749–57; discussion 757–8.
109. Freedland SJ, deGregorio F, Sacoolidge JC, et al. Preoperative p27 status is an independent predictor of prostate specific antigen failure following radical prostatectomy. J Urol 2003;169(4):1325–30.
110. Vis AN, Noordzij MA, Fitoz K, Wildhagen MF, Schroder FH, van der Kwast TH. Prognostic value of cell cycle proteins p27(kip1) and MIB-1, and the cell adhesion protein CD44s in surgically treated patients with prostate cancer. J Urol 2000;164(6):2156–61.
111. Diaz JI, Mora LB, Austin PF, et al. Predictability of PSA failure in prostate cancer by computerized cytometric assessment of tumoral cell proliferation. Urology 1999;53(5):931–8.
112. Oxley JD, Winkler MH, Parry K, Brewster S, Abbott C, Gillatt DA. p53 and bcl-2 immunohistochemistry in preoperative biopsies as predictors of biochemical recurrence after radical prostatectomy. BJU Int 2002;89(1):27–32.
113. Brewster SF, Oxley JD, Trivella M, Abbott CD, Gillatt DA. Preoperative p53, bcl-2, CD44 and E-cadherin immunohistochemistry as predictors of biochemical relapse after radical prostatectomy. J Urol 1999;161(4):1238–43.
114. Pollack A, Cowen D, Troncoso P, et al. Molecular markers of outcome after radiotherapy in patients with prostate carcinoma: Ki-67, bcl-2, bax, and bcl-x. Cancer 2003;97(7):1630–8.
115. Lee WH, Isaacs WB, Bova GS, Nelson WG. CG island methylation changes near the GSTP1 gene in prostatic carcinoma cells detected using the polymerase chain reaction: a new prostate cancer biomarker. Cancer Epidemiol Biomarkers Prev 1997;6(6):443–50.
116. Lee WH, Morton RA, Epstein JI, et al. Cytidine methylation of regulatory sequences near the pi-class glutathione S-transferase gene accompanies human prostatic carcinogenesis. Proc Natl Acad Sci USA 1994;91(24):11733–7.
117. Harden SV, Guo Z, Epstein JI, Sidransky D. Quantitative GSTP1 methylation clearly distinguishes benign prostatic tissue and limited prostate adenocarcinoma. J Urol 2003;169(3):1138–42.
118. Jeronimo C, Usadel H, Henrique R, et al. Quantitation of GSTP1 methylation in non-neoplastic prostatic tissue and organ-confined prostate adenocarcinoma. J Natl Cancer Inst 2001;93(22):1747–52.
119. Zhou M, Tokumaru Y, Sidransky D, Epstein JI. Quantitative GSTP1 methylation levels correlate with Gleason grade and tumor volume in prostate needle biopsies. J Urol 2004;171(6 Pt 1):2195–8.
120. Epstein JI, Walsh PC, Sanfilippo F. Clinical and cost impact of second-opinion pathology. Review of prostate biopsies prior to radical prostatectomy. Am J Surg Pathol 1996;20(7):851–7.
121. Nguyen PL, Schultz D, Renshaw AA, et al. The impact of pathology review on treatment recommendations for patients with adenocarcinoma of the prostate. Urol Oncol 2004;22(4):295–9.
122. Chan TY, Epstein JI. Patient and urologist driven second opinion of prostate needle biopsies. J Urol 2005;174(4 Pt 1):1390–4; discussion 1394; author reply 1394.

18
Complications of Transrectal Ultrasound–Guided Prostate Biopsy

Sam S. Chang and Michael S. Cookson

Abstract

Refinements in transrectal ultrasound biopsy over the last 25 years have led to improved cancer detection, fewer risks, and reduced morbidity. Hematuria, hematospermia, hematochezia, and rectal bleeding are common, but generally resolve without treatment. Anticoagulant medications should be stopped before planned biopsy unless contraindicated. For patients taking antithrombolytic therapy after cardiac stenting, the urologist should consult with the patient's cardiologist to determine the best course of treatment. Infection complications are significantly reduced with prophylactic antibiotics. However, clinical studies show wide variances for optimal antibiotic regimen. Pain is a source of anxiety for many patients. Periprostatic nerve block is an established method for reducing discomfort. Patients should be educated about common postbiopsy conditions with low morbidity and be able to differentiate these from medical emergencies.

Keywords: prostate biopsy, complications, hematuria, infection, urinary retention

An estimated 1 million patients will undergo transrectal ultrasound–guided needle biopsy (TRUS-Bx) of the prostate annually, and this number will undoubtedly increase in the foreseeable future as the number of men at risk for the development of prostate cancer in the United States continues to increase. Although TRUS-Bx of the prostate is generally safe and reasonably well tolerated in the outpatient setting, it is an invasive procedure associated with some potential risks and morbidity. Over the past 25 years, TRUS-Bx has undergone refinements in technique designed to both

From: *Current Clinical Urology: Prostate Biopsy: Indications, Techniques, and Complications*
Edited by J.S. Jones © Humana Press, Totowa, NJ

improve cancer detection and reduce discomfort. These modifications include increasing the number of needle biopsies obtained in a single session, directing the needle cores more posteriorly and laterally to accentuate the peripheral zone, and incorporating local anesthesia in the form of a periprostatic block. These modifications have impacted the potential morbidity of the procedure. Fortunately, the periprocedural management of patients undergoing TRUS-Bx has also evolved to meet the challenge of maintaining an acceptably low rate of complications. Herein, we review the morbidity associated with contemporary TRUS-Bx of the prostate, risk factors associated with specific complications, and outline strategies designed to reduce them. This information will hopefully aid in patient counseling, and serve as a guide in perioperative management of patients undergoing this procedure.

Overview of Complications

Most of what has been reported historically with respect to complications of TRUS-Bx of the prostate has been derived from studies designed to evaluate either cancer detection or technical aspects of the biopsy itself. Although the rates of various complications were recorded in these largely retrospective reports, variances in the definition of complications, highly variable methods of data collection, differences in patient characteristics and biopsy technique, and wide variances in practices such as antibiotic prophylaxis are partially responsible for a wide variation in rates of specific complications and further confound comparisons among series. More recently, studies have focused specifically on complications of the procedure itself and this has provided a more accurate and comprehensive accounting of the true morbidity of TRUS-Bx. From these studies, risk factors for complications have also been identified and strategies designed to reduce specific complications have been evaluated.

Bleeding

Bleeding is the most common complication reported after TRUS-Bx and may occur in up to 75% of patients.[1-3] Bleeding complications directly related to the biopsy include hematuria, hematospermia, and hematochezia. Most bleeding-related complications after TRUS-Bx are minor and usually resolve without intervention or at most require conservative measures. Approximately 50% of patients experience some mild hematuria that may persist for up to 7 days after the biopsy.[4] Although the risk of hematuria may increase with increasing number of cores[5,6] or transurethral biopsies,[7] most problematic bleeding has occurred when the biopsy strategy included midline biopsies.[8] Eskew et al.,[8] using a five-region biopsy that included midline biopsies—which often penetrate the urethra, reported self-limited hematuria in 80% of patients. However, avoidance of the midline is the best strategy because of the low yield for cancer detection coupled with increased risk of bleeding. Instead, needle biopsies should be directed at the posterior and lateral peripheral zone to improve cancer detection without increasing morbidity.[9]

Rectal bleeding has been reported in up to 30% of patients in some series.[1,3,10] At the time of biopsy, immediate brisk bleeding caused by puncture of a hemorrhoidal vessel can be managed with manual compression. In rare circumstances, additional maneuvers such as suturing or fulguration will be required. In general, hematochezia is minor and relatively short in duration, lasting only a couple of days. However, hematospermia, which occurs in 50%–80% of sexually active men after TRUS-Bx may persist for 4–6 weeks.[3] Although the incidence of hematochezia and hematospermia is increased with an extended biopsy regimen, in most circumstances, the bleeding is mild and resolves with conservative management.[5,6,11] In a prospective evaluation of bleeding-related complications in 760 men, Ghani et al.[1] found that extended core biopsies (8–12 cores) were associated with significantly more rectal bleeding than traditional sextant biopsies; however, the duration of bleeding was similar and only a single patient required hospitalization. In addition, Naughton et al.[6] found in a prospective, randomized study no significant increase in pain or major morbidity associated with a 12-core versus a 6-core biopsy scheme. They did, however, report that in the 12-core group there was a statistically significant increase in hematochezia and hematospermia (24% vs. 10%, p = 0.04 and 89% vs. 71%, p = 0.01, respectively) but no significant difference between groups reporting morbidity as a moderate or major problem. Similarly, in a prospective evaluation of 115 patients who reported sexual activity after biopsy, the incidence of hematospermia was 78.3% among men using a 10-core biopsy scheme.[5]

Avoidance of complications is optimal and it is generally recommended to discontinue any medications or supplements (e.g., Vitiman E) that can interfere with coagulation or platelet function before any procedure with an associated risk of bleeding. When possible, aspirin can be discontinued 10 days before the planned procedure because of its permanent platelet dysfunction and most nonsteroidal antiinflammatory agents 3–5 days before.[2] However, several studies have demonstrated that TRUS-Bx can be performed with relative safety in patients taking low-dose aspirin.[12-14] In a telephone survey of 1810 patients after TRUS-Bx, aspirin use was determined before the procedure and patients were surveyed for bleeding complications. Overall, 46 patients (2.5%) had bleeding complications. Of the 54 patients reporting use of aspirin, 2 patients (3.7%) reported bleeding that was not significantly different from those without aspirin use. The authors concluded that there was no evidence of an association between the use of aspirin and postbiopsy bleeding. In their study, Rodriquez and

Terris[13] found that none of the hemorrhagic complications were related to previous aspirin or nonsteroidal antiinflammatory drug use and concluded that recent use of these drugs is not an absolute contraindication for this procedure.

In a prospective cohort study of 200 patients who underwent TRUS-Bx, those routinely taking low-dose aspirin were encouraged to continue to do so before and after biopsy.[14] In all, 36 patients took aspirin. There were no major complications in either group. Of the patients taking aspirin, 20 (56%) had hematuria, compared with 83 (59%) of those not taking aspirin. Overall bleeding (hematuria, rectal bleeding, and hematospermia) occurred in 22 patients (61%) in the aspirin group and 105 (74%) in the other group. There was no statistically significant difference in the incidence of hematuria or overall bleeding after biopsy between the groups. Thus, it seems that although it may be optimal to discontinue any medications associated with an increased risk of bleeding before TRUS-Bx, the use of aspirin is a relative but not an absolute contraindication and will not significantly increase bleeding complications. However, this relative safety cannot be extrapolated to more potent anticoagulants.

In addition to the use of aspirin, it has become increasingly common to encounter patients taking various forms of anticoagulation including the use of warfarin (Coumadin). It has been our policy not to biopsy patients if they are currently taking warfarin, but rather to follow established guidelines for the management of these patients. Patients in special circumstances, including those at high risk for thromboembolic complications taking warfarin, should be managed in accordance with the American College of Chest Physicians guidelines.[15] However, there has been a recent report from the United Kingdom that found no increased bleeding complications among 49 patients undergoing TRUS-Bx while taking warfarin compared with those not receiving anticoagulation.[16] Although the absence of any statistically significant bleeding in this study is noteworthy, it would seem prudent to discontinue this medication in a procedure with a known risk of blood loss, especially when the medication could precipitate severe or life-threatening bleeding.

Another increasingly common situation is the patient who presents for consideration of a TRUS-Bx while taking antiplatelet therapy such as clopidogrel (Plavix) or ticlopidine hydrochloride (Ticlid). These drugs interfere with platelet function and are associated with an increased risk of bleeding as well. If medically acceptable to temporarily discontinue these medications, such as patients taking prophylaxis for stroke prevention, a biopsy could be safely performed after 10–14 days. However, the increasing use of drug-eluting cardiac stents, now used in up to 50% of cases, has further complicated the matter.[17] Although 4 weeks of antiplatelet therapy combined with aspirin has been recommended for patients after percutaneous coronary intervention with bare-metal stent implantation, the high rate of stent thrombosis with these drug-eluting cardiac stents has led some to recommend continued combination therapy with aspirin and clopidogrel for up to 1 year afterward.[18] At this point, there are no established guidelines for the urologist regarding the optimal strategy in this setting. Therefore, we recommend serious consideration to postponing the TRUS-Bx until safely outside of the critical time for risk of stent thrombosis. If there is an urgent need to perform the TRUS-Bx for histologic confirmation, such as need for confirmation of primary in the setting of metastatic disease, consultation with the cardiologist and consideration of the risk versus benefit are recommended.

Not only are bleeding complications the most frequently encountered side effect after TRUS-Bx, but they are also a major potential source of distress to patients. These complications are particularly disturbing to patients if they are not properly prepared for such events. Accordingly, patients should be counseled regarding the incidence, relative degree of anticipated bleeding, and the anticipated duration of symptoms. It is important for the patient to be instructed to alert the physician in the event of severe or persistent rectal bleeding or gross hematuria. The differentiation between significant rectal or urinary bleeding compared with hematospermia, which is often visually disturbing but of minor consequence, is critical. Informing patients about hematospermia before the procedure, and its 4- to 6-week duration, is often reassuring and significantly reduces both patient anxiety and unnecessary phone calls.

Infectious Complications

Infections are the second most frequently encountered complication of prostate biopsy. Most infections associated with TRUS-Bx are minor, although some are potentially serious. Among patients not receiving prophylactic antibiotics, asymptomatic bacteriuria and transient bacteremia are not uncommon after prostate biopsy with a reported incidence of 20%–53% and 16%–73%, respectively.[13,19] In one prospective study in which patients did not undergo prophylactic antibiotics, the incidence of infectious complications was about 3%.[10] Fortunately, with the use of preoperative antibiotics, the incidence of transient bacteremia is relatively low and the risk of serious complications requiring hospitalization is quite rare (<1%).[3] Nevertheless, severe, life-threatening complications including bacterial sepsis resulting in death have been reported.[20]

There is general consensus among clinicians that the use of antibiotic prophylaxis reduces, but does not completely eliminate, infectious complications associated with TRUS-Bx.[21–23] This has been validated in several placebo-controlled studies demonstrating the benefit of antibiotic prophylaxis compared with placebo to significantly reduce urinary tract infections.[24,25] Multiple periprocedural antibiotic regimens have been proposed to reduce the incidence of infectious complications. However, currently there are no published guidelines that have clearly demonstrated the optimal drug type, dose, or duration for antibiotic prophylaxis during TRUS-Bx.

In fact, surveys of practice patterns have revealed at least 19 different types of antibiotics and 48 different dosage and schedules, underscoring the wide variability and lack of consensus among clinicians.[23,26,27] One such survey regarding prebiopsy protocols was sent to 900 practicing American urologists randomly selected from the American Urological Association computer files.[27] Approximately 63% (568 of 900) of the surveys were returned and showed considerable differences in prebiopsy protocol among those urologists. The prebiopsy regimens included prophylactic antibiotics in 98.6% and a cleansing rectal enema in 81%. In this study alone, 11 different antibiotics were used, with 20 different doses and 23 different timing-duration regimens.

Several studies have demonstrated benefit from as little as a single pre-procedural dose of antibiotics.[25,28,29] In a prospective, randomized, multi-center trial, 537 patients received either oral ciprofloxacin 500 mg or placebo before TRUS-Bx.[25] Repeated urine cultures and urinalysis were obtained at 2–6 days after biopsy and 9–15 days after biopsy. The primary determinant of efficacy was bacteriologic response [bacteriuria ($>10^4$ colony-forming units (CFU)/mL) vs. no bacteriuria] at the 9- to 15-day follow-up evaluation. Three percent of ciprofloxacin-treated patients and 8% of total patients had bacteriuria ($>10^4$ CFU/mL) after the procedure (p = 0.009). Six ciprofloxacin recipients (3%) and 12 placebo recipients (5%) had clinical signs and symptoms of a urinary tract infection (p = 0.15). In addition, no ciprofloxacin-treated patients compared with four placebo-treated patients (2%) were admitted to the hospital for febrile urinary tract infection after the procedure. Another randomized trial, using a single dose of ciprofloxin 500 mg and tinidazole 600 mg, the same regimen twice daily for 3 days or placebo, was performed.[24] There was a significant reduction in infections among the antibiotic-treated patients, but no difference in infections based on a single versus 3-day course, showing single-dose prophylaxis to be adequate. Others have recommended both a preprocedural and postprocedural antibiotic dose because of low rates of infectious complications (2.5%–3.5%).[3,13]

It is important to remember that in absence of prospective, randomized trials, the choice of antibiotic, dose, duration, and schedule will remain a subject of controversy. In such situations, expert opinion and clinical judgment will influence practice patterns. Currently, most authors recommend a 3- to 5-day course of oral antibiotics beginning the day before the planned biopsy and continuing them for up to 3 days after the biopsy. In the setting of prophylaxis, an oral regimen is more cost effective than parenteral dosing with no clear benefit to the latter. The practice of extended prophylactic antibiotics, although not without its critics, is based on literature demonstrating an even further reduction in infectious complications compared with a single dose or single-day dosing.[10,30] Further evidence for this is based on the results of several studies demonstrating the lowest rates of infectious complications (<1%) with extended prophylaxis for at least 4 days.[2,4,26,31] In a retrospective study by Sieber et al.,[26] 4439 biopsies were performed using ciprofloxacin twice daily for eight doses beginning the day before biopsy with an overall infectious complication rate of 0.1% with only three patients requiring hospitalization. Extending antibiotics beyond this duration should be reserved for special circumstances and high-risk patients because of the risk of promoting resistant bacterial strains. Patients with valvular heart disease or mechanical prosthesis should undergo additional antibiotic coverage as recommended by the American Heart Association.[32]

The transrectal route for obtaining prostate needle biopsies is undoubtedly the source for the majority of infectious complications because of seeding of the needle tract with rectal flora. This has raised further controversy regarding the benefit of some form of bowel preparation or cleansing enema to decrease the rectal flora at the time of the procedure. Accordingly, some have recommended enemas[19,28,33,34] whereas others dispute the need for a preprocedural enema.[35,36] Similar to the use of antibiotics, there exists no current standards with which urologists can rely on for guidance. In a survey of more than 600 urologists in the late 1990s, 81% stated they administered enemas as part of their patient preparation.[27] In one study by Lindert et al.,[19] 50 men undergoing TRUS-Bx were randomized to receive a preoperative or no enema. Preoperatively, urine was obtained for culture, and the initial prostate biopsy, biopsy needle, and postoperative urine and blood specimens were cultured. Bacteriuria was noted in 44% of the cases and bacteremia was present in 16% of the patients, of whom 87.5% did not receive an enema (p = 0.0003). Of note, these patients were not administered antibiotics before the biopsy which limits application of these findings in the setting of current antibiotic regimens. Finally, the authors concluded that bacteremia and bacteriuria after multiple biopsies are common but usually asymptomatic.

In contrast, a retrospective review of 448 TRUS-Bx patients was performed.[36] There were 38 patients excluded from the study secondary to alternate antibiotic prophylaxis. A total of 225 patients received enemas before biopsy, whereas 185 did not. Overall, clinically significant complications developed in 4.4% (10 of 225) of patients who had versus 3.2% (6 of 185) of those who did not have an enema (p = 0.614). Of the patients who received enemas, two were hospitalized for urinary retention and complicated urinary tract infection. One patient in the group without an enema was hospitalized for hematuria and clot urinary retention. No patients who did not receive an enema were hospitalized for infectious complications. The authors concluded that an enema before biopsy provided no clinically significant reduction in infectious complications. A large retrospective series of 4439 patients who underwent TRUS-Bx without enemas showed acceptably low rates of infectious complications with only five symptomatic urinary tract infections noted, of which three were complicated.[26] All patients in this series were treated with 500 mg of ciprofloxacin twice daily for 8 doses beginning the day before biopsy. The authors concluded that these data demonstrate the low infection rate associated with this prophylaxis regimen, further questioning the need for cleansing enemas. In addition, Vallancien et al.[35] suggested that enemas may actually increase the risk of infections associated with TRUS-Bx. In their series, which was not randomized, 20% of patients (3 of 15) who received an enema developed a fever after the biopsy compared with 9% (4 of 44) who did not receive an enema.

Early recognition and prompt intervention are critical factors in the successful treatment of infectious complications and to prevent the development of life-threatening sepsis. Accordingly, patients should be informed of the signs and symptoms of these infectious complications, and provided with instructions including contact information in the event of an emergency. Because the majority of these procedures are performed in an office-based setting, patients should also be provided with the information of a hospital to which they should report if such an emergency arises.

In summary, the administration of as little as a single dose of prophylactic antibiotics has significantly reduced infectious complications associated with TRUS-Bx. However, the lowest rates of clinically significant infections have occurred among patients who began their antibiotics the day before the planned biopsy and continued it for 3 days after the biopsy. Most contemporary series have demonstrated these acceptably low rates of infectious complications using oral fluoroquinolone. The addition of an enema may further reduce transient bacteremia and bacteriuria although its true benefit when combined with the fluoroquinolone-based antibiotic prophylaxis is unproven. Patients with valvular heart disease or mechanical prosthesis should undergo additional antibiotic coverage as recommended by the American Heart Association.[32]

Urinary Retention

The incidence of urinary retention after TRUS-Bx is relatively low, with most series reporting rates of less than 2%, although some as high as 10% have been reported.[3,7,37] Risk factors include moderate to severe preexisting obstructive voiding symptoms (high international prostate symptom score), larger prostate volumes, the volume of the increased ratio of the transition zone to the peripheral zone, and increasing numbers of cores. The incidence of urinary retention in recent reports of men treated with saturation biopsies was between 4.5%–10%.[7,37] In the series by Borboroglu et al.,[37] an average of 22.5 cores were obtained and included the transition zone. In this series, urinary retention was reported in six patients (10%) and resolved within 72 hours. In most cases of urinary retention immediately after TRUS-Bx, urinary retention is usually short-lived and easily managed with either a temporary indwelling catheter or self-intermittent catheter. If the patient is at high risk for acute urinary retention, the addition of an alpha-blocker may prevent its occurrence or hasten the recovery of spontaneous voiding.

Vasovagal Episodes

Vasovagal episodes are not uncommon after office-based procedures and TRUS-Bx is no exception. However, the literature regarding this complication is sparse. Rodriguez and Terris[13] reported the first series addressing the incidence at 8% and found at least 5.3% had at least a moderate episode defined as a systolic blood pressure of less than 90 mm Hg, diaphoresis, and bradycardia requiring intravenous fluids. Included in their series was a single patient who required hospital admission because of a severe vasovagal response that induced seizures. Although anxiety and discomfort caused by rectal dilation may contribute, hypoglycemia is also a risk factor and accordingly patients should be encouraged to eat a light meal or snack before the procedure.[2] Additionally, it may be of benefit for the patient to remain lying down for a few minutes after the completion of the procedure to avoid postural hypotension and minimize the risk of fainting. Subsequently, it has been reported that the incidence of vasovagal episodes may actually decrease with repeat biopsy, suggesting the significant impact of anxiety as an etiology.[38] In this prospective series, the incidence of moderate to severe vasovagal episodes was 2.8% on initial biopsy and 1.4% on rebiopsy performed only 6 weeks later.

Pain

Despite the fact that TRUS-Bx has been in vogue since its introduction by Hodge et al. in 1989, the focus of patient discomfort and pain associated with this procedure actually was not emphasized until more than a decade later.[39,40] Unquestionably, anxiety, discomfort, and some degree of pain is experienced by almost all men undergoing this procedure. In patient surveys, pain to some degree has been reported ranging from severe in 7%,[4] "painful" in 22%,[41] to "acceptable discomfort" in up to 80%.[42] However, Irani et al.[43] found that 19% of 81 patients questioned would refuse to undergo further TRUS-Bx without analgesia, underscoring patient dissatisfaction with an anesthesia-free procedure. Clearly, variances in reporting may be attributable to the definition of pain used in the study, the method, instrument, and timing in which the question was asked, patient characteristics including age and baseline anxiety, and the technique in which the biopsy was obtained. Risk factors that seem to predict a higher rate of subjective pain include increasing the number of cores, repeat biopsy sessions, and patient age, with more pain associated with younger patients.[40]

Various analgesic strategies have been reported in an attempt to reduce the pain associated with TRUS-Bx. Intrarectal lidocaine gel is frequently used for this purpose. Advantages of this technique include easy administration and essentially no associated morbidity. However, randomized studies comparing this technique to placebo have been mixed. Some authors have found a significant benefit in pain reduction with the use of lidocaine gel over placebo,[44,45] whereas others have failed to demonstrate any significant reduction in pain.[46–48] Thus, although some patients may benefit from this technique, the results are inconsistent and investigators have subsequently turned to more effective alternatives.

An increasing common mode of analgesia administered during prostate biopsy is the periprostatic nerve block (PNB). This was first described by Nash et al.[49] who initially recommended PNBs after randomizing patients to receive a unilateral injection of 5 mL 1% lidocaine or 5 mL saline (0.9% sodium chloride) or placebo at the vascular pedicle located at the junction of the base of the prostate and the seminal vesicles. They demonstrated statistically significant reductions in pain on the side of the nerve block. However, it was not until subsequent studies, including that of Soloway and Obek,[50] demonstrating the significant reduction in pain associated with PNB that its use became more widely accepted. Soloway and Obek modified the original technique, recommending additional injections not only at the base but between the base and apex and at the apex as well. Subsequently, a variety of subtle modifications in the sites of injection, the concentration, and type of analgesic have been reported with generally favorable results, confirming the efficacy of PNB in reducing pain associated with the biopsy. Several randomized, placebo-controlled studies have also confirmed the results.[40]

There has been some concern regarding a potentially greater morbidity associated with the use of local anesthesia. Obek et al.[51] assessed morbidity associated with lidocaine PNB. In this study of 100 consecutive patients randomized to receive a PNB or no anesthesia, the amount of urethral bleeding was slight and similar in the two groups whereas rectal bleeding was significantly less in the patients who received anesthesia. Bacteriuria in postbiopsy urine cultures was significantly more common in the PNB group. High fever (>37.8°C) was more frequent in the PNB group, and two patients in this group required rehospitalization. Others, however, have noted no increase in infectious complications associated with PNB.[52] Similar to the findings by Obek et al., there does not seem to be an increased risk of bleeding in patients receiving PNB, including those who undergo an increasing number of injections to accomplish the nerve block.[53]

Conclusions

TRUS-Bx of the prostate remains one of the most frequently performed office-based procedures with an acceptably low rate of complications. Bleeding complications including hematuria, hematochezia, and hematospermia remain a potential source for morbidity but are generally minor and resolve with conservative measures. Medications that induce platelet dysfunction or prolong bleeding times should be avoided if possible, although several series have demonstrated the relative safety of TRUS-Bx in patients currently taking aspirin. Major infectious complications including serious life-threatening sepsis have been reported but are fortunately rare. In general, infection rates remain quite low because of the widespread use of effective and potent periprocedural antibiotics. Although variance exists regarding the optimal antibiotic regimen, the literature supports the use of oral antibiotics administered before the TRUS-Bx to reduce infectious complications. Furthermore, a regimen that extends the antibiotics 3 days postbiopsy has the lowest risk of infection compared with a single dose or single-day regimen. Cleansing enemas are considered optional and may further reduce the risk of transient bacteremia when combined with oral antibiotics.

Reducing patient discomfort and pain associated with the procedure has been accomplished by incorporating local analgesia in the form of either lidocaine gel or PNB. Patients should be made aware of the potential risks and side effects of TRUS-Bx before the procedure and provided with information and instructions regarding postbiopsy management. In general, a proactive approach aimed at prevention of the complications is preferred. Identification of high-risk features with modifications aimed at these special circumstances is also critical. Finally, prompt recognition and early intervention of potentially serious side effects are the best strategy to reduce major morbidity.

References

1. Ghani KR, Dundas D, Patel U. Bleeding after transrectal ultrasonography-guided prostate biopsy: a study of 7-day morbidity after a six-, eight- and 12-core biopsy protocol. BJU Int 2004;94:1014.
2. Rodriguez LV, Terris MK. Risks and complications of transrectal ultrasound. Curr Opin Urol 2000;10:111.
3. Raaijmakers R, Kirkels WJ, Roobol MJ, et al. Complication rates and risk factors of 5802 transrectal ultrasound-guided sextant biopsies of the prostate within a population-based screening program. Urology 2002;60:826.
4. Aus G, Hermansson CG, Hugosson J, et al. Transrectal ultrasound examination of the prostate: complications and acceptance by patients. Br J Urol 1993;71:457.
5. Peyromaure M, Ravery V, Messas A, et al. Pain and morbidity of an extensive prostate 10-biopsy protocol: a prospective study in 289 patients. J Urol 2002;167:218.
6. Naughton CK, Ornstein DK, Smith DS, et al. Pain and morbidity of transrectal ultrasound guided prostate biopsy: a prospective randomized trial of 6 versus 12 cores. J Urol 2000;163:168.

 7. Stewart CS, Leibovich BC, Weaver AL, et al. Prostate cancer diagnosis using a saturation needle biopsy technique after previous negative sextant biopsies. J Urol 2001;166:86.
 8. Eskew LA, Bare RL, McCullough DL. Systematic 5 region prostate biopsy is superior to sextant method for diagnosing carcinoma of the prostate. J Urol 1997;157:199.
 9. Presti JC Jr, Chang JJ, Bhargava V, et al. The optimal systematic prostate biopsy scheme should include 8 rather than 6 biopsies: results of a prospective clinical trial. J Urol 2000;163:163.
10. Enlund AL, Varenhorst E. Morbidity of ultrasound-guided transrectal core biopsy of the prostate without prophylactic antibiotic therapy. A prospective study in 415 cases. Br J Urol 1997;79:777.
11. Berger AP, Gozzi C, Steiner H, et al. Complication rate of transrectal ultrasound guided prostate biopsy: a comparison among 3 protocols with 6, 10 and 15 cores. J Urol 2004;171:1478.
12. Herget EJ, Saliken JC, Donnelly BJ, et al. Transrectal ultrasound-guided biopsy of the prostate: relation between ASA use and bleeding complications. Can Assoc Radiol J 1999;50:173.
13. Rodriguez LV, Terris MK. Risks and complications of transrectal ultrasound guided prostate needle biopsy: a prospective study and review of the literature. J Urol 1998;160:2115.
14. Maan Z, Cutting CW, Patel U, et al. Morbidity of transrectal ultrasonography-guided prostate biopsies in patients after the continued use of low-dose aspirin. BJU Int 2003;91:798.
15. Hirsh J, Dalen J, Guyatt G. The sixth (2000) ACCP guidelines for antithrombotic therapy for prevention and treatment of thrombosis. American College of Chest Physicians. Chest 2001;119:1S.
16. Ihezue CU, Smart J, Dewbury KC, et al. Biopsy of the prostate guided by transrectal ultrasound: relation between warfarin use and incidence of bleeding complications. Clin Radiol 2005;60:459.
17. Tamberella MR, Furman MI. The role of platelet inhibition in the drug-eluting stent era. Coron Artery Dis 2004;15:327.
18. Zimarino M, Renda G, De Caterina R. Optimal duration of antiplatelet therapy in recipients of coronary drug-eluting stents. Drugs 2005;65:725.
19. Lindert KA, Kabalin JN, Terris MK. Bacteremia and bacteriuria after transrectal ultrasound guided prostate biopsy. J Urol 2000;164:6.
20. Brewster SF, Rooney N, Kabala J, et al. Fatal anaerobic infection following transrectal biopsy of a rare prostatic tumour. Br J Urol 1993;72:977.
21. Crawford ED, Haynes AL Jr, Story MW, et al. Prevention of urinary tract infection and sepsis following transrectal prostatic biopsy. J Urol 1982;127:449.
22. Davison P, Malament M. Urinary contamination as a result of transrectal biopsy of the prostate. J Urol 1971;105:545.
23. Taylor HM, Bingham JB. The use of prophylactic antibiotics in ultrasound-guided transrectal prostate biopsy. Clin Radiol 1997;52:787.
24. Aron M, Rajeev TP, Gupta NP. Antibiotic prophylaxis for transrectal needle biopsy of the prostate: a randomized controlled study. BJU Int 2000;85:682.
25. Kapoor DA, Klimberg IW, Malek GH, et al. Single-dose oral ciprofloxacin versus placebo for prophylaxis during transrectal prostate biopsy. Urology 1998;52:552.

26. Sieber PR, Rommel FM, Agusta VE, et al. Antibiotic prophylaxis in ultrasound guided transrectal prostate biopsy. J Urol 1997;157:2199.

27. Shandera KC, Thibault GP, Deshon GE Jr. Variability in patient preparation for prostate biopsy among American urologists. Urology 1998;52:644.

28. Shandera KC, Thibault GP, Deshon GE Jr. Efficacy of one dose fluoroquinolone before prostate biopsy. Urology 1998;52:641.

29. Bates TS, Porter T, Gingell JC. Prophylaxis for transrectal prostatic biopsies: a randomized controlled study of intravenous co-amoxiclav given as a single dose compared with an intravenous dose followed by oral co-amoxiclav for 24 h. Br J Urol 1998;81:529.

30. Kraklau DM, Wolf JS Jr. Review of antibiotic prophylaxis recommendations for office-based urologic procedures. Tech Urol 1999;5:123.

31. Cooner WH, Mosley BR, Rutherford CL Jr, et al. Prostate cancer detection in a clinical urological practice by ultrasonography, digital rectal examination and prostate specific antigen. J Urol 1990;143:1146.

32. Dajani AS, Taubert KA, Wilson W, et al. Prevention of bacterial endocarditis. Recommendations by the American Heart Association. JAMA 1997;277:1794.

33. Melekos MD. Efficacy of prophylactic antimicrobial regimens in preventing infectious complications after transrectal biopsy of the prostate. Int Urol Nephrol 1990;22:257.

34. Jeon SS, Woo SH, Hyun JH, et al. Bisacodyl rectal preparation can decrease infectious complications of transrectal ultrasound-guided prostate biopsy. Urology 2003;62:461.

35. Vallancien G, Prapotnich D, Veillon B, et al. Systematic prostatic biopsies in 100 men with no suspicion of cancer on digital rectal examination. J Urol 1991;146:1308.

36. Carey JM, Korman HJ. Transrectal ultrasound guided biopsy of the prostate. Do enemas decrease clinically significant complications? J Urol 2001;166:82.

37. Borboroglu PG, Comer SW, Riffenburgh RH, et al. Extensive repeat transrectal ultrasound guided prostate biopsy in patients with previous benign sextant biopsies. J Urol 2000;163:158.

38. Djavan B, Waldert M, Zlotta A, et al. Safety and morbidity of first and repeat transrectal ultrasound guided prostate needle biopsies: results of a prospective European prostate cancer detection study. J Urol 2001;166:856.

39. Hodge KK, McNeal JE, Terris MK, et al. Random systematic versus directed ultrasound guided transrectal core biopsies of the prostate. J Urol 1989;142:71.

40. Autorino R, De Sio M, Di Lorenzo G, et al. How to decrease pain during transrectal ultrasound guided prostate biopsy: a look at the literature. J Urol 2005;174:2091.

41. Collins GN, Lloyd SN, Hehir M, et al. Multiple transrectal ultrasound-guided prostatic biopsies—true morbidity and patient acceptance. Br J Urol 1993;71:460.

42. Bastide C, Lechevallier E, Eghazarian C, et al. Tolerance of pain during transrectal ultrasound-guided biopsy of the prostate: risk factors. Prostate Cancer Prostatic Dis 2003;6:239.

43. Irani J, Fournier F, Bon D, et al. Patient tolerance of transrectal ultrasound-guided biopsy of the prostate. Br J Urol 1997;79:608.

44. Issa MM, Bux S, Chun T, et al. A randomized prospective trial of intrarectal lidocaine for pain control during transrectal prostate biopsy: the Emory University experience. J Urol 2000;164:397.

45. Saad F, Sabbagh R, McCormack M, et al. A prospective randomized trial comparing lidocaine and lubricating gel on pain level in patients undergoing transrectal ultrasound prostate biopsy. Can J Urol 2002;9:1592.

46. Chang SS, Alberts G, Wells N, et al. Intrarectal lidocaine during transrectal prostate biopsy: results of a prospective double-blind randomized trial. J Urol 2001;166:2178.

47. Cevik I, Ozveri H, Dillioglugil O, et al. Lack of effect of intrarectal lidocaine for pain control during transrectal prostate biopsy: a randomized prospective study. Eur Urol 2002;42:217.

48. Desgrandchamps F, Meria P, Irani J, et al. The rectal administration of lidocaine gel and tolerance of transrectal ultrasonography-guided biopsy of the prostate: a prospective randomized placebo-controlled study. BJU Int 1999;83:1007.

49. Nash PA, Bruce JE, Indudhara R, et al. Transrectal ultrasound guided prostatic nerve blockade eases systematic needle biopsy of the prostate. J Urol 1996; 155:607.

50. Soloway MS, Obek C. Periprostatic local anesthesia before ultrasound guided prostate biopsy. J Urol 2000;163:172.

51. Obek C, Onal B, Ozkan B, et al. Is periprostatic local anesthesia for transrectal ultrasound guided prostate biopsy associated with increased infectious or hemorrhagic complications? A prospective randomized trial. J Urol 2002;168:558.

52. Seymour H, Perry MJ, Lee-Elliot C, et al. Pain after transrectal ultrasonography-guided prostate biopsy: the advantages of periprostatic local anaesthesia. BJU Int 2001;88:540.

53. Ozden E, Yaman O, Gogus C, et al. The optimum doses of and injection locations for periprostatic nerve blockade for transrectal ultrasound guided biopsy of the prostate: a prospective, randomized, placebo controlled study. J Urol 2003;170:2319.

19

Management and Controversies of High-Grade Prostatic Intraepithelial Neoplasia and Atypical Small Acinar Proliferation on Prostate Biopsy

Alon Z. Weizer, Scott M. Gilbert, Rajal B. Shah, and
David P. Wood, Jr.

Abstract

High-grade prostatic intraepithelial neoplasia (HGPIN) and atypical small acinar proliferation (ASAP) are concerning pathologic findings. HGPIN is the most likely lesion precursor of prostate cancer. ASAP is not a diagnosis, but a statement of concern by the pathologist implying concomitant prostate cancer not sampled on biopsy. The likelihood of prostate cancer on repeat biopsy is greater in cases of ASAP than in cases of HGPIN. Repeat extended biopsy is recommended for ASAP. Repeat extended biopsy for a diagnosis of HGPIN is recommended only if the initial biopsy was undersampled, or if the clinical situation based on examination and prostate-specific antigen results dictates doing so. Parameters used for risk stratification do not aid in the diagnosis of cancer after detection of HGPIN of ASAP.

Chemoprevention may hold promise for patients diagnosed with HGPIN. The results of phase III clinical studies will prove very insightful in evaluating the use of chemoprevention. Currently, there are no studies on the use of chemoprevention for ASAP.

Keywords: high-grade prostatic intraepithelial neoplasia, prostate biopsy, chemoprevention, atypical small acinar proliferation

High-grade prostatic intraepithelial neoplasia (HGPIN) and atypical small acinar proliferation (ASAP) are potentially concerning findings on prostate

From: *Current Clinical Urology: Prostate Biopsy: Indications, Techniques, and Complications*
Edited by J.S. Jones © Humana Press, Totowa, NJ

biopsy and typically prompt further evaluation. HGPIN is considered the most likely precursor to prostate cancer, and when found on biopsy, has traditionally been associated with an increased likelihood of prostate cancer. ASAP, or atypical glands, is not a diagnosis but rather a statement of concern by the pathologist that implies the presence of concomitant prostate cancer not sampled on biopsy. Detection rates are variable according to different retrospective studies, and uncertainty regarding the management of HGPIN and ASAP on prostate biopsy, including rebiopsy and chemopreventive strategies, exists.

At the microscopic level, HGPIN is characterized by atypical cellular proliferations within architecturally normal preexisting ducts and glands.

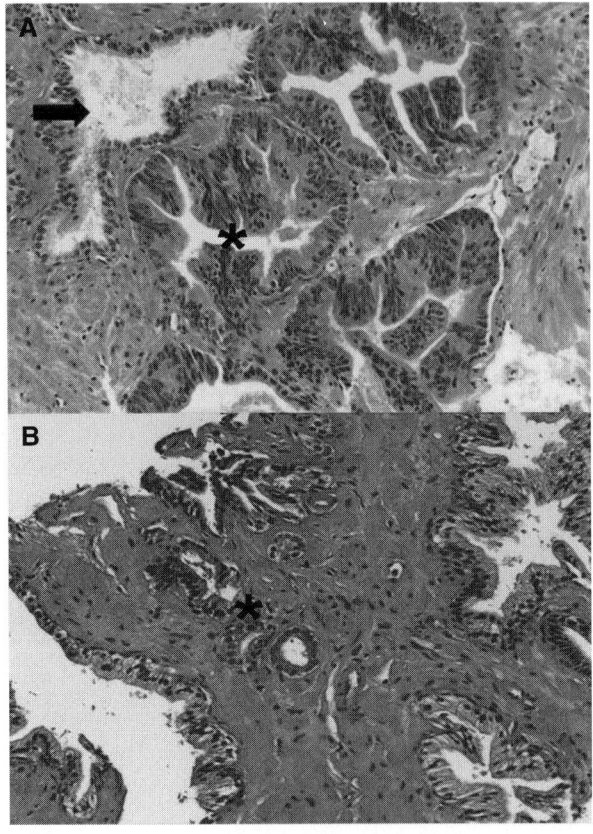

FIGURE 19.1. Representative images of typical histologic pattern of high-grade prostatic intraepithelial neoplasia (HGPIN) and atypical small acinar proliferation (ASAP). **A**: Low-power image of common papillary/tufting pattern of HGPIN (*) with adjacent benign prostate gland (arrow). **B**: Low-power image of ASAP demonstrating focus of three small glands with features highly suspicious for prostate cancer (*) but without sufficient amount to diagnose as prostate cancer.

In addition, HGPIN coexists with cancer in greater than 85% of cases. Unlike cancer, PIN is characterized by an intact or fragmented basal cell layer. Previously, PIN, and in particular HGPIN, have been associated with clinical concern secondary to its association with prostate cancer, and therefore the detection of HGPIN on prostate biopsy has resulted in additional evaluation and in some cases therapy. Many believe that the presence of HGPIN on prostate biopsy warrants further investigation for concomitant prostate cancer. In contrast, ASAP or atypical glands implies that the suspicious glands have some but not all of the features consistent with prostate cancer. Figure 19.1 demonstrates representative images of the most common patterns of HGPIN and ASAP.

In recent years, management questions and issues related to HGPIN found on needle biopsy have been reexamined based on extended follow-up and new data. Recent progress in our understanding of the role HGPIN may have in prostate cancer development and the frequency with which it is found on initial and rebiopsy using extended biopsy techniques have helped to address this controversial question.

In this chapter, our goal is to 1) analyze and describe the clinical implication of PIN and ASAP on prostate biopsy, 2) suggest an evidence-based approach to management after the detection of PIN and ASAP on prostate biopsy, and 3) discuss the current role of chemoprevention in the management of HGPIN and ASAP.

Detection and Clinical Implications of High-Grade Prostatic Intraepithelial Neoplasia

Detection of High-Grade Prostatic Intraepithelial Neoplasia

The reported detection rate of HGPIN varies considerably, ranging from 0% to 24.6% (Table 19.1). The average rate is 7.7%.[1] Interestingly, the detection of HGPIN on needle biopsy does not seem to be related to the number of biopsy cores sampled. In addition, the rate of detecting HGPIN does not differ substantially according to practice setting nor does there seem to be significant variation in the detection of HGPIN with time.[1]

Variation in reported detection rates may be related to several factors associated with pathologic classification and processing. Currently, there are no quantitative measures used to distinguish between low-grade PIN (LGPIN) and HGPIN. Lack of a quantitative assessment of nucleoli prominence, the principal histologic feature that differentiated HGPIN from LGPIN, allows for differential interpretation and interobserver variation. The pathologic criteria are, therefore, susceptible to misclassification that may contribute to variation in reporting HGPIN. The appearance of

TABLE 19.1. Detection of high-grade prostatic intraepithelial neoplasia (HGPIN) on initial biopsy and cancer detection on repeat biopsy stratified according to initial biopsy pathology (HGPIN or negative).

| Study | Year | Detection of HGPIN on initial biopsy Cases/total (%) | Cancer detection on repeat biopsy by initial biopsy finding | | No. of cores | |
			HGPIN Cases/total (%)	Benign Cases/total (%)	Initial biopsy	Repeat biopsy
Kamoi et al.[18]	2000	63/611 (10.3)	10/45 (22.2)	n/a	n/a	n/a
O'Dowd et al.[5]	2000	4902/132,426 (3.7)	295/1306 (22.6)	702/3544 (19.8)	n/a	n/a
Alsikafi et al.[64]	2001	21/485 (4.3)	3/21 (14.3)	n/a	n/a	n/a
Borboroglu et al.[17]	2001	76/1391 (5.5)	20/45 (44.4)	n/a	n/a	n/a
Lefkowitz et al.[26]	2001	119/1223 (9.7)	1/43 (2.3)	n/a	12	12
Goeman et al.[12]	2003	63/562 (11.2)	14/63 (22.2)	n/a	6	6
San Francisco et al.[20]	2003	49/389 (12.6)	5/21 (23.8)	1/43 (2.3)	≥10	≥10
Abdel-Khalek et al.[13]	2004	83/3081 (2.7)	30/83 (36.1)	n/a	6	11
Naya et al.[7]	2004	226/1086 (20.8)	5/47 (10.6)	13/75 (17.3)	≥10	≥10
Postma et al.[8]	2004	46/1840 (2.5)	4/30 (13.3)	79/739 (10.7)	6	6
Roscigno et al.[19]	2004	91/2314 (3.9)	21/47 (44.7)	n/a	≥10	≥10
Moore et al[14]	2005	30/1188 (2.5)	1/22 (4.5)	n/a	≥10	≥10

nucleoli prominence is affected by specimen processing, so that accurate interpretation may be influenced by technical processing factors.[1]

Association and Risk of Prostate Cancer after Detection of High-Grade Prostatic Intraepithelial Neoplasia

Although the relationship between HGPIN and prostate cancer has not been completely elucidated, HGPIN is currently considered the leading candidate precursor of prostate cancer.[2,3] In addition to sharing similar cellular morphologic, histochemical, and genetic changes, the precursor relationship of HGPIN with prostate cancer has been definitively demonstrated in a mouse model.[4] Questions regarding the risk of developing or detecting prostate cancer in the presence of HGPIN are therefore important and clinically relevant considerations.

The association between HGPIN and prostate cancer has broad implications that impact clinical decision making and subsequent patient management. Several issues relating to the presence of HGPIN on prostate biopsy remain, including: 1) the risk of developing prostate cancer once HGPIN is detected, 2) the risk of having unrecognized prostate cancer concomitant to the detection of HGPIN, and 3) the clinical management once HGPIN has been diagnosed.

As with the detection rate of HGPIN, prostate cancer detection on repeat biopsy varies considerably. Although early studies reported relatively high rates of cancer detection on repeat biopsy after an initial biopsy finding of HGPIN, more recent studies have reported substantially lower rates. The average risk of cancer detection on repeat biopsy is approximately 25% when 50 or more patients are considered. This does not differ considerably from reported cancer detection rates on repeat biopsy after an initial negative biopsy. For example, O'Dowd and colleagues[5] reported cancer detection in approximately 20% of cases on second biopsy after a negative first biopsy in a large cohort of men. Similarly, Gokden et al.[6] reported that 26% of men with an initial negative biopsy were subsequently diagnosed with prostate cancer on repeat biopsy. Although others have reported lower rates of cancer detection among men with an initial negative biopsy, several studies have reported the same risk of cancer detection on repeat biopsy in men with either HGPIN or negative findings on first biopsy.[5–11] To date, there is no compelling evidence to suggest that a significant difference in subsequent cancer detection exists after the detection of HGPIN compared with negative findings on first prostate biopsy.

The value of multiple repeat biopsies after an initial diagnosis of HGPIN is limited. Most studies indicate that the majority of cancer cases are detected on the first repeat biopsy, and that unless indicated for other reasons [increasing prostate specific antigen (PSA), abnormal digital rectal examination (DRE)], these patients should not be subjected to multiple repeat biospies.[12–16]

Risk Factors for the Development of Prostate Cancer in Men with High-Grade Prostatic Intraepithelial Neoplasia

Although several studies have attempted to identify risk factors associated with HGPIN and risk of subsequent prostate cancer, there are currently no clinical parameters that are useful in this regard. Factors such as PSA, PSA determinants, and PSA kinetics do not reliably stratify cancer cases from noncancer cases when repeat biopsy is performed for HGPIN.[8,13,16–22] In addition, other demographic and clinical parameters, including age, family history of prostate cancer, and DRE, have not been shown to reliably differentiate HGPIN cases that progress to cancer on subsequent biopsy from those that do not.[5,8,13,16,18–20,23–25] Despite the usefulness of these clinical parameters in defining risk of cancer in screening populations, there does not seem to be the same prognostic relationship in men with HGPIN detected on initial for-cause prostate biopsy.

Increased prostate sampling has likely had an impact on the detection of prostate cancer on repeat biopsy in the HGPIN population. In several studies, low rates of prostate cancer were reported on repeat biopsy when 10 or more cores were initially sampled.[7,14,20,26] Herawi and colleagues[27] recently demonstrated the relationship of sampling and subsequent prostate cancer detection by stratifying cases according to the number of cores obtained on initial biopsy. In cases of sextant biopsies for both initial and repeat biopsies, the risk of cancer detection was 14.1% on repeat biopsy. In those with sextant biopsies initially and eight or more cores on repeat biopsy, the cancer detection rate was 31.9% on second (repeat) biopsy. In cases with eight cores or more for both the initial and repeat biopsy, the second biopsy detected cancer in 14.6% of cases. The variation in cancer detection likely results from more extensive prostate sampling with greater number of prostate cores obtained on biopsy. Given that improved cancer detection rates have been demonstrated using extended prostate biopsy strategies, rates of cancer detection on repeat biopsy for HGPIN might be expected to continue to remain relatively low.

Others have researched the impact of the number of cores containing HGPIN and the subsequent risk of prostate cancer on repeat biopsy. Although Abdel-Khalek et al.[13] reported that the number of HGPIN-involved cores was predictive of subsequent prostate cancer detection, most studies have not found an association.[15,17,18,20,27] Similarly, the architectural pattern of HGPIN also has not been associated with cancer detection on subsequent biopsies. This may again be related to prostate sampling, and as contemporary practice moves toward more universal use of extended biopsy techniques, using clinical and initial biopsy parameters to predict risk of prostate cancer on repeat biopsy may become less relevant.

Atypical Small Acinar Proliferation and Its Potential Misinterpretation

ASAP reflects a broad group of lesions of varying clinical significance, and oftentimes may include cases that demonstrate focal carcinoma that do not contain sufficient cytologic or architectural atypia to establish the diagnosis of prostate cancer definitively. In other words, ASAP, or atypical glands, are not a biologic entity but rather a means for the pathologist to convey uncertainty regarding the diagnosis. The likelihood of finding cancer on repeat biopsy is greater in cases of ASAP than with HGPIN. As indicated by Epstein and colleagues,[1] however, many urologists are misinformed regarding differences between HGPIN and ASAP. In a survey of urologic oncologists, more than half considered HGPIN and ASAP representative of equivalent precancerous lesions, and an additional 12% considered HGPIN to be worse than ASAP.[28] The misinformation regarding the difference between ASAP and HGPIN is further evidenced in that men with HGPIN undergo repeat biopsy at earlier follow-up intervals than men with ASAP.[16]

This is a potentially concerning issue, and currently expert urologic pathologists believe that the use of terminology such as ASAP may undermine appropriate follow-up and repeat prostate biopsy recommendations. According to several studies, a substantial proportion of men with an atypical diagnosis are not evaluated further with a repeat biopsy, even when it is recommended in the pathology report.[29,30] The incidence of atypical glands suspicious for carcinoma has been reported at approximately 5%.[5,7,8,17,29–42] The risk of cancer detection on repeat biopsy ranges from 17% to 70% (Table 19.2), although the majority of studies consist of small patient numbers.[1] In large studies, the cancer detection rate on repeat

TABLE 19.2. Detection of atypical glands suspicious for carcinoma on initial prostate biopsy and subsequent detection of prostate cancer on repeat biopsy.

Study	Year	Detection of atypia on initial biopsy Cases/total (%)	Detection of cancer on repeat biopsy Cases/total (%)
Cheville et al.[29]	1997	48/1009 (4.8)	15/25 (60.0)
Renshaw et al.[34]	1998	204/2219 (9.0)	20/59 (33.9)
Hoedemaeker et al.[41]	1999	43/1824 (2.4)	15/39 (38.5)
O'Dowd et al.[5]	2000	3709/132,426 (2.8)	640/1530 (41.8)
Borboroglu et al.[17]	2001	61/1391 (4.4)	27/54 (50.0)
Ouyang et al.[42]	2001	21/331 (6.3)	9/17 (52.9)
Iczkowski et al.[39]	2002	184/7081	51/129 (39.5)
Brausi et al.[38]	2004	71/1327 (5.3)	6/23 (26.1)
Fadare et al.[30]	2004	36/1964 (1.8)	9/24 (37.5)
Postma et al.[8]	2004	108/4117 (2.6)	8/47 (17.0)

biopsy is approximately 40%. For example, Iczkowski et al.[43] reported a prostate cancer detection rate of 38.5% in 295 patients diagnosed with atypical glands on initial biopsy. In a larger study, O'Dowd and colleagues[5] reported a diagnosis of prostate cancer in 41.8% on repeat biopsy after the detection of atypical glands on initial biopsy. As with HGPIN, few, if any, clinical parameters are predictive of subsequent prostate cancer with the atypical gland diagnosis.[8,14,16,17,30,43-46] Although the presence of atypical glands suspicious for malignancy is associated with subsequent detection of prostate cancer in a substantial proportion of cases, the majority of cancers detected will be favorable risk. In several studies, more than 70% of cancers detected on rebiopsy were Gleason score 6 or less.[41,43,46]

Management of High-Grade Prostatic Intraepithelial Neoplasia and Atypical Small Acinar Proliferation

Rebiopsy and Surveillance after a Diagnosis of High-Grade Prostatic Intraepithelial Neoplasia and/or Atypical Small Acinar Proliferation

High-Grade Prostatic Intraepithelial Neoplasia

Because of the growing use of extended transrectal ultrasound–guided biopsy techniques, there has been a shift in the recommendation for rebiopsy of HGPIN. Recently, the National Comprehensive Cancer Network (NCCN) published guidelines for rebiopsy in men including those diagnosed with HGPIN and/or ASAP on a transrectal ultrasound biopsy.[47] Based on several series that have demonstrated a lower rate of detection of cancer on a second biopsy after a diagnosis of HGPIN, this report does not recommend immediate repeat biopsy for men with an initial diagnosis of HGPIN if an extended biopsy pattern was used. However, in cases in which HGPIN is detected using a sextant biopsy technique, a repeat biopsy *is* recommended. Furthermore, the NCCN recommends evaluation with an extended biopsy technique, including sampling of the transition zone based on several studies demonstrating a high percentage of cancers detected in other locations than the original site of PIN on a sextant needle biopsy (Figure 19.2).

If no cancer is found on the subsequent biopsy or the patient had HGPIN diagnosed on an initial extended-pattern biopsy, the NCCN recommends close follow-up with PSA and DRE (Figure 19.2). The interval of follow-up has not been well defined. There are few studies that have evaluated patients with third and fourth biopsies after an initial diagnosis of HGPIN. Obviously, the diagnostic rate in those circumstances becomes exceedingly

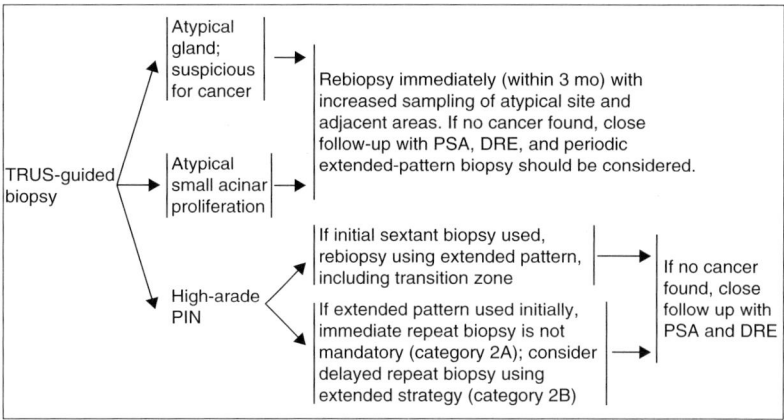

FIGURE 19.2. Management recommendations for atypical small acinar proliferation (ASAP) or high-grade prostatic intraepithelial neoplasia (HGPIN) on initial biopsy. TRUS = transrectal ultrasound, PSA = prostate-specific antigen, DRE = digital rectal examination. (Reproduced with permission from the National Comprehensive Cancer Network [NCCN] (1.2005) Prostate Cancer Early Detection Guidelines, The Complete Library of NCCN Clinical Practice Guidelines in Oncology [CD-ROM]. Jenkintown, PA: © National Comprehensive Cancer Network, March 2006. To view the most recent and complete version of the guideline, go online to www.nccn.org. These guidelines are a statement of consensus of its authors regarding their views of currently accepted approaches to judgment in the context of individual clinical circumstances to determine any patient's care or treatment. The NCCN makes no warranties of any kind whatsoever regarding their content, use, or application and disclaims any responsibility for their application or use in any way. These guidelines are copyrighted by the National Comprehensive Cancer Network. All rights reserved. These guidelines and illustrations herein may not be reproduced in any form for any purpose without the express written permission of the NCCN.)

low.[14,48] It has therefore been suggested that patients with HGPIN on an initial biopsy be treated no differently than screened patients in general as described above. This implies that patients with a diagnosis of HGPIN on an initial extended-pattern biopsy have annual screening with PSA and DRE and that these parameters should drive the indication for repeat biopsy. However, it is not unreasonable to consider a semiannual approach in this population considering they were high enough risk to warrant an initial biopsy. As reviewed above, the literature indicates that there are no clinical parameters that can predict patients with HGPIN that will have cancer on a subsequent biopsy, so the decision to rebiopsy should ultimately be based on either objective clinical indications or an informed, shared decision between the patient and physician.

Atypical Glands or Atypical Small Acinar Proliferation

The recommendations for ASAP differ primarily because ASAP is not a diagnosis but rather terminology that pathologists use to describe a variety of pathologic findings that are concerning for malignancy. Patients with a combination of ASAP and HGPIN should be treated similar to patients with ASAP alone. Again, the NCCN guidelines published in 2005 recommended that all patients with a diagnosis of ASAP undergo a repeat extended-pattern biopsy within 3 months of the initial biopsy because of the approximately 40%–50% chance of cancer diagnosis on a repeat biopsy (Figure 19.2).[47] A recent study reported that initial extended-pattern biopsies with ASAP do not have a lower detection rate of cancer on subsequent biopsies.[14] Several studies have shown significant interobserver variability among pathologists in assigning ASAP on pathology reports. Epstein et al.[1] suggest that cases of ASAP be reviewed by a second pathologist to assess for the presence of undetected prostate cancer. This suggestion stems from results of re-review of 376 ASAP cases indicating that a total of 67 biopsies (18%) were reinterpreted as cancer and 14 (4%) were interpreted as negative, thus avoiding the need for rebiopsy in these patients.[1] Whereas this may be a useful strategy for urologists who have their pathology interpreted by a pathologist who does not see a large volume of prostate biopsies, this may have less of an impact for those specimens interpreted by pathologists seeing large volumes.

If a patient has a negative biopsy after an initial biopsy with ASAP, the NCCN guidelines recommend more rigorous follow-up, including periodic PSA, DRE, and repeat extended-pattern biopsies (Figure 19.2). Although there is no clear evidence regarding the interval for PSA, DRE, and repeat biopsy, the high likelihood of cancer in this group of men warrants at least semiannual PSA and DRE, and likely a repeat biopsy within 1 year of the second negative biopsy.

Chemoprevention and High-Grade Prostatic Intraepithelial Neoplasia

Chemoprevention is defined as a pharmacologic intervention intended to delay the development of cancer or retard its progression. Prostate cancer represents an ideal target for chemoprevention for several reasons. First, it is a common disease affecting almost 230,000 men according to the American Cancer Society in 2005.[49] Second, many prostate cancers are slow growing, so there is an opportunity to alter the natural history of the disease in low-risk patients without compromising cancer control and survival. This is predicated on the belief that men with low-risk cancers (Gleason score 6 or less, low-volume disease on prostate biopsy, and no clinical signs of significant disease) represent good candidates for an active surveillance protocol, which is now being addressed by several prospective trials in the

United States, Canada, and England.[50,51] Third, HGPIN is known to be a precancerous lesion that precedes the diagnosis of cancer by up to 10 years by some estimates. This provides clinicians a window of opportunity to intervene before the presumed development of prostate cancer. The Prevention Trials Decision Network, a branch of the National Cancer Institute, has identified PIN as a biomarker of increased risk for the development of prostate cancer which represents a target for chemoprevention trials.[52,53]

A second issue for chemoprevention strategies is the identification of markers to evaluate response to treatment. Although several studies have shown that HGPIN does not significantly alter PSA levels, there are intriguing data that suggest that certain treatments can reduce the extent of PIN in a prostate. Much of this evidence is derived from prostates removed after radiation therapy or androgen deprivation therapy which have shown a reduction or eradication of HGPIN in these pathologic specimens.[54–56]

Whereas radiation therapy and androgen deprivation may alter the natural history of PIN, a second goal of chemoprevention is the identification of active, nontoxic agents that alter the natural history of cancer. Both androgen deprivation as well as radiation have significant toxicities that likely preclude their use as chemoprevention strategies in patients with HGPIN. Additional problems with these treatment strategies include the cost and possible limited number of patients that would benefit from these approaches.

A review of chemoprevention strategies for prostate cancer is beyond the scope of this chapter. However, there have been several studies that have evaluated the use of these chemoprevention strategies in patients diagnosed with HGPIN on initial prostate biopsy. As an end point, most of these studies have relied on repeat prostate biopsies to evaluate the impact of treatment.

- Toremifene citrate is an oral selective estrogen receptor modulator. An initial study evaluated the safety of this oral agent (60 mg daily for 4 months) in 21 men with a diagnosis of HGPIN on a prostate biopsy. Thirteen of 18 men (72%) had no evidence of HGPIN or invasive cancer on a repeat biopsy compared with 18% of historical controls.[57] A phase IIb randomized, double-blinded, controlled study of 514 men compared three doses of the medication (20, 40, and 60 mg) with placebo taken over 12 months in men with a diagnosis of HGPIN on prostate biopsy. The incidence of prostate cancer was reduced by 48% in men in the 20-mg group compared with placebo at 12 months (9.1% vs. 17.4%, p = 0.05). The relative risk reduction for the two higher doses was not statistically significant.[58] This medication was well tolerated, and is currently undergoing evaluation in a phase III study.
- Lycopene, a red carotenoid pigment found in a variety of fruits (especially tomatoes) has been studied in a chemoprevention study for men diagnosed with HGPIN on biopsy. Forty men identified as having HGPIN

on transurethral resection of prostate chips were randomized to 4 mg of lycopene (Lyc-O-Mato, LycoRed Natural Products Industries, Ltd., Beer-Sheva, Israel) twice daily versus placebo (who were asked to reduce lycopene intake). After 2 years of follow-up, the study demonstrated a reduction of PSA from 6.07 ng/mL in the treatment group to 3.5 ng/mL and an increase in the control group from 6.55 to 8.06 ng/mL. A higher serum lycopene level indicated a lower PSA. Also, of six patients rebiopsied in the treatment group, two were found to have cancer compared with 6 of 9 patients with cancer who were rebiopsied in the control group.[59] Although the cause of the reduction of PSA is not clear in the treatment group, McDonald and colleagues[60] found that men given multivitamin supplementation with or without lycopene had reductions in the PSA level that returned to baseline after stopping therapy, concurring with the PSA-lowering effect of lycopene described above. This report is part of a National Cancer Institute–sponsored trial. Kucuk and colleagues[61] demonstrated that lycopene reduced the volume of HGPIN in prostatectomy specimens compared with controls, which similarly concurs with the impact seen on prostate biopsies in the first study. Although the role of lycopene in prostate cancer prevention seems promising, results of current phase III studies will provide more information regarding the benefit of this approach.

- Green tea catechins (GTCs) were tested in a phase I/II study in 60 patients diagnosed with HGPIN on prostate biopsy randomized to 600 mg of GTCs compared with placebo. GTCs have been shown to be effective in inhibiting cancer growth in several experimental models. There were no adverse events, and only 1 of 30 patients given GTCs was diagnosed with prostate cancer on prostate biopsy at 1 year compared with nine men in the control arm. Although this intriguing approach seems safe, further studies are needed to elucidate the value of this therapy.[62]

- Clinical trials: Multiple clinical trials recently completed or underway are evaluating the role of chemoprevention in patients diagnosed with HGPIN on prostate biopsy. Below is a summary of studies listed at ClinicalTrials.gov and their status. Studies mentioned above are not included here.
  - Randomized Study of Flutamide for Prostate Cancer Prevention in Patients with High Grade Prostatic Intraepithelial Neoplasia, sponsored by North Central Cancer Treatment Group and National Cancer Institute (no longer recruiting).
  - Phase II Randomized Chemoprevention Study of Calcitriol in Patients with High-Grade Prostatic Intraepithelial Neoplasia, sponsored by Cancer Institute of New Jersey and National Cancer Institute (recruiting).
  - Phase II Randomized Study of Vitamin E, Selenium, and Soy Protein Isolate in Patients with High-Grade Prostatic Intraepithelial Neopla-

sia, sponsored by National Cancer Institute of Canada and National Cancer Institute (no longer recruiting).

- Phase III Randomized Study of Selenium as Chemoprevention of Prostate Cancer in Patients with High-Grade Prostatic Intraepithelial Neoplasia, sponsored by Southwest Oncology Group, National Cancer Institute (NCI), Eastern Cooperative Oncology Group, Cancer and Leukemia Group B (recruiting).
- Randomized Study of Fish Oil Supplements and/or Simvastatin in Preventing Prostate Cancer in Patients with Prostatic Intraepithelial Neoplasia or Who Are at Risk for Developing Prostate Cancer, sponsored by Oregon Health and Science University and National Cancer Institute (recruiting).

There are several studies underway evaluating the role of selenium and vitamin E in preventing the progression of HGPIN, and the rationale behind these studies is based on the initial work by Clark and colleagues[63] at the Arizona Cancer Center and the finding of prostate cancer reduction in a study evaluating the role of selenium in preventing nonmelanoma skin cancer. There are currently no published studies evaluating the impact of selenium on the natural history of PIN. The studies listed above will likely provide insight into the impact of this promising chemoprevention strategy.

Alternate Strategies for Atypical Small Acinar Proliferation

Although no reports of chemoprevention strategies exist for patients diagnosed with ASAP, a single report from Brausi et al.[38] identified 71 patients with ASAP on prostate biopsy. Of twenty-five men undergoing immediate radical retropubic prostatectomy, all were found to have cancer including one patient with extracapsular extension (pT3a) and one with a single positive lymph node (pT4). Of the other 45 patients with ASAP, 12 were lost to follow-up or were unable to undergo a second biopsy. Of the remaining 33 patients, nine (27%) were diagnosed with prostate cancer and four are awaiting subsequent biopsies for suspicious pathology. While prostate cancer was identified in 36 of 71 patients with ASAP ultimately undergoing radical prostatectomy in this series, the potential for overtreatment should caution against this approach. The summation of available re-search indicates that ASAP should be treated as a probable marker of undetected prostate cancer for which patients should be reevaluated with repeat prostate biopsy or pathologic review of the initial prostate biopsy.[38]

Conclusions

HGPIN is the most likely precursor lesion of prostate cancer. Atypical glands, defined as ASAP, are a concerning biopsy finding because it may indicate that concurrent prostate cancer exists, but that the pathologic features of the prostate sample are not definitive. The clinical implications and management of these separate pathologic entities is different. Whereas the risk of prostate cancer detection after a diagnosis of HGPIN is likely not substantially different from cases with negative findings on initial biopsy, ASAP may be associated with concomitant undetected prostate cancer in up to half of cases. In addition, clinical parameters used to risk-stratify in screening populations do not aid the diagnosis of cancer after detection of HGPIN or ASAP on prostate biopsy. An evidence-based and best-practice approach to further evaluation suggests that in adequately sampled cases (extended biopsy), HGPIN is not an independent indication for rebiopsy. Cases of undersampled prostate biopsies, however, should undergo rebiopsy to assess for undetected prostate cancer. Significantly greater risk of concomitant prostate cancer makes timely reevaluation of ASAP cases mandatory. While several promising strategies have been evaluated for chemoprevention in patients diagnosed with HGPIN, the results of phase III studies that are recently completed or underway will shed light on the value of these strategies in patients with HGPIN. Using NCCN recommendations to guide standard practice, the management of these cases may be improved.

References

1. Epstein JI, Herawi M. Prostate needle biopsies containing prostatic intraepithelial neoplasia or atypical foci suspicious for carcinoma: implications for patient care. J Urol 2006;175:820.
2. Bostwick DG, Qian J. High-grade prostatic intraepithelial neoplasia. Mod Pathol 2004;17:360.
3. Haggman MJ, Macoska JA, Wojno KJ, et al. The relationship between prostatic intraepithelial neoplasia and prostate cancer: critical issues. J Urol 1997; 158:12.
4. Garabedian EM, Humphrey PA, Gordon JI. A transgenic mouse model of metastatic prostate cancer originating from neuroendocrine cells. Proc Natl Acad Sci USA 1998;95:15382.
5. O'Dowd GJ, Miller MC, Orozco R, et al. Analysis of repeated biopsy results within 1 year after a noncancer diagnosis. Urology 2000;55:553.
6. Gokden N, Roehl KA, Catalona WJ, et al. High-grade prostatic intraepithelial neoplasia in needle biopsy as risk factor for detection of adenocarcinoma: current level of risk in screening population. Urology 2005;65:538.
7. Naya Y, Ayala AG, Tamboli P, et al. Can the number of cores with high-grade prostate intraepithelial neoplasia predict cancer in men who undergo repeat biopsy? Urology 2004;63:503.

8. Postma R, Roobol M, Schroder FH, et al. Lesions predictive for prostate cancer in a screened population: first and second screening round findings. Prostate 2004;61:260.
9. Fowler JE Jr, Bigler SA, Miles D, et al. Predictors of first repeat biopsy cancer detection with suspected local stage prostate cancer. J Urol 2000;163: 813.
10. Rabets JC, Jones JS, Patel A, et al. Prostate cancer detection with office based saturation biopsy in a repeat biopsy population. J Urol 2004;172:94.
11. Stewart CS, Leibovich BC, Weaver AL, et al. Prostate cancer diagnosis using a saturation needle biopsy technique after previous negative sextant biopsies. J Urol 2001;166:86.
12. Goeman L, Joniau S, Ponette D, et al. Is low-grade prostatic intraepithelial neoplasia a risk factor for cancer? Prostate Cancer Prostatic Dis 2003;6:305.
13. Abdel-Khalek M, El-Baz M, Ibrahiem el-H. Predictors of prostate cancer on extended biopsy in patients with high-grade prostatic intraepithelial neoplasia: a multivariate analysis model. BJU Int 2004;94:528.
14. Moore CK, Karikehalli S, Nazeer T, et al. Prognostic significance of high grade prostatic intraepithelial neoplasia and atypical small acinar proliferation in the contemporary era. J Urol 2005;173:70.
15. Bishara T, Ramnani DM, Epstein JI. High-grade prostatic intraepithelial neoplasia on needle biopsy: risk of cancer on repeat biopsy related to number of involved cores and morphologic pattern. Am J Surg Pathol 2004;28:629.
16. Park S, Shinohara K, Grossfeld GD, et al. Prostate cancer detection in men with prior high grade prostatic intraepithelial neoplasia or atypical prostate biopsy. J Urol 2001;165:1409.
17. Borboroglu PG, Sur RL, Roberts JL, et al. Repeat biopsy strategy in patients with atypical small acinar proliferation or high grade prostatic intraepithelial neoplasia on initial prostate needle biopsy. J Urol 2001;166:866.
18. Kamoi K, Troncoso P, Babaian RJ. Strategy for repeat biopsy in patients with high grade prostatic intraepithelial neoplasia. J Urol 2000;163:819.
19. Roscigno M, Scattoni V, Freschi M, et al. Monofocal and plurifocal high-grade prostatic intraepithelial neoplasia on extended prostate biopsies: factors predicting cancer detection on extended repeat biopsy. Urology 2004;63: 1105.
20. San Francisco IF, Olumi AF, Kao J, et al. Clinical management of prostatic intraepithelial neoplasia as diagnosed by extended needle biopsies. BJU Int 2003;91:350.
21. Keetch DW, Humphrey P, Stahl D, et al. Morphometric analysis and clinical followup of isolated prostatic intraepithelial neoplasia in needle biopsy of the prostate. J Urol 1995;154:347.
22. Kronz JD, Allan CH, Shaikh AA, et al. Predicting cancer following a diagnosis of high-grade prostatic intraepithelial neoplasia on needle biopsy: data on men with more than one follow-up biopsy. Am J Surg Pathol 2001;25:1079.
23. Langer JE, Rovner ES, Coleman BG, et al. Strategy for repeat biopsy of patients with prostatic intraepithelial neoplasia detected by prostate needle biopsy. J Urol 1996;155:228.
24. Raviv G, Janssen T, Zlotta AR, et al. Prostatic intraepithelial neoplasia: influence of clinical and pathological data on the detection of prostate cancer. J Urol 1996;156:1050.

25. Davidson D, Bostwick DG, Qian J, et al. Prostatic intraepithelial neoplasia is a risk factor for adenocarcinoma: predictive accuracy in needle biopsies. J Urol 1995;154:1295.

26. Lefkowitz GK, Sidhu GS, Torre P, et al. Is repeat prostate biopsy for high-grade prostatic intraepithelial neoplasia necessary after routine 12-core sampling? Urology 2001;58:999.

27. Herawi M, Kahane H, Cavallo C, et al. Risk of prostate cancer on first re-biopsy within 1 year following a diagnosis of high grade prostatic intraepithelial neoplasia is related to the number of cores sampled. J Urol 2006;175:121.

28. Rubin MA, Bismar TA, Curtis S, et al. Prostate needle biopsy reporting: how are the surgical members of the Society of Urologic Oncology using pathology reports to guide treatment of prostate cancer patients? Am J Surg Pathol 2004; 28:946.

29. Cheville JC, Reznicek MJ, Bostwick DG. The focus of "atypical glands, suspicious for malignancy" in prostatic needle biopsy specimens: incidence, histologic features, and clinical follow-up of cases diagnosed in a community practice. Am J Clin Pathol 1997;108:633.

30. Fadare O, Wang S, Mariappan MR. Practice patterns of clinicians following isolated diagnoses of atypical small acinar proliferation on prostate biopsy specimens. Arch Pathol Lab Med 2004;128:557.

31. Kahane H, Sharp JW, Shuman GB, et al. Utilization of high molecular weight cytokeratin on prostate needle biopsies in an independent laboratory. Urology 1995;45:981.

32. Kobayashi T, Nishizawa K, Watanabe J, et al. Effects of sextant transrectal prostate biopsy plus additional far lateral cores in improving cancer detection rates in men with large prostate glands. Int J Urol 2004;11:392.

33. Novis DA, Zarbo RJ, Valenstein PA. Diagnostic uncertainty expressed in prostate needle biopsies. A College of American Pathologists Q-probes Study of 15,753 prostate needle biopsies in 332 institutions. Arch Pathol Lab Med 1999;123:687.

34. Renshaw AA, Santis WF, Richie JP. Clinicopathological characteristics of prostatic adenocarcinoma in men with atypical prostate needle biopsies. J Urol 1998;159:2018.

35. Weinstein MH, Greenspan DL, Epstein JI. Diagnoses rendered on prostate needle biopsy in community hospitals. Prostate 1998;35:50.

36. Wills ML, Hamper UM, Partin AW, et al. Incidence of high-grade prostatic intraepithelial neoplasia in sextant needle biopsy specimens. Urology 1997;49:367.

37. Roehrborn CG, Pickens GJ, Sanders JS. Diagnostic yield of repeated transrectal ultrasound-guided biopsies stratified by specific histopathologic diagnoses and prostate specific antigen levels. Urology 1996;47:347.

38. Brausi M, Castagnetti G, Dotti A, et al. Immediate radical prostatectomy in patients with atypical small acinar proliferation. Over treatment? J Urol 2004; 172:906.

39. Iczkowski KA, Chen HM, Yang XJ, et al. Prostate cancer diagnosed after initial biopsy with atypical small acinar proliferation suspicious for malignancy is similar to cancer found on initial biopsy. Urology 2002;60:851.

40. Gupta C, Ren JZ, Wojno KJ. Individual submission and embedding of prostate biopsies decreases rates of equivocal pathology reports. Urology 2004;63:83.

41. Hoedemaeker RF, Kranse R, Rietbergen JB, et al. Evaluation of prostate needle biopsies in a population-based screening study: the impact of borderline lesions. Cancer 1999;85:145.

42. Ouyang RC, Kenwright DN, Nacey JN, et al. The presence of atypical small acinar proliferation in prostate needle biopsy is predictive of carcinoma on subsequent biopsy. BJU Int 2001;87:70.

43. Iczkowski KA, Bassler TJ, Schwob VS, et al. Diagnosis of "suspicious for malignancy" in prostate biopsies: predictive value for cancer. Urology 1998;51: 749.

44. Levine MA, Ittman M, Melamed J, et al. Two consecutive sets of transrectal ultrasound guided sextant biopsies of the prostate for the detection of prostate cancer. J Urol 1998;159:471.

45. Iczkowski KA, MacLennan GT, Bostwick DG. Atypical small acinar proliferation suspicious for malignancy in prostate needle biopsies: clinical significance in 33 cases. Am J Surg Pathol 1997;21:1489.

46. Chan TY, Epstein JI. Follow-up of atypical prostate needle biopsies suspicious for cancer. Urology 1999;53:351.

47. National Comprehensive Cancer Network. Prostate cancer early detection. In: Clinical Practice Guidelines in Oncology. v.1.2005. Jenkintown, PA: National Comprehensive Cancer Network; 2005.

48. Yanke BV, Gonen M, Scardino PT, et al. Validation of a nomogram for predicting positive repeat biopsy for prostate cancer. J Urol 2005;173:421.

49. Jemal A, Siegel R, Ward E, et al. Cancer statistics, 2006. CA Cancer J Clin 2006;56:106.

50. Donavan J, Lane A, Hamdy M, et al. Evaluating screening and treatment for localised prostate cancer concurrently: the ProtecT study. Presented at the American Society of Clinical Oncology, Orlando, 2005.

51. Klotz LH. Active surveillance with selective delayed intervention: walking the line between overtreatment for indolent disease and undertreatment for aggressive disease. Can J Urol 2005;12(Suppl 1):53.

52. Kelloff GJ, Boone CW, Crowell JA, et al. Risk biomarkers and current strategies for cancer chemoprevention. J Cell Biochem Suppl 1996;25:1.

53. Greenwald P. Cancer risk factors for selecting cohorts for large-scale chemoprevention trials. J Cell Biochem Suppl 1996;25:29.

54. Wheeler TM. Influence of irradiation and androgen ablation on prostatic intraepithelial neoplasia. Eur Urol 1996;30:261.

55. Alberts SR, Blute ML. Chemoprevention for prostatic carcinoma: the role of flutamide in patients with prostatic intraepithelial neoplasia. Urology 2001;57:188.

56. Balaji KC, Rabbani F, Tsai H, et al. Effect of neoadjuvant hormonal therapy on prostatic intraepithelial neoplasia and its prognostic significance. J Urol 1999;162:753.

57. Steiner MS, Pound CR. Phase IIA clinical trial to test the efficacy and safety of toremifene in men with high-grade prostatic intraepithelial neoplasia. Clin Prostate Cancer 2003;2:24.

58. Price D, Stein B, Goluboff E, et al. Double-blind placebo-controlled trial of toremifene for the prevention of prostate cancer in men with high-grade prostatic intraepithelial neoplasia. Presented at the American Society of Clinical Oncology, Dallas, TX, 2005.

59. Mohanty NK, Saxena S, Singh UP, et al. Lycopene as a chemopreventive agent in the treatment of high-grade prostate intraepithelial neoplasia. Urol Oncol 2005;23:383.

60. McDonald AC, Bunker CH, De la Rosa N, et al. Serum PSA response to lycopene supplementation along with multivitamin does not differ from response to multivitamin alone in men with high grade intraepithelial neoplasia in randomized trial. Presented at the American Association of Cancer Research, Washington, DC, 2006.

61. Kucuk O, Sarkar FH, Sakr W, et al. Phase II randomized clinical trial of lycopene supplementation before radical prostatectomy. Cancer Epidemiol Biomarkers Prev 2001;10:861.

62. Bettuzzi S, Brausi M, Rizzi F, et al. Chemoprevention of human prostate cancer by oral administration of green tea catechins in volunteers with high-grade prostate intraepithelial neoplasia: a preliminary report from a one-year proof-of-principle study. Cancer Res 2006;66:1234.

63. Clark LC, Combs GF Jr, Turnbull BW, et al. Effects of selenium supplementation for cancer prevention in patients with carcinoma of the skin. A randomized controlled trial. Nutritional Prevention of Cancer Study Group. JAMA 1996;276:1957.

64. Alsikafi NF, Brendler CB, Gerber GS, et al. High-grade prostatic intraepithelial neoplasia with adjacent atypia is associated with a higher incidence of cancer on subsequent needle biopsy than high-grade prostatic intraepithelial neoplasia alone. Urology 2001;57:296.

20
Future Directions in Prostate Cancer Diagnosis

Nicholas J. Fitzsimons, Lionel L. Bañez, Leon L. Sun, and Judd W. Moul

Abstract

In our aging society, the incidence of prostate cancer will continue to increase, and improvements in detection and treatment of this prevalent yet extremely treatable and curable disease are needed. Research into new molecular markers described in this chapter is especially promising. These markers will improve specificity and sensitivity of screening and will serve to supplement or supplant current prostate-specific antigen screening. Targeted biopsy utilizing new radiographic techniques such as Doppler ultrasound, magnetic resonance imaging, and magnetic resonance spectroscopy can reduce the number of needle cores and improve pathologic specimen quality. Improvements in anesthetic agents and techniques decrease discomfort and improve patient readiness to undergo prostate biopsy. As emerging research continues to elucidate the pathology of prostate cancer, diagnostic screening expands into genetic and even viral etiologies that may offer the possibility of a vaccine against prostate cancer.

Keywords: prostate cancer, screening, PSA, biopsy, ultrasound, bioimaging, biomarker

New Diagnostic Screening Tools

Complementary to the development of novel techniques in performing the procedure of prostate gland biopsy, the discovery of clinically-significant biomarkers for the early and accurate detection of prostate cancer has been the focus of research for a majority of institutions seeking to redefine current standards of care which hope to decrease worldwide mortality from prostate cancer as well as morbidity from prostate biopsy. Current data

From: *Current Clinical Urology: Prostate Biopsy: Indications, Techniques, and Complications*
Edited by J.S. Jones © Humana Press, Totowa, NJ

from recently concluded chemoprevention trials[1] underscore the less-than-optimal nature of the current molecular marker of choice, serum prostate-specific antigen (PSA), for identifying men with prostate cancer. Poor specificity and positive predictive value (25%–30%) observed for this test are further aggravated by findings from the Prostate Cancer Prevention Trial demonstrating that 15% of men with a negative PSA test (<4 ng/mL) and normal digital rectal examination (DRE) have prostate cancer and 15% of these undiagnosed prostate cancer cases have potentially lethal high-grade tumors.[2] Although PSA is prostate disease–specific, it is not prostate cancer–specific, and for this reason, a vacuum remains for other molecular markers that may serve to supplement or supplant the serum PSA test leading not only to increased detection of clinically significant disease, but reduced number of unnecessary prostate biopsies.

Among the score of biomarkers being studied, several markers and techniques deserve attention because of the published data showing promise that better prostate cancer screening methods will be available in the near future that will maintain noninvasiveness and acceptability for both patients and urologists in clinical practice.

uPM3/DD3

A notable shift from the traditional blood-based human biologic specimens such as serum and plasma has characterized the noteworthy advances in prostate screening tools currently being developed around the world. A prototypical and very promising biomolecular test for prostate cancer, the uPM3 (DiagnoCure, Quebec, Canada), is conducted on urine specimens from men after they have undergone a vigorous prostate examination or an *attentive* DRE.[3] This particular method of extracting a test specimen for laboratory examination takes advantage of expulsion of prostate epithelial cellular material expressed in the urine after manipulation of the prostate gland. The molecular basis for the test lies in assaying for *DD3*, a prostate cancer–specific gene that was shown to be strongly overexpressed in more than 95% of primary prostate cancer specimens and in metastatic prostate cancer.[4,5] Compared with benign prostate tissue, *DD3* was noted to be up-regulated 66-fold in malignant prostate tissue that hinted to a diagnostic potential for this non-protein coding gene.[6]

In an initial study, it was found that mRNA transcripts of the *DD3* gene could be detected in cell lysates from urinary sediments of men after attentive DRE using a time-resolved florescence-based quantitative reverse transcription-polymerase chain reaction (RT-PCR) assay.[6] Using measured *PSA* transcripts to correct for the number of prostate cells in the urinary specimen, an optimal cut-off value for this *DD3*-based RT-PCR assay garnered a specificity of 83% and a negative predictive value of 90%. To further refine the technique, the uPM3 test was developed utilizing a nucleic acid sequence-based amplification assay that simultaneously quantifies both *DD3* mRNA transcripts and *PSA* mRNA transcripts and uses the relative expression levels between the two to determine the presence of disease.[3,7] In a single-institution study, the uPM3 test had an overall sensitivity of 82% and specificity of 76%.[7] In men with serum PSA levels between 4–10 ng/mL, the uPM3 test predicted the presence of prostate cancer in 84% of the biopsy-proven cases and correctly identified 80% of the men who had a negative biopsy result. In a multicenter study involving five institutions, uPM3 demonstrated an astounding 89% overall specificity and a positive predictive value of 75% superior to serum PSA (38% in the study population).[3] Most promising was the noted maintenance of high specificity of the test observed in men with PSA<4 ng/mL (91%) and in those with PSA between 4–10 ng/mL (91%) suggesting that this new molecular urine test may serve as an important adjunct to current methods of prostate cancer diagnosis.

One rather obvious disadvantage of the uPM3 test stems from the question, How attentive is an *attentive* DRE? The technique for expressing prostatic secretions into the urine would no doubt vary among urologists and its effects on the results of the uPM3 test have not been carefully studied, demanding a need for standardization of prostate gland manipulation performed before collection of the specimen. Another important issue to be considered is increasing the adequacy rate (portion of assessable specimens with an adequate number of prostate cells in the voided specimen for the assay), which for the initial studies ranged from 79% to 86%.[3,7] Developers of this promising urine-based molecular test are currently addressing these and other minor disadvantages.

Serum Protein Profiling

The technique of utilizing serum protein profiles as resolved by mass spectrometry as a diagnostic tool for prostate cancer and as a platform for the discovery of prostate cancer biomarkers has garnered much attention because of very promising results that have been tempered by close scrutiny and criticism by the scientific community. Serum protein profiling using surface-enhanced laser/desorption ionization time-of-flight mass spectrometry (SELDI-TOF-MS) profiling relies on affinity-based chromatographic separation of proteins in minute amounts of serum applied to arrays that are subjected to matrix-assisted laser desorption/ionization time-of-flight mass spectrometry (MALDI-TOF-MS) producing mass spectral profiles dependent on proteins found in the sera.[3,7] Bioinformatics analyses of these serum proteomic signatures generate classification algorithms predictive of diseases ranging from ovarian, prostate, and breast cancer in blinded serum samples with very favorable accuracy.[8–10] Deriving diagnostic information from patterns of proteins hidden in human serum elucidated through SELDI-TOF-MS for detection of prostate adenocarcinoma was first reported by Adam et al.,[9] wherein serum protein signatures generated from a copper-metal affinity array (Ciphergen Biosystems, Fremont, CA) were used to generate decision tree algorithms that could accurately identify prostate cancer patients with a sensitivity of 83% and specificity of 97%. Comparable successes were reported by other institutions that used modifications in their methodologies such as utilizing other protein array types and methods of spectral data analyses.[11–13]

The popularity elicited when serum protein profiling was first introduced has led to close scrutiny by critics of serum protein profiling technology.[14–16] Much of the criticism focused on controlling potential sources of bias in the experiments as well as drifting mass calibration of the mass spectrometer used. To address these issues, a multicenter trial consisting by eight institutions was constructed and aimed at validating the utility of serum SELDI-TOF-MS profiling and assessing the reproducibility of this technology.[17] The initial phase of validation focused on standardization of serum processing and optimization of spectral data generated in all mass spectrometers consistently throughout the study while providing quality assurance among all laboratories. Robotic handling was used to minimize human error and further enhance mass spectral quality and reproducibility. The reproducibility of serum SELDI-TOF-MS profiles across laboratories was found to be closely comparable with acceptably low variability.[18] This reduction of variation was successfully preserved across all institutions over a 6-month period and was attributed to strict adherence to standard operating procedures while maintaining optimal calibration of instruments. This multicenter trial has now progressed to its second phase wherein serum samples from multiple institutions will be used to refine the classification algorithms generated from serum protein profiles.

Efforts to further improve serum protein profiling technology range from improvements in instrumentation to identification of candidate biomarkers as a means of validation. Higher-resolution mass spectrometers such as the QSTAR (Applied Biosystems, Foster City, CA), a hybrid quadrupole time-of-flight mass spectrometer have expanded the number of candidate biomarkers by resolving a greater number of data points compared with SELDI-TOF-MS. Serum profiles generated with the QSTAR have shown to discriminate men with increased PSA attributed to benign conditions from men with prostate cancer even when PSA levels were within the diagnostic gray zone of 2.5–15 ng/mL.[19]

Critics of serum protein profiling technology have pushed for identification of candidate protein markers derived from studies to validate the results. By using liquid chromatography, gel electrophoresis, and tandem mass spectrometry, an isoform of apolipoprotein A-II (ApoA-II) was identified as one of the discriminatory SELDI-TOF-MS proteins by one of the pioneering laboratories.[20] This finding not only validated the technique of serum protein profiling by showing a correlation between serum levels of ApoA-II and its corresponding peak on the protein spectral profile but it also yielded a novel biomarker that could detect prostate cancer in patients whose PSA is within normal limits (0–4 ng/mL). Another laboratory reported serum amyloid A as a potential biomarker for metastatic prostate cancer using SELDI-TOF-MS as an initial screening tool then using two-dimensional gel electrophoresis, in-gel trypsin digestion, and tandem mass spectrometry for protein identification.[21] Breakthroughs in engineering exhibited by constant upgrading of mass spectrometry platforms giving rise to high-performance hardware resources capable of fairly rapid protein identification that will lead to the development of a platform that provides very high resolution, robust spectra, and easy identification of protein markers, which does not sacrifice ease of use and portability, seems to be the compromise that will eventually translate into clinical practice.

Alpha Methylacyl-CoA Racemase/Autoantibody Signatures

Among the prostate cancer markers recently discovered through tissue and gene microarray technology, alpha methylacyl-CoA racemase (AMACR) seems to be one of the biomarkers whose overexpression in malignant prostate epithelial cells has the potential to yield a novel clinically-usable test for diagnosis of prostate cancer.[22,23] AMACR protein has been assayed for using Western blot in urine specimens after transrectal ultrasound (TRUS)-guided prostate biopsy and was detected in the urine of all patients with biopsy-confirmed prostate cancer in a pilot study.[24] Similar to the forerunner of the uPM3 test, mRNA transcripts of the *AMACR* gene have been measured in prostatic secretions in urine voided after prostatic massage using quantitative RT-PCR.[25] Relative *AMACR* value scores calculated by normalizing *AMACR* transcript levels with *PSA* mRNA transcript measurements correlated well with disease status, correctly identifying all cancer-free participants including men with benign prostatic hyperplasia in this preliminary investigation.

The presence of autoantibodies to AMACR protein has also been investigated in its ability to detect adenocarcinoma of the prostate. Screening through protein microarrays and later development of high-throughput immunoblot analysis and enzyme-linked immunosorbent assays for sera using AMACR as a target molecule yielded positive results.[26] In this study, immune response against AMACR was observed to be more sensitive (77.8%) and specific (80.6%) than PSA in distinguishing sera from prostate cancer patients relative to control specimens. Furthermore, by assaying for autoantibodies directed at Huntingtin interacting protein-1 (HIP-1), another bait molecule, reactivity of sera also correlated well with the presence of prostate cancer.[27] Interestingly, when the humoral response information from HIP-1 is supplemented to the AMACR autoantibody assay, the overall specificity of the combined test may be increased further, up to 97%.

These proof-of-principle studies on AMACR and HIP-1 have led to a more global approach of autoantibody profiling that further exploits the humoral immune response to amplify otherwise undetectable molecular signals that are characteristic of disease and may prove to be diagnostic for prostate malignancy.[28] To assay for autoantibodies in serum, phage protein microarrays were developed using a phage-display library derived from prostate cancer tissue. By iterative purification and isolation of phages carrying high affinity and specificity for autoantibodies and by subjecting humoral response information to bioinformatics analyses, a 22-phage-peptide detector elicited an autoantibody signature predictive of disease. In a blinded validation, 49 of 60 (81.6%) prostate cancer serum samples and 60 of 68 (88.2%) controls were correctly identified according to their autoantibody signature. This humoral reactive panel even performed better than serum PSA in this investigation. Further refinements to the technology along with prospective trials and evaluation of these autoantibody signatures in subjects with inflammatory conditions such as prostatitis, rheumatic and autoimmune disease should be forthcoming.

ERG/*Biomarker Panel*

Synergism by combining multiple biomarkers may hold the solution in attaining a truly superior diagnostic test for prostate cancer. Following microarray analysis of micro-dissected prostate cancer tissue samples, ETS-related gene (*ERG*) was recently reported as the most frequently overexpressed protooncogene in the transcriptome of malignant prostate epithelial cells.[29] *ERG* codes for transcription factors which through molecular signaling regulate cellular differentiation and proliferation.[30] Recurrent fusion of *ERG* with another gene, *TMPRSS2*, was also reported to be associated with prostate cancer, validating *ERG* as a potential biomarker for prostate cancer and implicating these genes in carcinogenesis and possible clinical use in molecular diagnostics.[31] By taking advantage of the high sensitivity of *AMACR* and the impressive specificity of *DD3* for prostate cancer, researchers demonstrated that the combined quantitative expression analysis in a novel three-gene panel (*ERG* + *AMACR* + *DD3*) can detect virtually all malignant prostate specimens.[29] This discovery emphasizes the advantage of multiplexing biomarkers to optimize the accuracy of prostate cancer detection. Investigators are on the cusp of translating these preliminary results and developing this biomarker panel into a new screening tool for prostate cancer.

These emerging technologies comprise the cutting-edge in noninvasive prostate cancer diagnostics. As limitations to current diagnostic screening procedures have come to light, it is not enough for screening tests to merely ascertain the presence of disease. Clinical tests developed for early detection of prostate cancer must also be able to differentiate slow-growing indolent tumors, which may be treated conservatively, from high-grade disease that warrants prompt intervention. The necessity for earliest possible diagnosis should be balanced against the potential morbidities of over-diagnosis and overtreatment. It is of paramount importance that a diagnostic test be able to elucidate the aggressive potential of a particular tumor as well as identify men who would benefit more from surveillance than repeat prostate biopsies. The information supplied by future diagnostic procedures should also be able to stratify patients according to risk for recurrence after treatment, bringing the practice of treatment for prostate cancer, whether surgical or nonsurgical, closer to the ideal therapy tailored to the individual patient. Use of novel biologic specimens, engineered technologic advances, and new paradigms incorporating multiplexed biomarker assays are forging the superior and more clinically-relevant prostate cancer tests for the future.

Advances in Biopsy Technique

Needle-core biopsy of the prostate for the diagnosis of prostate cancer has been a continually evolving field since the advent of the sextant biopsy technique in 1989.[32] In recent years, a multitude of new advances have arisen that aim to improve both the sensitivity and specificity of diagnosis, to decrease the morbidity associated with biopsy, and to increase the pathologic quality of biopsy specimens.

Although the sextant biopsy scheme has attained worldwide acceptance, many urologists have begun advocating 10–12 extended-core schemes in recent years, and others use "saturation" protocols. However, both patient morbidity and pathology costs increase with the number of cores taken. Several new radiologic tests allow for visual identification of tumors, thereby permitting directed tumor biopsy with the goal of improved biopsy yield and decreased false-negative rates. These tests hold the prospect of improving the sensitivity of diagnosis and increasing overall cancer detection with fewer biopsy cores, thus decreasing both costs and morbidity.

Periprostatic nerve block is now generally considered the standard for biopsy anesthesia, but the procedure is often as uncomfortable as the biopsy itself. Topical anesthetics and analgesic suppositories aim to reduce the pain and discomfort of the procedure without the need for an additional injection. In addition, short-acting anesthetic agents have been investigated for use in prostate biopsy after their successful application during female labor.

The most frequently used prostate biopsy needle employs a side-cutting technique. End-cutting devices have been developed which increase the length and weight of the sample and improve the pathologic quality of the biopsy specimen.

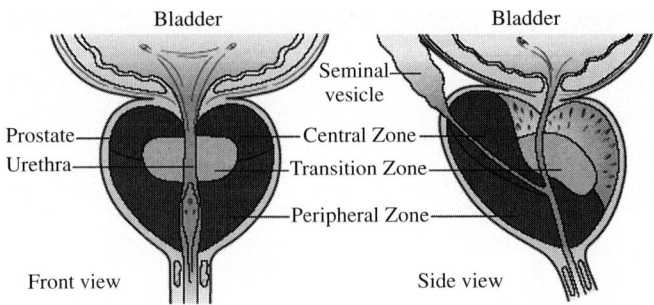

FIGURE 20.1. Anatomy of the prostate. (Reprinted with permission from Prostate Research Campaign, UK. Kirby RS. The Prostate: Small Gland, Big Problem. 2nd ed. London: Prostate Research Campaign; 2002)

Anatomy of the Prostate

The prostate gland is often divided into peripheral, transitional, and central zones with differing structural and functional characteristics (Figure 20.1). The peripheral zone accounts for about 70% of prostate glandular tissue and a similar percentage of carcinomas. The transition zone makes up only approximately 5% of glandular tissue in younger men and grows markedly with age because of benign prostatic hyperplasia. The central zone is a conical region with its base constituting the greater part of the base of the gland and its apex at the proximal verumontanum of the urethra.

Radiographic Advances

Since its introduction in the early 1980s, TRUS has been the mainstay of prostate imaging for the purposes of biopsy. Traditional grayscale TRUS is sometimes able to identify cancerous foci, which may appear as hypoechoic lesions. Yet, most hypoechoic areas are not cancers,[33] and some tumors can be hyperechoic or isoechoic. As such, lesion-directed biopsies using TRUS provide little unique cancer detection.[34,35] Therefore, although TRUS is useful in obtaining prostate-volume information as well as an overall view of the prostate for biopsy, it is suboptimal for identifying likely tumors and allowing the physician to perform directed biopsies.

The field of radiology, however, has experienced a multitude of recent advances, many of which apply directly to prostate biopsy. These include three-dimensional ultrasound (3D US), color Doppler ultrasound (CDU), contrast-enhanced ultrasound, and, perhaps most notably, magnetic resonance imaging (MRI).

Three-Dimensional Ultrasound

Three-dimensional ultrasound is a method of producing whole volume images of solid structures. Although it was first used for utero-fetal imaging, 3D US has since been applied to imaging of the liver,[36] breast,[37] and cardiovascular system.[38] It has also demonstrated improved detection of intraprostatic lesions when compared with 2D US (Figure 20.2).[39] Although 3D

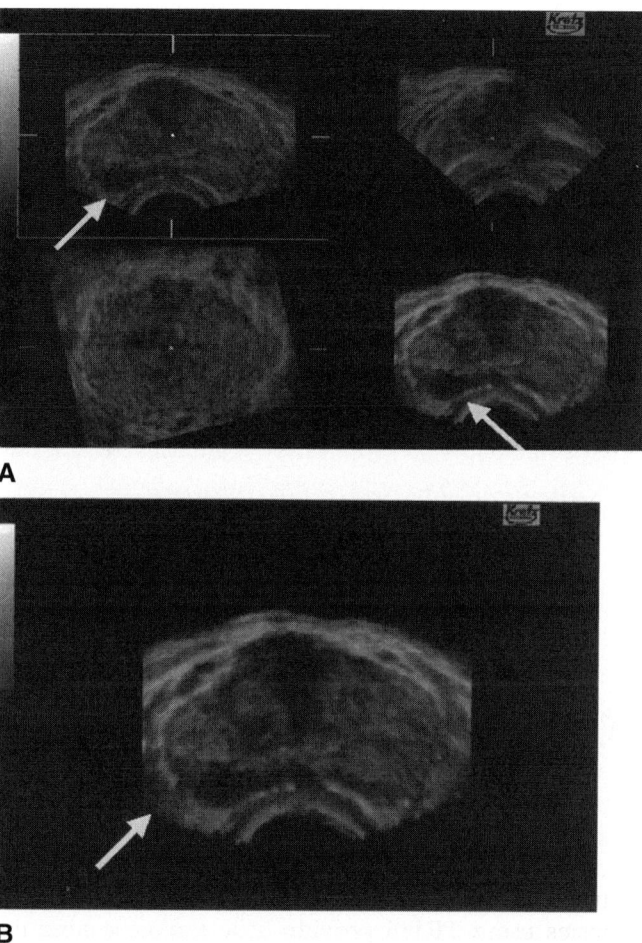

A

B

FIGURE 20.2. **A**: Three-dimensional (3D) ultrasound volume set. Top left image is a transverse section through the prostate; top right image is a longitudinal section through the prostate; and bottom left image is the cranial section (composed of the transverse and longitudinal sections). Reference lines indicate the position of the different planes. Bottom right image is the reconstructed 3D image. **B**: Enlarged 3D reconstruction of the same prostate. White arrow indicates hypoechoic lesion, which is clearer on the 3D reconstruction. In particular, the tissue surrounding the prostate is more hyperechoic, giving more contrast to the prostate and the hypoechoic lesion. (Reprinted from Sedelaar et al.[40])

US showed a significant improvement in prostate cancer detection by ultrasound experts when compared with 2D, it did not show significant clinical improvement for detection and staging.[40]

Doppler Ultrasound

CDU techniques add the component of perfusion imaging which could improve the detection of prostate cancer (Figure 20.3). By demonstrating tumor blood flow, CDU has been shown to improve the positive predictive value of hypervascular nodule detection.[41,42] However, a hypervascular nodule is not always malignant because benign conditions such as benign prostatic hyperplasia or prostatitis can also result in increased vascularity.[43]

Power Doppler ultrasound (PDU) offers several advances over CDU. It is angle independent, does not alias, and can be used at a high gain level, therefore detecting blood flow at much lower levels and with higher sensitivity than CDU.[44] PDU-guided lesion-targeted biopsy in conjunction with random sextant biopsy has been shown to improve cancer detection, but was insufficient for cancer detection when used alone.[45]

Contrast-Enhanced Doppler Ultrasound

Because of the relative limitations of CDU in displaying necessary information about microvessel perfusion around tumors, ultrasound contrast agents have been introduced. Most contrast agents consist of gas-encapsulated microbubbles with a diameter smaller than 10 μm, which enables penetration of the microvascular system. The mismatch of acoustic properties of these agents relative to the surrounding blood components result in signal enhancement.[46,47] This allows for detection of the signal in even smaller vessels than are detectable with Doppler alone (Figure 20.4). Bogers et al.[48] found that this combination improved the sensitivity of prostate cancer detection from 38% for unenhanced power Doppler to 85% for contrast-enhanced images, while maintaining specificity of 80%.

However, others have demonstrated that although contrast-enhanced PDU enabled analysis of the vascular network of a hypoechoic nodule seen on TRUS, it was not reliable enough to discriminate malignant from benign.[49] Similarly, Pelzer et al.[50] showed comparable rates of prostate cancer detection between standard TRUS-guided biopsy and contrast-enhanced CDU-targeted biopsies (27.6% vs. 27.4%, respectively) in patients with a PSA between 4 and 10 ng/mL. However, overall detection improved to 37.6% when using a combination of random sextant biopsy and contrast-enhanced CDU-targeted biopsy.

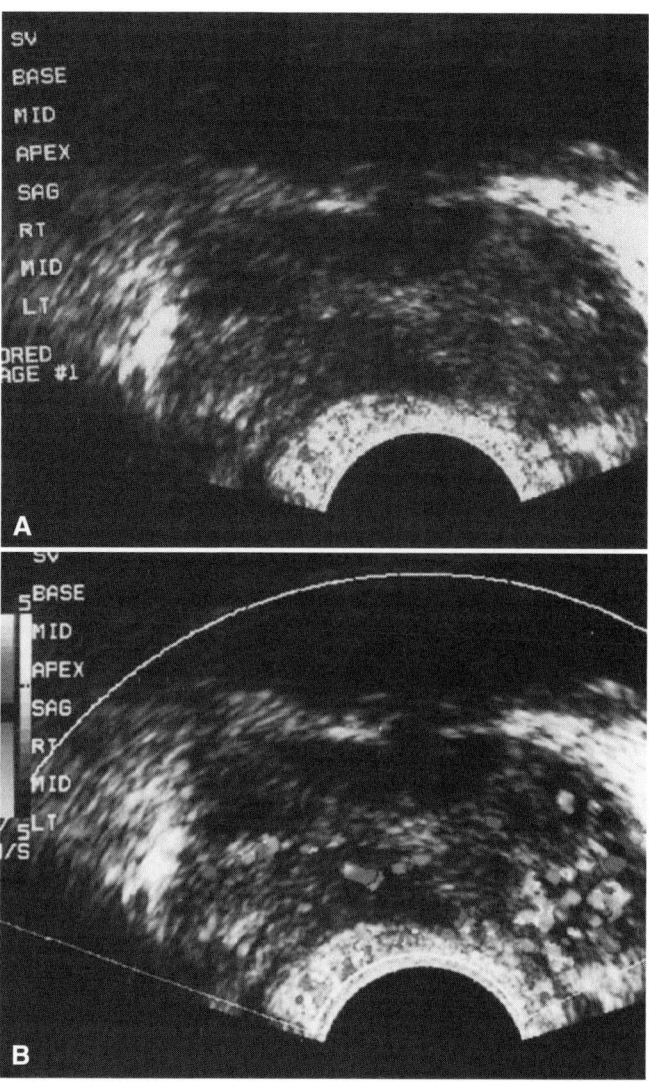

FIGURE 20.3. A grayscale image **(A)** shows mild hypoechoic changes but with distinct increased color Doppler flow at the left base **(B)**. A biopsy core from this sextant revealed 5 mm of tumor with a Gleason score of 7. (Reprinted from Louvar et al.[43])

Intermittent/Harmonic Imaging

Intermittent imaging techniques use contrast agents in conjunction with bursts of high-intensity ultrasound and periods of low-intensity ultrasound in succession.[51] The high-intensity bursts destroy the contrast agents in the scan plane, and during low-intensity periods reperfusion occurs. By

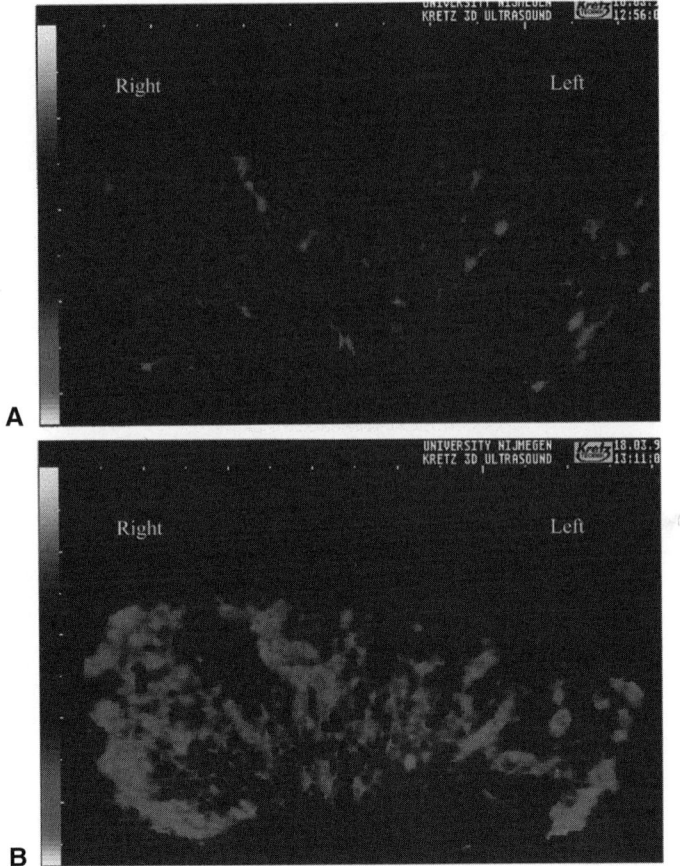

FIGURE 20.4. Three-dimensional images of a histologically malignant prostate **(A)** before and **(B)** 1 minute after administration of microbubble contrast agent. A clear asymmetry (right side more than left side) is seen after enhancement of the flow signals. Two of three biopsies on the right side showed malignancy (Gleason score 7). (Reprinted from Bogers et al.[48])

comparing images right before a high-intensity burst and immediately after this burst, the distribution of contrast can be measured in a very sensitive manner (Figure 20.5). Although this method showed a significant improvement in discrimination between benign and malignant biopsy sites over grayscale US, there was a minimal advantage over standard contrast-enhanced CDU.[52]

Magnetic Resonance Imaging

MRI allows concomitant detailed evaluation of prostatic, periprostatic, and pelvic anatomy.[51] Shortly after the introduction of MRI, it was established that prostate cancer lesions are characterized by low T2 signal intensity in the normally high T2 signal peripheral zone.[53] However, this is of limited sensitivity presumably because some tumors are isointense. In addition, there are many other causes of low T2 signal intensity including hemorrhage, prostatitis, scarring, radiotherapy, cryosurgery, and hormonal therapy.[54,55] Therefore, although use of an endorectal coil has been shown to significantly improve accuracy of prostate cancer localization over TRUS

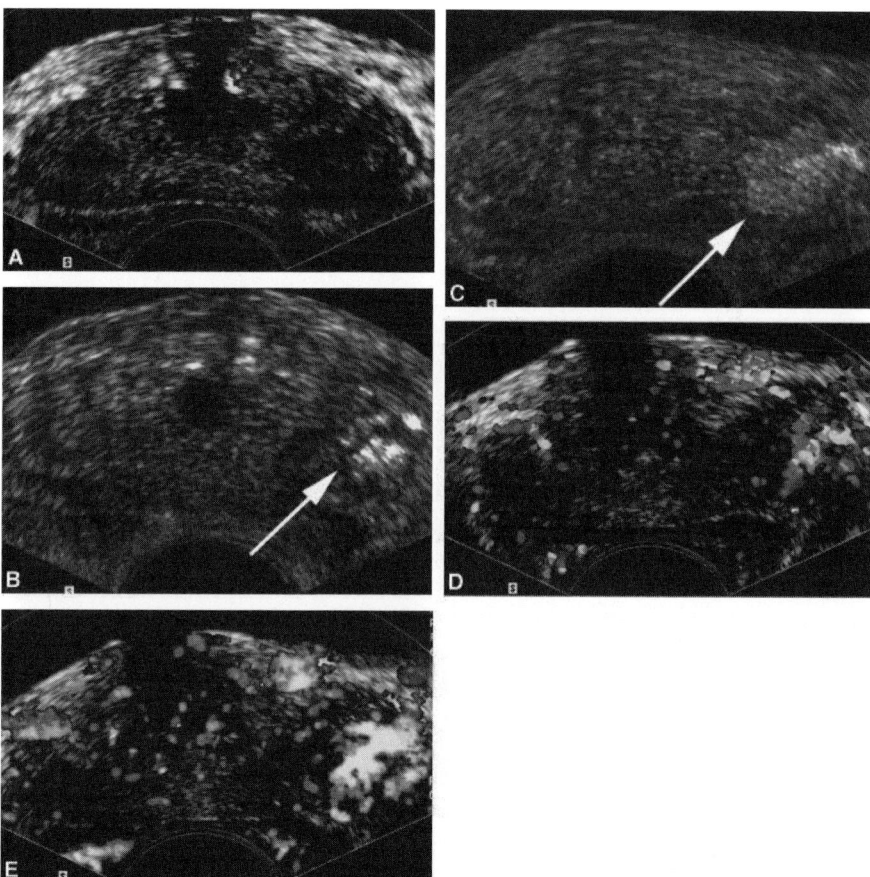

FIGURE 20.5. Imaging from a 75-year-old man with Gleason 8 carcinoma in the left midgland. **A**: Baseline color Doppler image demonstrates a hypoechoic mass in the left midgland. **B**: Postcontrast continuous harmonic imaging demonstrates enhancement of the carcinoma (arrow). **C**: Postcontrast intermittent harmonic imaging with 1.0-second interscan delay demonstrates larger blush of tumor enhancement (arrow). **D**: Postcontrast color Doppler demonstrates enhancement of tumor. **E**: Postcontrast power Doppler demonstrates enhancement of tumor. (Reprinted from Halpern et al.[52])

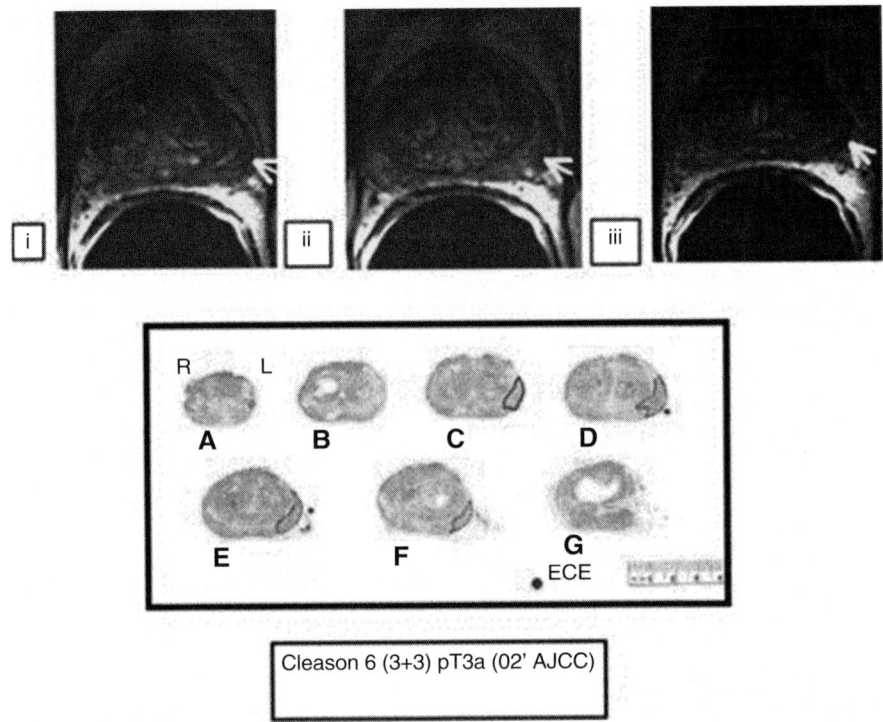

Cleason 6 (3+3) pT3a (02' AJCC)

FIGURE 20.6. Impalpable left posterior tumor in mid and base of prostate detected by endorectal coil magnetic resonance imaging (erMRI) in a 57-year-old patient presenting with prostate-specific antigen 5.37 ng/mL and negative digital rectal examination. Biopsy was positive on left side with Gleason grade 3 + 3. Axial T2-weighted erMRI demonstrated low-signal-intensity lesion in posterior left mid **(i)** and base **(ii and iii)** of gland, consistent with tumor, whereas posterior left mid and base of gland were categorized as 4/5 (arrow). (Reprinted from Mullerad et al.[56])

and DRE (Figure 20.6),[56] there is still low overall specificity when using MRI as a diagnostic tool.

Three-Dimensional Magnetic Resonance Spectroscopy

Three-dimensional magnetic resonance spectroscopy (3D MRS) permits precise measurement of intracellular resonances of specific metabolites within the prostate. Three-dimensional MRS has demonstrated significantly higher levels of choline relative to creatine, and low levels of citrate in prostate cancers. By measuring the choline-plus-creatine-to-citrate ratio, prostate malignancies can be differentiated from normal tissue.[57] Casciani et al.[58] demonstrated that combining 3D MRS with endorectal MRI improved sensitivity from 76% to 95% and specificity from 56% to 81%.

Furthermore, 3D MRS imaging examinations and metabolic data can be transferred to TRUS images to sample regions of cancer (Figure 20.7).[59]

Three-dimensional MRS holds particular promise in patients who have an elevated PSA, but prior negative TRUS-guided biopsies. Three-dimensional MRS targeting of cancer in these patients has been shown to increase the positive yield of subsequent TRUS biopsies.[60] This technology may be especially helpful for targeting biopsies in men with larger prostates, because there is an inverse relationship between prostate size and the likelihood of detecting prostate cancer with TRUS.[61]

Although many of the above radiographic advances have demonstrated an improvement in overall cancer detection when used in conjunction with standard TRUS-guided sextant biopsy, few (if any) have been able to improve cancer detection when used alone. The goal of many of these technologies, as mentioned above, is to minimize the number of cores taken while still improving overall detection of clinically significant cancers.

Individualized Biopsy Protocol

Since the advent of the classic sextant biopsy scheme, a number of investigators have recommended a variety of expanded biopsy patterns to improve cancer detection.[62–64] However, others have shown that the cancer detection rate of sextant biopsies decreases with increasing prostate gland volume.[65,66] Another technique designed to increase detection of prostate cancer is individualization of the biopsy protocol according to prostate gland volume. Addition of lateral peripheral biopsies (10-core scheme) increased detection from 14% to 38% over the classic sextant scheme in increasing prostate volumes.[35]

Pain During Prostate Biopsy

Pain during prostate biopsy can result from anal discomfort from the ultrasound probe as well as from insertion of the needles. Because the biopsy needles penetrate the rectal wall above the dentate line in an area of decreased sensorium, most of the pain is attributable to penetration of the prostatic capsule.[67] Pain increases with the number of cores taken, which is significant given the widespread adoption of expanded biopsy schemes in recent years. Therefore, patient discomfort during biopsy is an increasingly recognized problem. Since the introduction of the classic sextant biopsy protocol in 1989 by Hodge et al.,[32] there have been multiple investigations into methods to decrease this pain, with conflicting results. Although Nash et al.[68] first demonstrated that injection of lidocaine into the nerve bundles adjacent to the prostate decreased patient reported pain, a recent survey[69] demonstrated that more than a third of urologists did not provide any analgesia at all during biopsy.

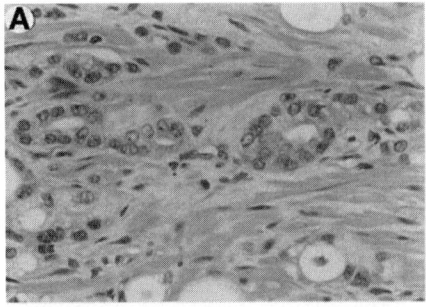

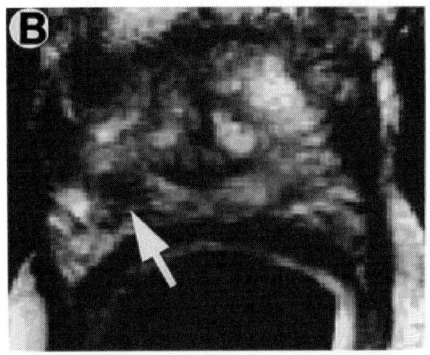

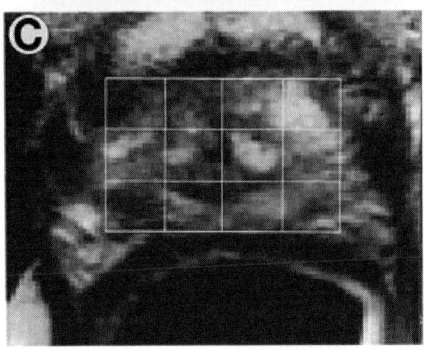

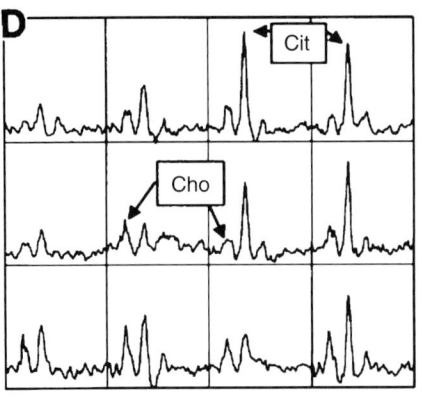

FIGURE 20.7. Gleason score 7 adenocarcinoma in right apex of 64-year-old man was detected by postprostatectomy step section histology. Magnetic resonance imaging and magnetic resonance spectroscopic imaging correctly identified tumor in right apex but sextant biopsy of right apex was negative. **A**: Photomicrograph shows prostate cancer in right apex peripheral zone specimen. Hematoxylin and eosin; reduced from 400× magnification. **B**: Axial fast spin-echo, T2-weighted, 4000/100 ms image of prostate demonstrates low T2 signal intensity in peripheral zone of right apex (arrow), consistent with tumor. **C**: Same image with overlying 0.24 cc magnetic resonance spectroscopic imaging spectral grid. **D**: Magnetic resonance spectroscopic imaging of prostatic apex peripheral zone reveals increased choline (Cho) and decreased citrate (Cit) in right apex voxels, consistent with tumor. (Reprinted from Wefer et al.[60])

Periprostatic Nerve Block

Cadaveric studies have shown that the neuroanatomic pathway originates from the inferior hypogastric plexus located at the tip of the seminal vesicles and passes between the prostate and rectum on the inferolateral border of the gland.[70] Based on these anatomic considerations, various injection schemes have been proposed in order to obtain a periprostatic nerve block, including bilateral injections at the junction of the base and seminal vesicles (Figure 20.8),[68] bilateral apical injections,[71] apical and midgland injections,[72] and lateral to the seminal vesicles.[73] Others have investigated direct intraprostatic lidocaine administration (Figure 20.9) and found it superior to nerve block in reducing biopsy-associated pain.[74]

Although each of these methods was effective at decreasing patient discomfort, they involve the painful insertion of two or more needles through the rectum to administer the anesthetic agents. Therefore, others have investigated less-invasive methods to reduce biopsy-associated discomfort.

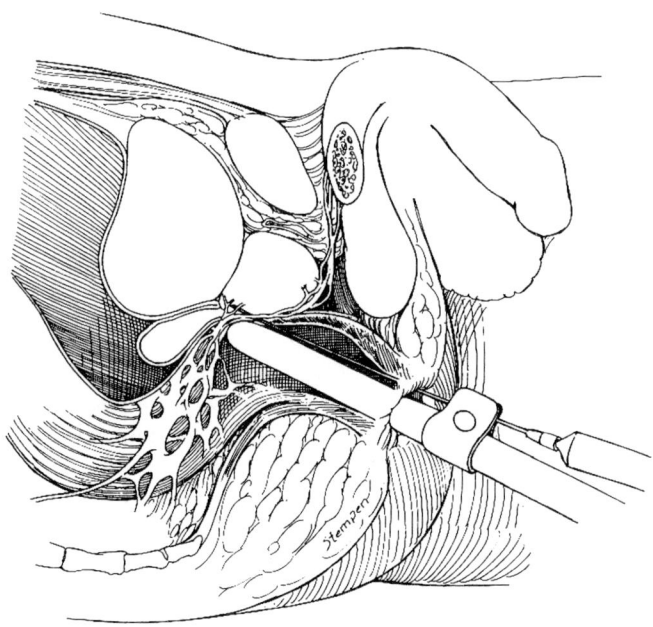

FIGURE 20.8. Ultrasound probe in situ and spinal needle placement within neurovascular bundle at base of prostate just lateral to junction between prostate and seminal vesicle. (Reprinted from Nash et al.[68])

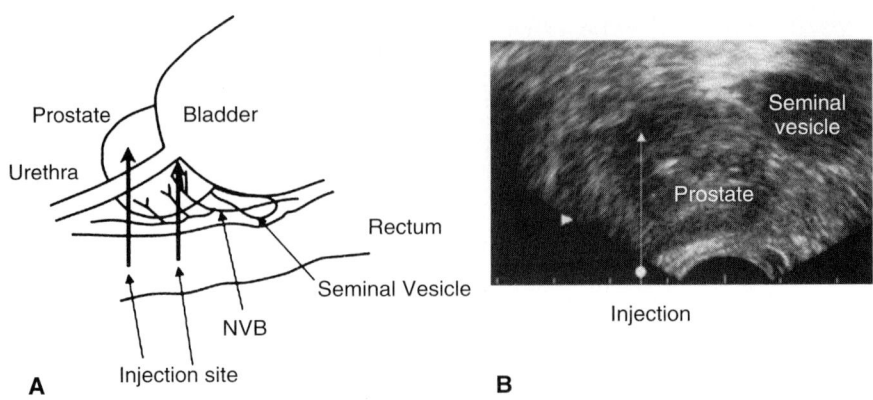

A Injection site   **B**

FIGURE 20.9. Intraprostatic lidocaine administration. **A**: Lidocaine is infiltrated in several portions directly into prostate at 2 or 3 sites at right and left sides from base to apex. NVB = neurovascular bundle. **B**: Injection is easily confirmed by formation of hypoechoic area under ultrasound monitoring. (Reprinted from Mutaguchi et al.[74])

Topical Agents

Lidocaine gel was one of the first topical agents investigated but has been met with mixed results. Some have found no efficacy whatsoever when using the topical gel,[75] whereas others have reported a significant improvement in pain score compared with placebo.[76] Stirling et al.[77] found that intrarectal lidocaine was effective at reducing discomfort with rectal probe insertion, but not with biopsy. Similarly, most studies have found lidocaine gel inferior to periprostatic lidocaine infiltration at reducing biopsy-associated discomfort.[78,79]

In a prospective analysis comparing types of analgesia, Obek et al.[80] randomized patients to one of four groups: periprostatic nerve block, lidocaine gel plus nerve block, tramadol (a centrally acting codeine analog), and controls. They concluded that lidocaine gel plus nerve block provided significantly better analgesia than the other methods.

However, lidocaine suppositories were found to be more effective than intrarectal lidocaine gel in a randomized, prospective trial of 100 patients.[81] Of note, the suppository was significantly more effective for patients when placed 2 hours before biopsy than 1 hour before. Similarly, diclofenac suppositories have been shown to improve patient tolerance when administered 1 hour before biopsy[82]; however, these findings have yet to be confirmed in other studies.

Finally, intrarectal administration of 40% dimethyl sulfoxide (DMSO) in association with perianal injection of 1% lidocaine demonstrated better tolerance of probe insertion.[83] The authors suggested that this method might be of particular value in patients with a history of anorectal surgery or other problems. Kravchick et al.[83] randomized patients to intrarectal lidocaine gel, 40% DMSO and lidocaine, perianal lidocaine injection, and nerve block. They found that nerve block only decreased pain during biopsy, not during probe insertion. DMSO, however, was safe and rapidly effective for both biopsy pain and probe insertion-related discomfort.

Short-Acting Anesthetic Agents

Short-acting gaseous anesthetic agents have also been investigated. Entonox (50% nitrous oxide and oxygen) provides analgesia within 3 minutes of inhalation and the effect disappears less than 4 minutes after cessation, a combination that makes it ideal for office-based procedures such as prostate biopsy.[67] It has been used extensively in the United Kingdom during labor and other minor procedures, such as resetting of fractured bones.

Masood et al.[84] randomized 96 men to receive either Entonox or air only via a breath-activated device before prostate biopsy. They found that patients in the Entonox group experienced significantly less pain based on visual analog pain scores. In addition, 96% of the men in the Entonox group said they would have the procedure again if necessary. This finding has been confirmed by others, and no side effects, respiratory problems, or prolonged drowsiness were demonstrated.[85] However, it should not be used in patients with congestive heart failure or chronic obstructive airway disease. Nitrous oxide is more soluble than oxygen and nitrogen, so will tend to diffuse into any air spaces within the body. This makes Entonox dangerous to use in patients with pneumothorax or who have recently been scuba diving, and there are cautions over its use with any bowel obstruction.

Biopsy Needles

Traditional biopsy needles operate in a side-cutting method and are able to retrieve samples 17–22 mm in length. A new instrument with an end-cutting technique and an adjustable stroke length (13, 23, and 33 mm) has been developed (BioPince®, Amedic, Sweden), and in a prospective, randomized trial, the end-cutting device was shown to obtain cylindrical cores that were significantly longer and heavier than those obtained with a standard side-cutting needle (Figure 20.10).[86] Furthermore, use of this device did not increase biopsy-associated complications or patient-perceived pain. However, despite the fact that the end-cutting technique was able to obtain pathologically superior cores, there was no difference in cancer detection between the two devices, a finding that was similar to that of an earlier trial.[87,88]

Conclusions

There are a wide variety of recent advances that offer the prospect of increasing prostate cancer detection, decreasing procedure-associated morbidity, and improving the overall quality of the biopsy specimens. New

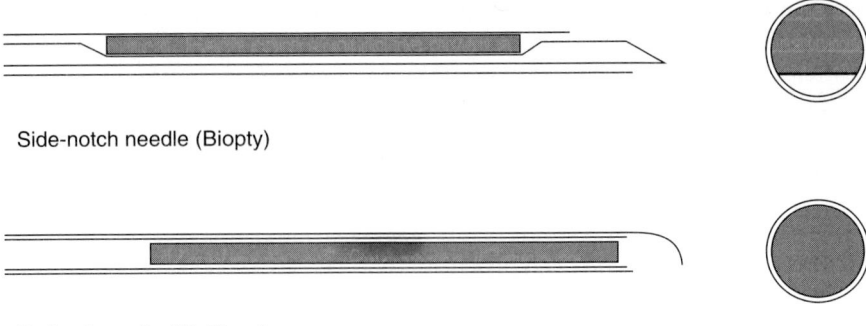

Side-notch needle (Biopty)

End-cut needle (BioPince)

FIGURE 20.10. The upper panel shows the side-notch needle and the lower panel shows the end-cut needle. Longitudinal sections of the needles with biopsy specimens (gray) are seen to the left and cross-sections are seen to the right. (Reprinted from Haggarth et al.[88])

radiographic techniques such as Doppler ultrasound, 3D US, contrast-enhanced Doppler, MRI, and MRS can help localize prostate cancer tumors. Using targeted biopsy, we may be able to reduce the number of cores taken while increasing cancer detection, thereby improving patient tolerance of the procedure. Similarly, although extended biopsy schemes have become increasingly popular, individualization of the biopsy protocol according to prostate volume may limit unnecessary biopsy while maintaining or increasing cancer detection.

A number of anesthetic agents and techniques have been introduced including periprostatic nerve block, intraprostatic lidocaine administration, intrarectal lidocaine gel, lidocaine suppositories, diclofenac suppositories, DMSO, and short-acting anesthetic agents. Use of these agents alone or in combination has been shown to decrease biopsy-associated discomfort. Finally, newer biopsy needles can improve pathologic specimen quality and eventually may be able to improve cancer detection.

Future Advances

Prostate cancer is an extremely prevalent problem, especially in our aging population. The field of prostate biopsy will undoubtedly continue to experience technologic advances with the ultimate goal of improving cancer detection while minimizing patient discomfort. Investigators will certainly continue to examine prostate cancer biomarkers for use in diagnostic tests. The ultimate such examination would be a serum or urine test that not only is highly sensitive and specific for prostate cancer, but could help differentiate clinically significant disease from indolent tumors. A similar procedure would involve testing the prostate biopsy specimens for genes that are associated with more aggressive disease. Such a method has been tested by Jhavar and associates,[89] who describe a simple and highly reliable technique, known as the "Checkerboard Tissue Microarray (TMA) Method." The checkerboard TMA method looks for multiple markers of various genes associated with prostate cancer, including the *E2F3* gene. Overexpression of the *E2F3* gene is a marker of how aggressive the prostate cancer will be.

Furthermore, researchers have identified a new virus, called XMRV, which was found 30 times more frequently in men with prostate cancer who had a particular genetic mutation than in men without this mutation.[90] Confirmation of this finding could lead to techniques designed to detect virus RNA in order to diagnose prostate cancer. Even more exciting is the possibility that a vaccine against prostate cancer could someday be developed.

A new technique, multimodality diagnostic imaging technique, is emerging. Fusion of a previously obtained high-resolution endorectal MRI with real-time ultrasound for stereotactic biopsy has shown the potential to improve prostate cancer detection and staging accuracy.[91] Using radical prostatectomy specimens, our group and others built 3D tumor distribution atlases and characterized the probability of anatomic location-associated tumor occurrence.[92] A system that integrates the images of MRI, TRUS, and the 3D tumor atlas with individualized biopsy protocol would be the next generation of machine intelligence for automatic tumor detection and tumor-targeted biopsy.

Clearly, there is a significant amount of attention given to prostate cancer within the scientific community. This will continue to lead to improvements in prostate cancer detection, treatment, and outcomes in this extremely prevalent, yet highly treatable and curable disease.

References

1. Thompson IM, Goodman PJ, Tangen CM, et al. The influence of finasteride on the development of prostate cancer [see comment]. N Engl J Med 2003;349:215.
2. Thompson IM, Pauler DK, Goodman PJ, et al. Prevalence of prostate cancer among men with a prostate-specific antigen level ≤4.0 ng per milliliter [see comment] [erratum appears in N Engl J Med 2004;351(14):1470]. N Engl J Med 2004;350 2239.
3. Fradet Y, Saad F, Aprikian A, et al. uPM3, a new molecular urine test for the detection of prostate cancer. Urology 2004;64:311.
4. Bussemakers MJ, van Bokhoven A, Verhaegh GW, et al. DD3: a new prostate-specific gene, highly overexpressed in prostate cancer. Cancer Res 1999;59: 5975.
5. de Kok JB, Verhaegh GW, Roelofs RW, et al. DD3(PCA3), a very sensitive and specific marker to detect prostate tumors [see comment]. Cancer Res 2002;62:2695.

6. Hessels D, Klein Gunnewiek JM, van Oort I, et al. DD3(PCA3)-based molecular urine analysis for the diagnosis of prostate cancer [see comment]. Eur Urol 2003;44:8.

7. Tinzl M, Marberger M, Horvath S, et al. DD3PCA3 RNA analysis in urine—a new perspective for detecting prostate cancer. Eur Urol 2004;46:182.

8. Petricoin EF, Ardekani AM, Hitt BA, et al. Use of proteomic patterns in serum to identify ovarian cancer [see comment]. Lancet 2002;359:572.

9. Adam BL, Qu Y, Davis JW, et al. Serum protein fingerprinting coupled with a pattern-matching algorithm distinguishes prostate cancer from benign prostate hyperplasia and healthy men [see comment]. Cancer Res 2002;62:3609.

10. Li J, Zhang Z, Rosenzweig J, et al. Proteomics and bioinformatics approaches for identification of serum biomarkers to detect breast cancer. Clin Chem 2002;48:1296.

11. Petricoin EF 3rd, Ornstein DK, Paweletz CP, et al. Serum proteomic patterns for detection of prostate cancer [see comment]. J Natl Cancer Inst 2002;94: 1576.

12. Bañez LL, Prasanna P, Sun L, et al. Diagnostic potential of serum proteomic patterns in prostate cancer [see comment]. J Urol 2003;170:442.

13. Li J, White N, Zhang Z, et al. Detection of prostate cancer using serum proteomics pattern in a histologically confirmed population [erratum appears in J Urol 2004;172(1):389]. J Urol 2004;171:1782.

14. Baggerly KA, Morris JS, Coombes KR. Reproducibility of SELDI-TOF protein patterns in serum: comparing datasets from different experiments. Bioinformatics 2004;20:777.

15. Sorace JM, Zhan M. A data review and re-assessment of ovarian cancer serum proteomic profiling. BMC Bioinformatics 2003;4:24.

16. Diamandis E. Mass spectrometry as a diagnostic and a cancer biomarker discovery tool: opportunities and potential limitations. Mol Cell Proteomics 2004;3:367.

17. Grizzle WE, Adam BL, Bigbee WL, et al. Serum protein expression profiling for cancer detection: validation of a SELDI-based approach for prostate cancer. Dis Markers 2003;19:185.

18. Semmes OJ, Feng Z, Adam BL, et al. Evaluation of serum protein profiling by surface-enhanced laser desorption/ionization time-of-flight mass spectrometry for the detection of prostate cancer: I. Assessment of platform reproducibility [see comment]. Clin Chem 2005;51:102.

19. Ornstein DK, Rayford W, Fusaro VA, et al. Serum proteomic profiling can discriminate prostate cancer from benign prostates in men with total prostate specific antigen levels between 2.5 and 15.0 ng/ml. J Urol 2004;172: 1302.

20. Malik G, Ward MD, Gupta SK, et al. Serum levels of an isoform of apolipoprotein A-II as a potential marker for prostate cancer. Clin Cancer Res 2005;11:1073.

21. Le L, Chi K, Tyldesley S, et al. Identification of serum amyloid A as a biomarker to distinguish prostate cancer patients with bone lesions. Clin Chem 2005;51: 695.

22. Rubin MA, Zhou M, Dhanasekaran SM, et al. Alpha-methylacyl coenzyme A racemase as a tissue biomarker for prostate cancer [see comment]. JAMA 2002;287:1662.

23. Luo J, Zha S, Gage WR, et al. Alpha-methylacyl-CoA racemase: a new molecular marker for prostate cancer. Cancer Res 2002;62:2220.
24. Rogers CG, Yan G, Zha S, et al. Prostate cancer detection on urinalysis for alpha methylacyl coenzyme, a racemase protein. J Urol 2004;172:1501.
25. Zielie PJ, Mobley JA, Ebb RG, et al. A novel diagnostic test for prostate cancer emerges from the determination of alpha-methylacyl-coenzyme, a racemase in prostatic secretions. J Urol 2004;172:1130.
26. Sreekumar A, Laxman B, Rhodes DR, et al. Humoral immune response to alpha-methylacyl-CoA racemase and prostate cancer [see comment] [erratum appears in J Natl Cancer Inst 2004;96(14):1112]. J Natl Cancer Inst 2004;96: 834.
27. Bradley SV, Oravecz-Wilson KI, Bougeard G, et al. Serum antibodies to huntingtin interacting protein-1: a new blood test for prostate cancer. Cancer Res 2005;65:4126.
28. Wang X, Yu J, Sreekumar A, et al. Autoantibody signatures in prostate cancer [see comment]. N Engl J Med 2005;353:1224.
29. Petrovics G, Liu A, Shaheduzzaman S, et al. Frequent overexpression of ETS-related gene-1 (ERG1) in prostate cancer transcriptome. Oncogene 2005;24: 3847.
30. Oikawa T, Yamada T. Molecular biology of the Ets family of transcription factors. Gene 2003;303:11.
31. Tomlins SA, Rhodes DR, Perner S, et al. Recurrent fusion of TMPRSS2 and ETS transcription factor genes in prostate cancer [see comment]. Science 2005;310:644.
32. Hodge KK, McNeal JE, Stamey TA. Ultrasound guided transrectal core biopsies of the palpably abnormal prostate. J Urol 1989;142:66.
33. Partin AW, Stutzman RE. Elevated prostate-specific antigen, abnormal prostate evaluation on digital rectal examination, and transrectal ultrasound and prostate biopsy. Urol Clin North Am 1998;25:581.
34. Presti JC Jr. Prostate biopsy: how many cores are enough? Urol Oncol 2003;21:135.
35. Eskicorapci SY, Guliyev F, Akdogan B, et al. Individualization of the biopsy protocol according to the prostate gland volume for prostate cancer detection [see comment]. J Urol 2005;173:1536.
36. Xu HX, Yin XY, Lu MD, et al. Estimation of liver tumor volume using a three-dimensional ultrasound volumetric system. Ultrasound Med Biol 2003;29:839.
37. Chen DR, Chang RF, Chen CJ, et al. Three-dimensional ultrasound in margin evaluation for breast tumor excision using Mammotome. Ultrasound Med Biol 2004;30:169.
38. Belohlavek M, Foley DA, Gerber TC, et al. Three-dimensional ultrasound imaging of the atrial septum: normal and pathologic anatomy. J Am College Cardiol 1993;22:1673.
39. Elliot TL, Downey DB, Tong S, et al. Accuracy of prostate volume measurements in vitro using three-dimensional ultrasound. Acad Radiol 1996;3:401.
40. Sedelaar JP, van Roermund JG, van Leenders GL, et al. Three-dimensional grayscale ultrasound: evaluation of prostate cancer compared with benign prostatic hyperplasia. Urology 2001;57:914.
41. Kelly IM, Lees WR, Rickards D. Prostate cancer and the role of color Doppler US. Radiology 1993;189:153.

42. el-Gabry EA, Halpern EJ, Strup SE, et al. Imaging prostate cancer: current and future applications. Oncology (Huntington) 2001;15:325.
43. Louvar E, Littrup PJ, Goldstein A, et al. Correlation of color Doppler flow in the prostate with tissue microvascularity. Cancer 1998;83:135.
44. Rubin JM, Bude RO, Carson PL, et al. Power Doppler US: a potentially useful alternative to mean frequency-based color Doppler US. Radiology 1994; 190:853.
45. Kimura G, Nishimura T, Kimata R, et al. Random systematic sextant biopsy versus power doppler ultrasound-guided target biopsy in the diagnosis of prostate cancer: positive rate and clinicopathological features. J Nippon Med School 2005;72:262.
46. Burns PN. Ultrasound contrast agents in radiological diagnosis. Radiol Med 1994;87:71.
47. Wijkstra H, Wink MH, de la Rosette JJ. Contrast specific imaging in the detection and localization of prostate cancer. World J Urol 2004;22:346.
48. Bogers HA, Sedelaar JP, Beerlage HP, et al. Contrast-enhanced three-dimensional power Doppler angiography of the human prostate: correlation with biopsy outcome. Urology 1999;54:97.
49. Karaman CZ, Unsal A, Akdilli A, et al. The value of contrast enhanced power Doppler ultrasonography in differentiating hypoechoic lesions in the peripheral zone of prostate. Eur J Radiol 2005;54:148.
50. Pelzer A, Bektic J, Berger AP, et al. Prostate cancer detection in men with prostate specific antigen 4 to 10 ng/ml using a combined approach of contrast enhanced color Doppler targeted and systematic biopsy. J Urol 2005;173:1926.
51. Roscigno M, Scattoni V, Bertini R, et al. Diagnosis of prostate cancer. State of the art. Minerva Urol Nefrol 2004;56:123.
52. Halpern EJ, Ramey JR, Strup SE, et al. Detection of prostate carcinoma with contrast-enhanced sonography using intermittent harmonic imaging. Cancer 2005;104:2373.
53. Hricak H, Williams RD, Spring DB, et al. Anatomy and pathology of the male pelvis by magnetic resonance imaging. AJR Am J Roentgenol 1983;141:1101.
54. Sommer FG, Nghiem HV, Herfkens R, et al. Gadolinium-enhanced MRI of the abnormal prostate. Magn Reson Imaging 1993;11:941.
55. Schiebler ML, Tomaszewski JE, Bezzi M, et al. Prostatic carcinoma and benign prostatic hyperplasia: correlation of high-resolution MR and histopathologic findings. Radiology 1989;172:131.
56. Mullerad M, Hricak H, Kuroiwa K, et al. Comparison of endorectal magnetic resonance imaging, guided prostate biopsy and digital rectal examination in the preoperative anatomical localization of prostate cancer. J Urol 2005;174:2158.
57. Kurhanewicz J, Vigneron DB, Hricak H, et al. Three-dimensional H-1 MR spectroscopic imaging of the in situ human prostate with high (0.24–0.7-cm3) spatial resolution. Radiology 1996;198:795.
58. Casciani E, Polettini E, Bertini L, et al. Prostate cancer: evaluation with endorectal MR imaging and three-dimensional proton MR spectroscopic imaging. Radiol Med 2004;108:530.
59. Prando A, Kurhanewicz J, Borges AP, et al. Prostatic biopsy directed with endorectal MR spectroscopic imaging findings in patients with elevated prostate specific antigen levels and prior negative biopsy findings: early experience. Radiology 2005;236:903.

60. Wefer AE, Hricak H, Vigneron DB, et al. Sextant localization of prostate cancer: comparison of sextant biopsy, magnetic resonance imaging and magnetic resonance spectroscopic imaging with step section histology [see comment]. J Urol 2000;164:400.
61. Vashi AR, Wojno KJ, Gillespie B, et al. A model for the number of cores per prostate biopsy based on patient age and prostate gland volume. J Urol 1998;159:920.
62. Eskew LA, Bare RL, McCullough DL. Systematic 5 region prostate biopsy is superior to sextant method for diagnosing carcinoma of the prostate [see comment]. J Urol 1997;157:199.
63. Eskicorapci SY, Baydar DE, Akbal C, et al. An extended 10-core transrectal ultrasonography guided prostate biopsy protocol improves the detection of prostate cancer. Eur Urol 2004;45:444.
64. Presti JC Jr, Chang JJ, Bhargava V, et al. The optimal systematic prostate biopsy scheme should include 8 rather than 6 biopsies: results of a prospective clinical trial [see comment]. J Urol 2000;163:163.
65. Uzzo RG, Wei JT, Waldbaum RS, et al. The influence of prostate size on cancer detection. Urology 1995;46:831.
66. Karakiewicz PI, Bazinet M, Aprikian AG, et al. Outcome of sextant biopsy according to gland volume. Urology 1997;49:55.
67. Autorino R, De Sio M, Di Lorenzo G, et al. How to decrease pain during transrectal ultrasound guided prostate biopsy: a look at the literature. J Urol 2005;174:2091.
68. Nash PA, Bruce JE, Indudhara R, et al. Transrectal ultrasound guided prostatic nerve blockade eases systematic needle biopsy of the prostate. J Urol 1996;155:607.
69. Davis M, Sofer M, Kim SS, et al. The procedure of transrectal ultrasound guided biopsy of the prostate: a survey of patient preparation and biopsy technique. J Urol 2002;167:566.
70. Hollabaugh RSJ, Dmochowski RR, Steiner MS. Neuroanatomy of the male rhabdosphincter. Urology 1997;49:426.
71. Rodriguez A, Kyriakou G, Leray E, et al. Prospective study comparing two methods of anaesthesia for prostate biopsies: apex periprostatic nerve block versus intrarectal lidocaine gel: review of the literature. Eur Urol 2003;44:195.
72. Alavi AS, Soloway MS, Vaidya A, et al. Local anesthesia for ultrasound guided prostate biopsy: a prospective randomized trial comparing 2 methods. J Urol 2001;166:1343.
73. Wu CL, Carter HB, Naqibuddin M, et al. Effect of local anesthetics on patient recovery after transrectal biopsy. Urology 2001;57:925.
74. Mutaguchi K, Shinohara K, Matsubara A, et al. Local anesthesia during 10 core biopsy of the prostate: comparison of 2 methods. J Urol 2005;173:742.
75. Desgrandchamps F, Meria P, Irani J, et al. The rectal administration of lidocaine gel and tolerance of transrectal ultrasonography-guided biopsy of the prostate: a prospective randomized placebo-controlled study. BJU Int 1999;83:1007.
76. Issa MM, Bux S, Chun T, et al. A randomized prospective trial of intrarectal lidocaine for pain control during transrectal prostate biopsy: the Emory University experience. J Urol 2000;164:397.

77. Stirling BN, Shockley KF, Carothers GG, et al. Comparison of local anesthesia techniques during transrectal ultrasound-guided biopsies. Urology 2002;60: 89.
78. Lynn NN, Collins GN, Brown SC, et al. Periprostatic nerve block gives better analgesia for prostatic biopsy. BJU Int 2002;90:424.
79. Adamakis I, Mitropoulos D, Haritopoulos K, et al. Pain during transrectal ultrasonography guided prostate biopsy: a randomized prospective trial comparing periprostatic infiltration with lidocaine with the intrarectal instillation of lidocaine-prilocain cream. World J Urol 2004;22:281.
80. Obek C, Ozkan B, Tunc B, et al. Comparison of 3 different methods of anesthesia before transrectal prostate biopsy: a prospective randomized trial. J Urol 2004;172:502.
81. Fink KG, Gnad A, Meissner P, et al. Lidocaine suppositories for prostate biopsy. BJU Int 2005;96:1028.
82. Haq A, Patel HR, Habib MR, et al. Diclofenac suppository analgesia for transrectal ultrasound guided biopsies of the prostate: a double-blind, randomized controlled trial. J Urol 2004;171:1489.
83. Kravchick S, Peled R, Ben-Dor D, et al. Comparison of different local anesthesia techniques during TRUS-guided biopsies: a prospective pilot study. Urology 2005;65:109.
84. Masood J, Shah N, Lane T, et al. Nitrous oxide (Entonox) inhalation and tolerance of transrectal ultrasound guided prostate biopsy: a double-blind randomized controlled study. J Urol 2002;168:116.
85. McIntyre IG, Dixon A, Pantelides ML. Entonox analgesia for prostatic biopsy. Prostate Cancer Prostatic Dis 2003;6:235.
86. Dogan HS, Eskicorapci SY, Ertoy-Baydar D, et al. Can we obtain better specimens with an end-cutting prostatic biopsy device? Eur Urol 2005;47:297.
87. Ozden E, Gogus C, Tulunay O, et al. The long core needle with an end-cut technique for prostate biopsy: does it really have advantages when compared with standard needles? Eur Urol 2004;45:287.
88. Haggarth L, Ekman P, Egevad L. A new core-biopsy instrument with an end-cut technique provides prostate biopsies with increased tissue yield. BJU Int 2002;90:51.
89. Jhavar S, Corbishley CM, Dearnaley D, et al. Construction of tissue microarrays from prostate needle biopsy specimens. Br J Cancer 2005;93:478.
90. Klein E, Urisman A, Molinaro R, et al. Identification of a novel retrovirus in prostate tumors of patients homozygous for the R462q mutation in the Hpc1 gene. Presented at ASCO Prostate Cancer Symposium, 2006.
91. Kaplan I, Oldenburg NE, Meskell P, et al. Real time MRI-ultrasound image guided stereotactic prostate biopsy. Magn Reson Imaging 2002;20:295.
92. Zhu Y, Williams S, Zwiggelaar R. Computer technology in detection and staging of prostate carcinoma: a review. Med Image Anal 2006;10:178–99.

Index

Printed in the United States of America